ATLAS OF
APPLIED HUMAN HISTOLOGY

ATLAS OF
APPLIED HUMAN HISTOLOGY

The Identification of Tissues by Light Microscopy
for
Students, Residents, and Pathologists

By

J.D. REID, M.D., F.R.A.C.P.

Professor of Pathology
Northeast Ohio Universities College of Medicine
Pathologist
Robinson Memorial Hospital
Ravenna, Ohio
Former Professor of Pathology
Case Western Reserve University
Former Director of Pathology
Cleveland Metropolitan General Hospital
Cleveland, Ohio

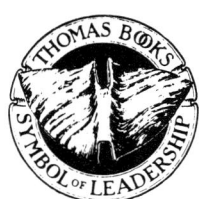

CHARLES C THOMAS • PUBLISHER
Springfield • Illinois • U.S.A.

Published and Distributed Throughout the World by
CHARLES C THOMAS • PUBLISHER
2600 South First Street
Springfield, Illinois 62717 U.S.A.

This book is protected by copyright. No part of it
may be reproduced in any manner without written
permission from the publisher.

© *1982 by* CHARLES C THOMAS • PUBLISHER
ISBN 0-398-04590-9
Library of Congress Catalog Card Number: 81-9328

With THOMAS BOOKS careful attention is given to all details of manufacturing and design. It is the Publisher's desire to present books that are satisfactory as to their physical qualities and artistic possibilities and appropriate for their particular use. THOMAS BOOKS will be true to those laws of quality that assure a good name and good will.

Printed in the United States of America
I-R-10

Library of Congress Cataloging in Publication Data

Reid, J. D. (John D.)
   Atlas of applied human histology.

   Bibliography: p.
   Includes index.
   1. Histology--Atlases. I. Title. [DNLM: 1. Histology--Atlases. QS 517 R356a]
   QM557.R38   611'.018'0222   81-9328
   ISBN 0-398-04590-9   AACR2

PREFACE

ANATOMY is the science that deals with the structure of the body as found by dissection and with the identification of different parts and organs according to their size, shape, situation, solidity, and other properties. Microscopic anatomy or histology arose in the last half of the seventeenth century, when van Leeuwenhoek and Malpighi began the study of biologic materials by light microscopy, and a new world of anatomic substructure was opened up. It was found that organs and parts were built of elementary fabrics, or tissues, which in turn were seen to be aggregates of cells. The cell became recognized as the basic unit of structure, and different types of cells were identified by variations in their size, shape, situation, and fine detail. The science of histology thus concerns the cellular composition of tissues and the way tissues participate in the formation of parts and organs.

In the midnineteenth century, from the work of Müller and Virchow and their concept that the basis of disease lay at cell level, histology expanded into histopathology, and various disorders were defined by abnormal microscopic appearances. At the present time, essentially all specimens of tissue removed from patients in duly accredited hospitals in this country must by regulation be submitted for pathologic examination, and in the great majority of instances, this involves light microscopic examination. Under these circumstances, structure is frequently obscured, the specimens are often tiny, and their origin may be uncertain. An ability to identify the part from which the sample came is thus invaluable. It provides an independent check on what is said to have been removed by the surgeon, and it adds a quality control on the accuracy of the labelling and identity of the specimen as it passes through a rather lengthy and complicated processing sequence. It also underwrites the competence of the histopathologist, who must know what is normal before he can reasonably describe what is abnormal.

Description by light microscopy has been greatly expanded in recent years by newer applications of fluorescence, phase, and polarizing microscopy. Histochemical and immunocytochemical techniques are providing new approaches, and electron microscopy has added new dimensions of knowledge. Nevertheless, the first approach to histology remains identification by light microscopy. This is an aspect that is not ordinarily taught in any systematic or objective fashion. Rather, both histology and histopathology texts begin with lists of different parts and organs, each of which is then described according to normal or abnormal appearances. In practice, examination begins with the microscopic preparation from which identification must first be made. Only then is it rational for histologists to study details of normal structure or for histopathologists to examine deviations from normal.

This work has been prompted first by the repeated question of students and residents, "How do I tell what I am looking at?" It is hoped that a brief discussion of the general principles by which a structure is identified and the demonstration of a simple and systematic practical approach will reduce their frustrations when faced with unknown slides. Second, it is an attempt to lift histologic identification above the accusation of mere picture matching and establish it as a rational scientific activity with principles that can be clearly stated and applied.

It is realized that most histopathologists and, it may be suspected, most histologists have learned to identify things by looking down a microscope and by the process known as recognizing your friend John Smith. For them, the method proposed here is probably unnecessary, but for those beginning histologic study, a key will hopefully prove useful.

ACKNOWLEDGMENTS

ALL of the material used here is human, chiefly surgical specimens and tissues obtained from young adults autopsied at the Cleveland Metropolitan General Hospital, but it includes some tissue blocks and slides received from colleagues in the community. For two slides of the adult inner ear, I am indebted to Dr. V. Hyams, Armed Forces Institute of Pathology. The slides demonstrating insulin and glucagon in pancreatic islet cells were kindly provided by Dr. R. Jaffe, Pittsburgh; the slide of thyroid C cells with argyrophil reaction by Dr. J. Crissman, Cincinnati; and the slide showing enzyme reactions in muscle by Dr. B. Banker. The great majority of the sections were prepared under the supervision of Mrs. L. Hrabak, and the photomicrographs were taken by Mr. R. A. McCashen on a Zeiss Ultraphot® with contrast process pan film. The manuscript was typed by Mrs. A. Nolan, and the figures are the work of Mrs. M. Bitans. To all of these sincere thanks are offered.

CONTENTS

Page

Preface v
  I PRINCIPLES AND METHODS OF IDENTIFICATION 3
 II PRACTICAL IDENTIFICATION 12
      1 Anuclear Materials, Bodies and Crystals 12
      2 Cells 15
      3 Tissues 18
      4 Parts 57
III SUMMARY 202
References 205
Index 207

ATLAS OF
APPLIED HUMAN HISTOLOGY

I
PRINCIPLES AND METHODS OF IDENTIFICATION

IDENTIFICATION is the process of comparing some newly discovered object to a previously defined prototype, matching them point for point, and concluding that they are the same. If the two structures are similar but not entirely identical, they may be regarded as variants of a single species, but if they are quite dissimilar, they are considered to be different types. The distinction between a variant and a type is thus often a matter of opinion, depending on what is taken to be a significant difference. Organs and parts that are highly organized and have a complex substructure offer a greater number of characteristics for comparison and are thus more confidently identified than more simple structures. A single feature that is known to occur infrequently may have a relatively high discriminatory value, but in general, identification depends on multiple features; the more that are the same, the more secure the identification and the less likely the possibility of a chance similarity. A good analogy is fingerprinting, where many points of identity are needed before accepting a positive identification.

In histology, the variables or parameters that can be compared relate to size, shape, and substructure, and each of these can be described objectively. However, tissues in their natural state are essentially transparent, and it is first necessary to make them visible by coloring their cells or by inducing precipitates to deposit on some particular constituent. The most common method is dyeing or staining. This involves the use of ionizable colored compounds, or chromogens, which have an affinity for tissues. The essential part of the dye conferring its color is termed a chromophore, and in the great majority of dyes in common use, this is a quinoid ring. Other chromophores involve an azo linkage or a nitro group. To bind as a dye, it is also necessary that ionizing groups be present, since it is cations or anions that form the links to protein and other tissue constituents. The molecular size of the dye, and the absorptive or adsoptive properties and permeability of the tissue elements are also important. By itself, the cytoplasm of a cell is amphoteric and may react with either acid or basic dyes, depending on the pH. The various proteins, carbohydrates, lipids, and other substances within a cell have different staining affinities. At ordinary pH, mucopolysaccharides and some mucoproteins are negatively charged and, consequently, react with cationic (basic) dyes such as hematoxylin. On the other hand, mitochondria and hemoglobin have a positive charge and will attach acidic dyes, such as eosin. In ordinary sections, with the usual hematoxylin and eosin stains, the net result is a basophilia of nuclei and a pink or eosinophilic reaction in cytoplasm. In coloring by lysochromes, the principle is that the colored substance is more soluble in tissue lipids than the solvent in which it had been prepared. The common example is Sudan red, used to demonstrate fat.

Visible precipitates can be induced by interacting various constituents with different chemical agents. Black deposits of metallic silver can be formed by the reducing properties of tissue acting on silver salts. Four or five modifications of silver reduction methods are used to demonstrate things as diverse as melanin, calcium, paracrine granules, axons, and reticulin fibers. Despite the general nonspecificity, the particular technique used enables reasonably precise identification of the reducing agent, when considered in relation to the type of tissue being examined. Blue precipitates of a complex iron salt (ferric ferrocyanide or Prussian blue) can be produced with hemosiderin in Perls' test. In enzyme reactions, colored formazan deposits are frequently used. Coloring procedures commonly used in the identification of cells and intercellular materials are listed in Table 1, and some of the more useful texts bearing on this subject are listed in the appended bibliography.

The thin slice of tissue used in histology represents an extremely small sample of the whole part, and identification thus resembles the method of identifying trees by their leaves. Just as the size, shape, color, and rib structure of an isolated leaf may indicate (from previous experience) the tree from which it came, so the elements in a section may accurately point to the organ from which it was derived. However, there are limitations to the method. Just as a single leaf could come from any one of a number of trees of the same kind, there are situations in which a section could have come from any number of parts. This applies particularly to nerves and muscles, which are so widely distributed that no specific anatomic origin can be assigned to any one of them. Glomeruli indicate that a section has come from the kidney but do not enable a distinction between right or left sides.

The elements (Figs. 1 through 4) to be identified range from parts and organs visible by naked eye, through smaller organized units seen only by microscopy (and which thus can be termed microparts), to the four major tissues or elementary fabrics (generally recognized as epithelium, neural tissue, muscle, and connective tissue) and the cells and matrix of which tissues may be composed. At whatever level of organization, size, shape, and substructure are the variables to be defined, taking due notice to variations relating to age, which must be accepted as normal in the sense that they are universally found.

Size

Size is commonly defined subjectively by terms such as large or small, assuming some known standard. It is preferable to make an objective measurement, which requires a calibrated eyepiece. As an alternative, it is possible to use the light pointer, which is now included in the optical pathway of some microscopes and which can be calibrated and used in much the same way. Less accurately, the ubiquitous red cell provides a basis for comparison; it is approximately 5μ in diameter in the fixed state.

Shape

Shape is defined by reference to regular geometric forms or to items of everyday knowledge. It is common practice to use terms such as spherical, cuboidal, columnar, pyramidal, or polyhedral, but these are three-dimensional descriptions. In fact, histologic sections are so thin that all structures are seen in essentially one plane. Thus they have two dimensions, and it is more accurate to refer to profiles, with words such as round, square, rectangular, or polygonal. Terms that refer to common, if much larger, objects such as kidneys (reniform), serpents (serpentine), spindles (fusiform), roots (dendrites), or stemmed drinking glasses (goblets) are more or less self-explanatory.

Substructure

Substructure refers to the position, size, shape, and arrangement of the different components that make up any structure. Size and shape can be defined as described previously for any discrete unit but are inapplicable to nondiscrete elements such as cytoplasm or intercellular ground substance. Here, terms such as texture, refractility, and staining properties are used, with more specific descriptive words such as smooth, granular, or vacuolated; bright or dull; and eosinophilic or basophilic.

Position

This can be described whenever the relation of one structure to another can be seen. In ordinary anatomy this is a matter of naked eye description, as when describing the situation of the liver, spleen, and so forth. In histology, the same principles apply. An organ may have

Table 1
COLORING PROCEDURES COMMONLY USED IN IDENTIFICATION

General tissue identification — Hematoxylin and eosin — nuclei blue; cytoplasm pink

Epithelial tissues

Keratin	Eosin (no specific stain)
Mucin	PAS (periodic acid-Schiff) diastase resistant — red
	Mayer's mucicarmine — pink
	Alcian blue PAS — green-blue-red
Glycogen	PAS — red (color removed by prior diastase)
Beta cells, pancreas	Gomori aldehyde fuchsin — purple granules
Endocrine granules	Pascual (argyrophil) — black
Lipids	Oil red O or Sudan red — red
Kulchitsky (argentaffin) cells	Masson-Fontana — black silver deposits
Melanocytes	Masson-Fontana — black silver deposits

Neural tissues

Axons	Bodian — black
Glial fibers	Phosphotungstic acid-hematoxylin (PTAH) — blue-gray
Myelin	Luxol fast blue — myelin sheaths blue
	Woelke — myelin sheaths blue

Connective tissues

Lipids	Oil red O or Sudan red — red
Collagen	Mallory — blue
	Masson — green
	Movat — yellow
Elastin	Verhoeff — blue-black
	Movat — black
Reticulin	Bielschowsky (modification) — black
Ground substance	Movat — green
	Abdul-Haz and Rhinehart — blue
Calcium	von Kossa — black
	Alizarin red S — red
Plasma cells	Methyl green-pyronin (MGP) — red cytoplasm
Mast cells	Toluidine blue O — metachromatic (purple) granules
Polymorphs	Wright-Giemsa — eosinophilic, basophilic, and neutrophilic granules
	Leder — neutrophil esterase giving a red color

Muscle tissues

Myosin	Mallory trichrome — red
	Masson trichrome — red
	Movat pentachrome — red

Other

Bile	Hall or Stein — green
Lipofuscin	AFIP method — reddish-brown
Hemosiderin	Perls-blue

LEVELS OF ORGANIZATION

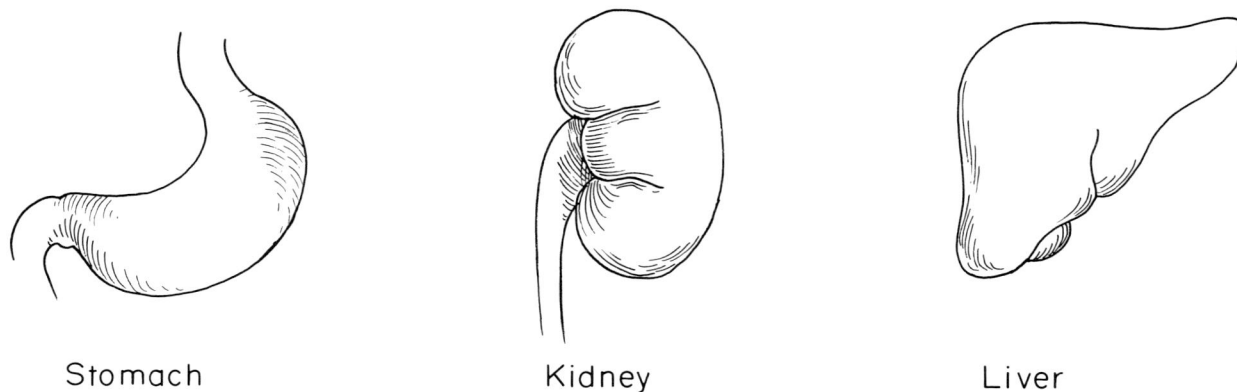

Figure 1. The body, as a whole, is constructed from parts and organs that can be separated by ordinary naked eye dissection. Some are single, others are paired; some are solid others are cavitary.

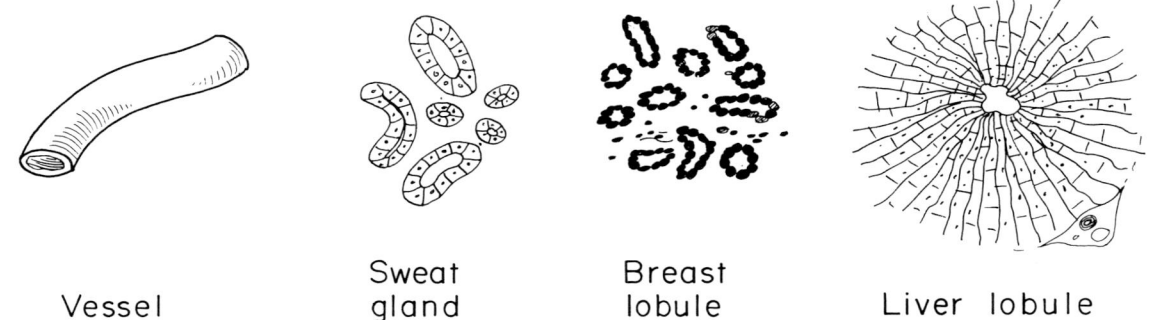

Figure 2. There are also smaller, solid or cavitary parts visible only by microscopy (microparts).

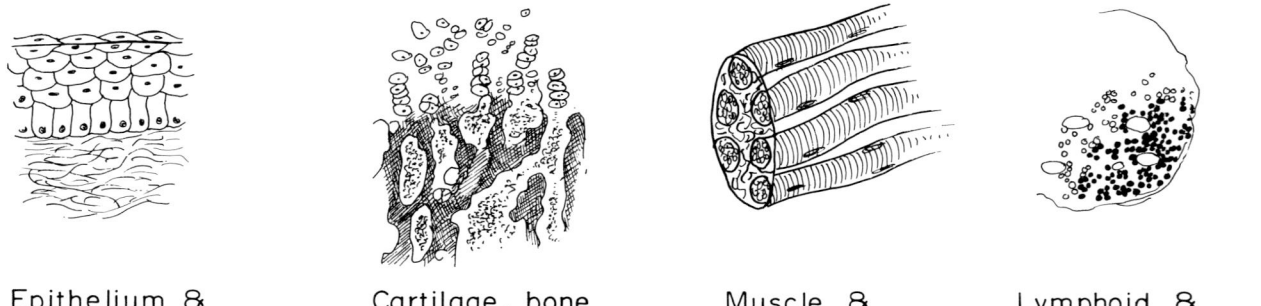

Figure 3. Each macropart and micropart is ultimately formed of tissues, of different kinds in differing arrangements.

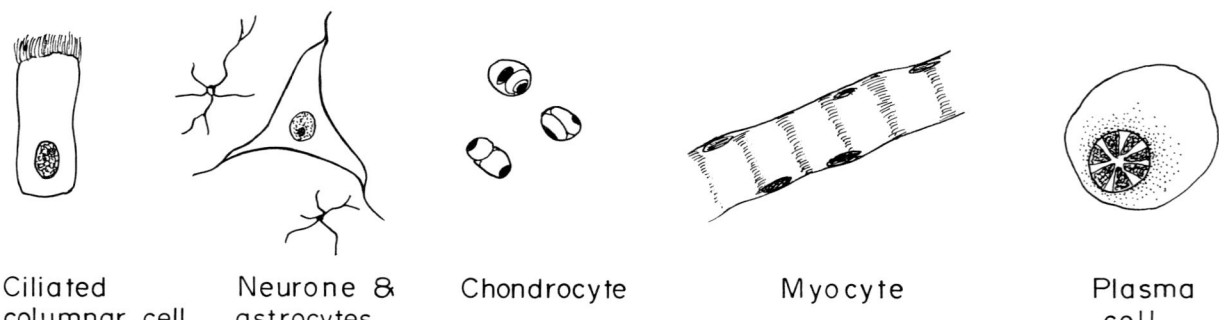

Figure 4. Within a tissue, different cells are identified by their particular cytoplasmic and nuclear characteristics.

recognizable cortical and medullary parts, as in the adrenal. In the central nervous system, identification relies heavily on the situation of various collections of neurones and fiber tracts as seen in relation to the surface, ventricles, or some other definable landmark. At tissue level, a layer of epithelium may be clearly forming the surface. At cell level, position may be described in terms such as juxtaglomerular, parafollicular, or basal, and in other ways, as listed later in Table 2, page 19.

Arrangement or Construction

Regarding arrangement and construction, it is helpful to consider how the body as a whole is put together before proceeding to examine the construction of organs and tissues. The body may be regarded as a number of cavities (skull, thorax, abdomen), each with its own walls, with which are various organs, hollow or solid — e.g. stomach and liver. There are also large external projections (limbs, ears, male genitalia) in whose substance, as well as within the body walls, are further cavitary or solid substructures, such as vessels and bones. Hollow or solid arrangements are still to be seen when a part is examined by microscopy, although now a variety of methods of construction is found (Figs. 5 through 8).

The simplest parts consist merely of a collection of cells isolated within connective tissue; more commonly they are demarcated by a condensation of connective tissue or a distinct fibrous capsule. The microscopic lymphoid structures that constitute Peyer's patches in the intestine fall in the first category; the parathyroid is an example of a single type of tissue within a capsule, although fat is a normal second component after puberty. Two different tissues are not uncommonly joined together to form a part. This may be a simple juxtaposition as in the pituitary, or one tissue may envelope another as in the adrenal and, in a more complex way, in the thymus. In a more complex organization, small microparts may be repeated over and over and grouped together to form the organ. This is frequently seen with simple cavitary units such as tubules, alveoli, follicles, saccules, and acini but also with epithelial cells in plates and with neural or connective tissues whose basic structure is a small bundle of fibers. This may be termed modular unit construction. In some parts, there is a diffuse collection of the basic units (as in testis), but in many structures, they form smaller and larger groups passing through stages recognized as sublobules and lobules or as fascicles of different sizes. Multiple cavitary microparts form the thyroid, kidneys, sweat glands, gonads, erectile tissues, and lung. Solid cylindroid structures in more or less parallel arrangement can be identified from the limbs downwards. Bones, muscles, and nerves all run the same general direction, and the entire limb is wrapped in skin. Individual muscles and nerves may be subdivided into smaller bundles, each essentially identical, down to the smallest fascicles. A further type of construction is lamination, in which sheets of different cells are layered one on top of another. This is seen in the walls of the hollow viscera but also in the walls of various tubes and vessels. The surface is always an epithelium of one sort or another supported by layers of fibrous and muscular tissue and not infrequently by cartilage or bone.

At tissue level, there are a number of variations in construction, related chiefly to the configuration of the constituent cells and to the kinds and amounts of intercellular matrix that may be present. Polyhedral cells may be found closely fitted together without any intervening matrix, which is the identifying characteristic of epithelium. As seen in sections, this arrangement resembles that of floor tiles and may be described as tessellated. When polyhedral cells are separated by small amounts of intercellular material, the general appearance resembles that of a mosaic, or tiles that are set in small amounts of mortar. If the matrix is abundant, the cells resemble isolated stones set in a bed of cement in what may be described as an inlaid pattern. At the other extreme, polyhedral cells without any close attachment to one another and without matrix (so that they appear to lie free) confer a punctate appearance on the section.

Cells of other shapes determine other arrangements. Those of a stellate configuration tend to form tangles, while elongated spindle or straplike cells are found in parallel arrays, giving a fibrillary appearance.

These general appearances may be termed the *format* of the tissue, and the five chief variants are tessellated, mosaic, inlaid, fibrillary, and punctate (Figs. 9 through 13). The tessellated format is used as the identifying characteristic of epithelium; within other formats, the tissue family is identified by cellular characteristics, chiefly the type of cytoplasm and matrix that may be present.

At cellular level, construction can also be described in terms of the general shape of the cell, the position of the nucleus within the cell, the composition of cytoplasm in terms of granules, vacuoles, and organelles, their relation to the nucleus, and the arrangement of chromatin within the nucleus itself. The last criterion is used as an identifying feature in plasma cells or Anitschkow's cells, for example. Nucleoli may be prominent or inconspicuous.

THE CONSTRUCTION OF PARTS

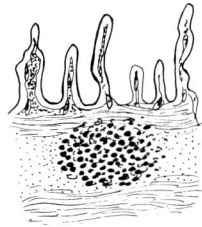
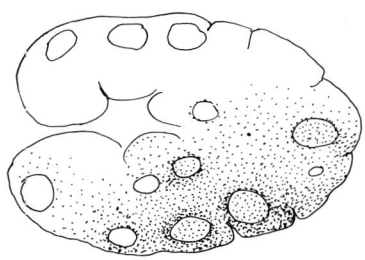
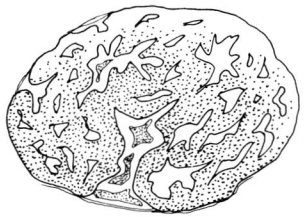

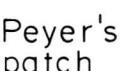
Peyer's patch

Lymph node

Parathyroid

Figure 5. Isolation. The simplest form of construction is isolation of a tissue or groups of cells within some other tissue; usually demarcated by a fibrous capsule.

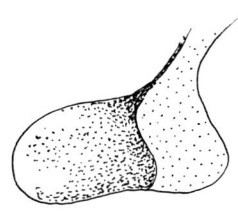
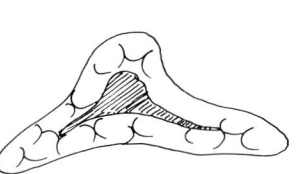
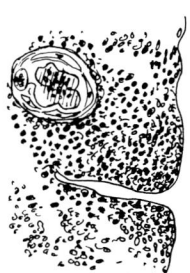

Pituitary

Adrenal

Thymus

Figure 6. Combination. Tissues from different families may be organized by simple juxtaposition (abutting) or by one enveloping another.

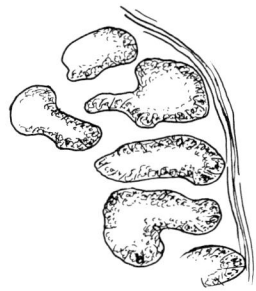
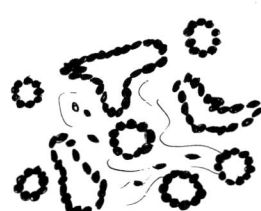
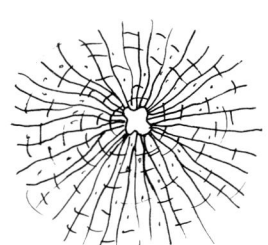
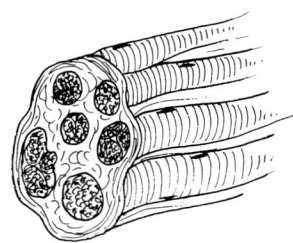

Testis

Breast

Liver

Nerve

Figure 7. Simple and modular-unit aggregation. Identical microparts (tubules, acini, bundles, or plates) may be diffusely massed or may be found in small repeating groups as lobules or fascicles.

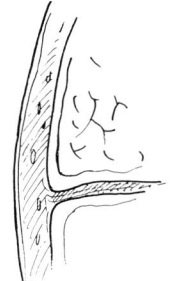
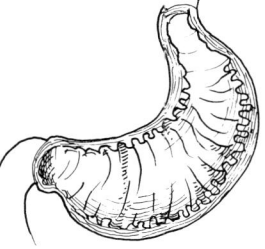
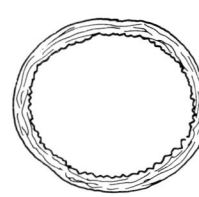
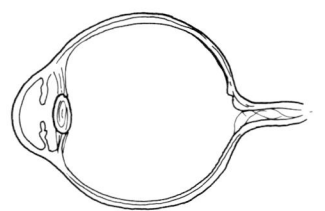

Body wall with diaphragm

Stomach

Aorta

Eye

Figure 8. Lamination. Sheets of different tissues may be layered to form walls and partitions.

TISSUE FORMATS

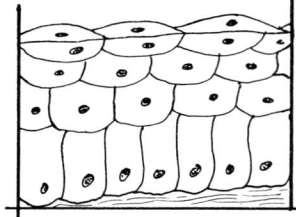 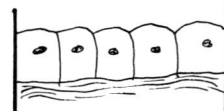 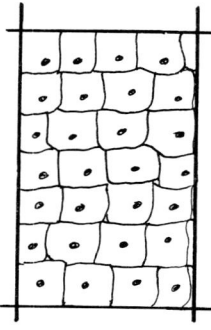

Figure 9. Tessellated. Formed of contiguous cells (epithelium) found in surface layers and also in some deep structures.

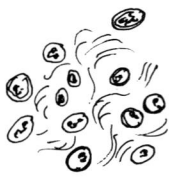 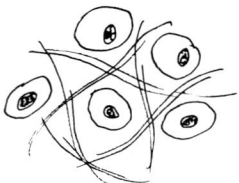

Figure 10. Mosaic. Polyhedral cells separated by small amounts of matrix forming neural or connective tissues according to the glial or mesenchymal material between cells.

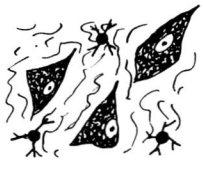 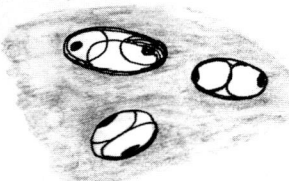 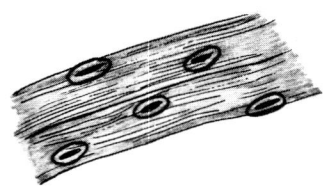

Figure 11. Inlaid. Cells isolated in an abundant matrix forming neural or connective tissue.

TISSUE FORMATS

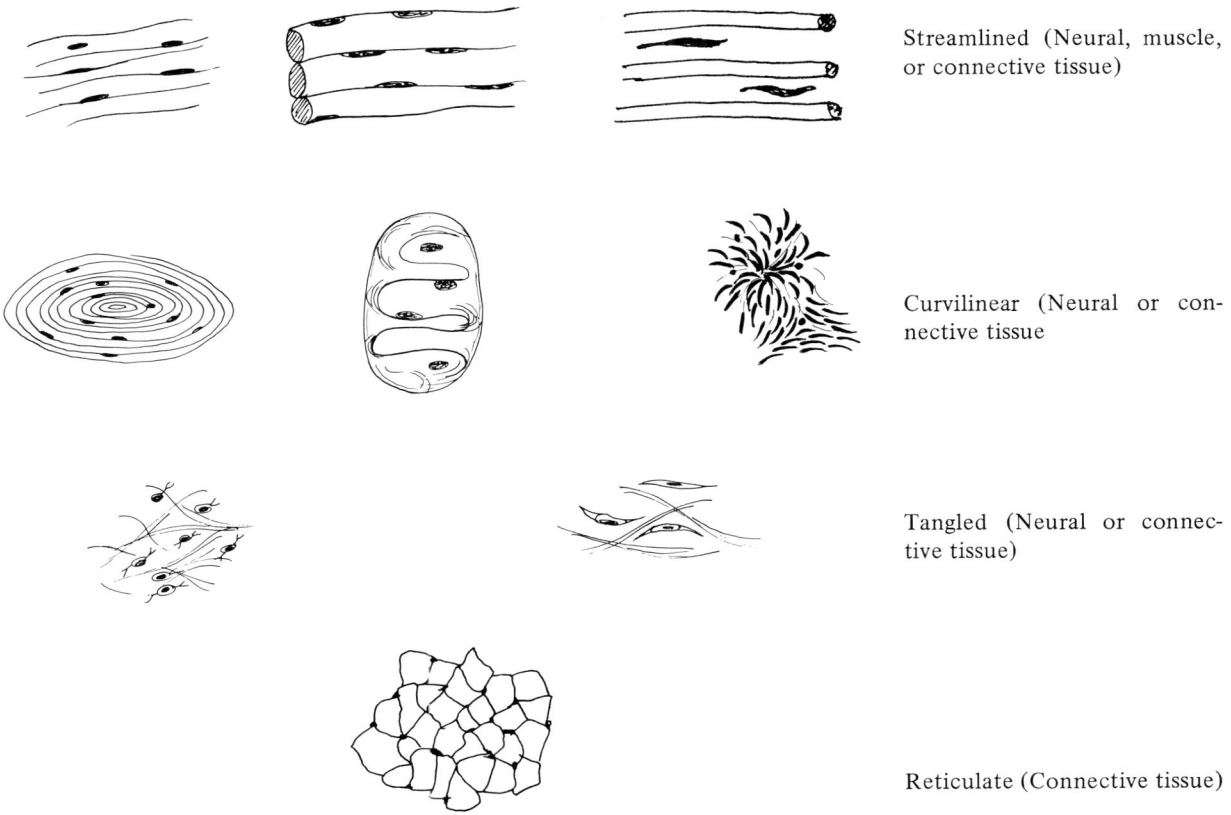

Streamlined (Neural, muscle, or connective tissue)

Curvilinear (Neural or connective tissue)

Tangled (Neural or connective tissue)

Reticulate (Connective tissue)

Figure 12. Fibrillary. Threadlike, due either to cell processes or to intercellular fibers.

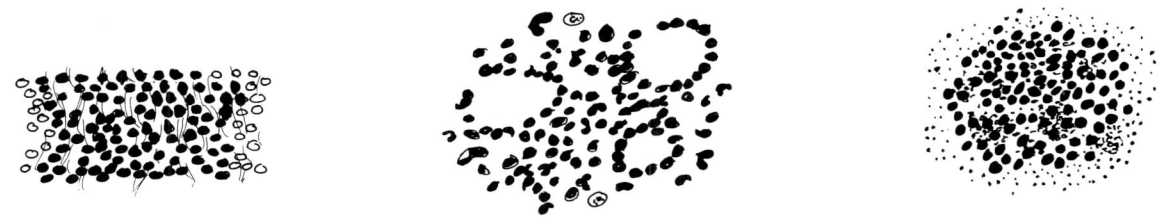

Figure 13. Punctate. Multiple dots representing nuclei, seen in neural, myeloid, and lymphoid tissues.

II

PRACTICAL IDENTIFICATION

HAVING briefly considered the principles that underline identification, the practical question is how different structures are identified as they are encountered in histologic preparations. Because of thinness of sections, size and shape can be defined in only two dimensions, and then only when the part is small enough to be completely cut across and mounted on an ordinary glass slide. This applies to parts that are less than 2.5 cm in one or other dimension and which consequently, appear as rings (if tubular), as seives (if multiple spaces are present), and as islands (if solid). Examples are arteries, bronchi, the ovary, seminal vesicles, endocrine glands, and lymph nodes. Microparts appear as small islands or enclaves within some other structure, as with arterioles, ductules, sweat glands, sebaceous glands, hair follicles, islets of Langerhans, Pacini's and Meissner's corpuscles. In all of these size, shape, and substructure may be described, and in some, position can also be defined.

When dealing with large organs such as the brain, kidney, or liver, where only small samples can be examined histologically, the blocks are selected and cut out by the prosector so that their size and shape is often quite unrelated to the natural appearance of the part. However, configuration may be so important in identification (as in the central nervous system) that special provision is made for examination of very large sections, using 3 inch by 2 inch glass slides to accommodate parts as large as the frontal or occipital poles.

In practice, examination begins by looking at the section as a whole and by defining the largest unit structure that can be seen. However, for teaching purposes, it is more convenient to begin with the simplest elements and work up to more complex structures. Those with least substructural detail are anuclear materials and bodies, and in increasing order of complexity are cells, the tissues formed from cells, and the microparts and macroparts that are formed from tissues.

1

ANUCLEAR MATERIALS, BODIES AND CRYSTALS

These are to a limited extent identifiable in their own right. Anuclear derivatives of epithelium may still retain distinctive characteristics, such as the mosaic shadow of cells in superficial keratin, or the linear appearance of hair and nail. Bodies also vary in their size and composition, although the organ in which they lie, e.g. brain, choroid plexus, pineal body, and prostate, enables their identification most easily. Crystals (Reinke) are found in the interstitial cells of the testis and ovary and crystalloids (almost invisible) in Sertoli cells.

Most bodies are small, round, basophilic structures without nuclei and are usually lamellated. Those seen in the brain are usually close to the ependyma or pia mater and are termed amyloid bodies or corpora amylacea; those in the choroid plexus are merely termed calcific bodies and are identified chiefly by their location. In the pineal are found sand granules or corpora arenacea, and bodies in the acini of the prostate, often calcified, are again termed calcific bodies or corpora amylacea.

BODIES

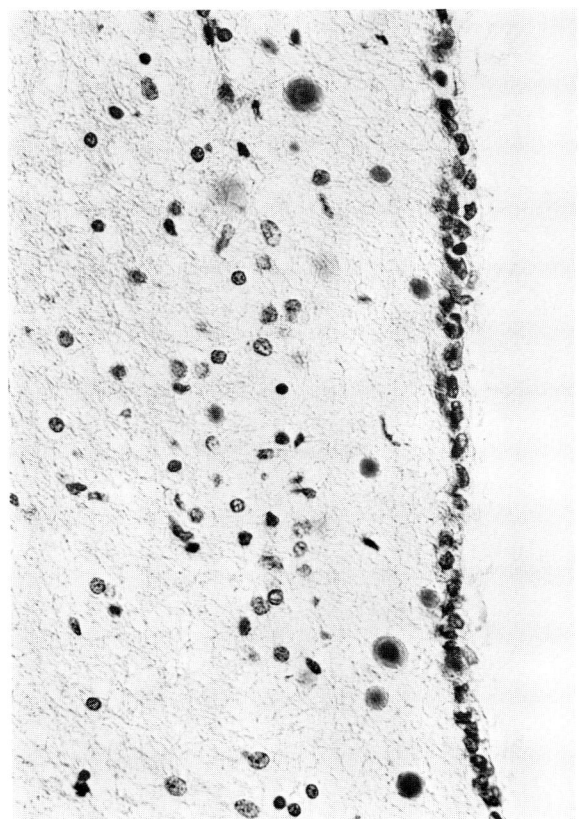

Figure 14. Corpora amylacea, brain. (×320)

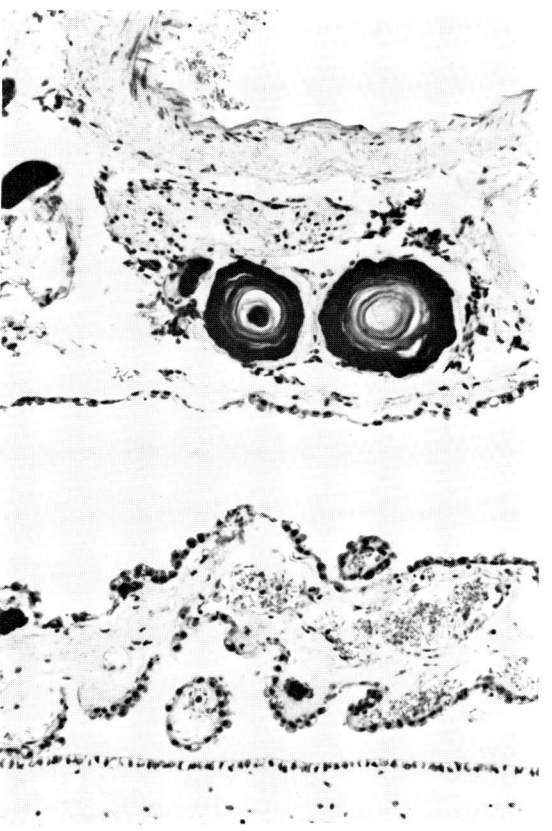

Figure 15. Calcific bodies, choroid plexus. (×120)

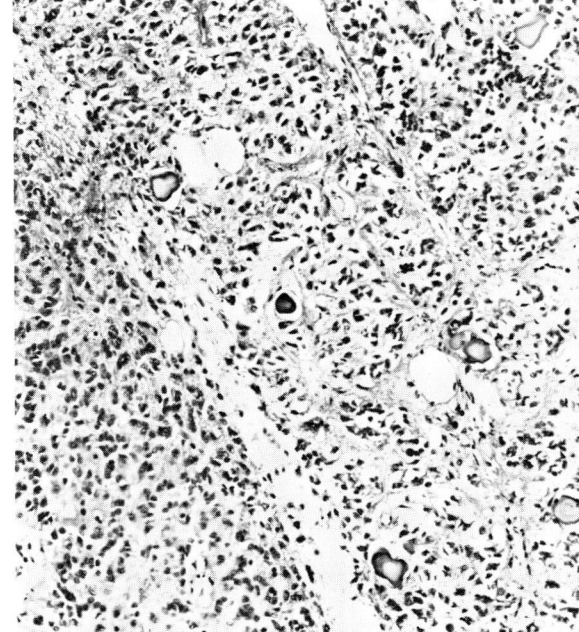

Figure 16. Corpora arenacea, pineal. (×120)

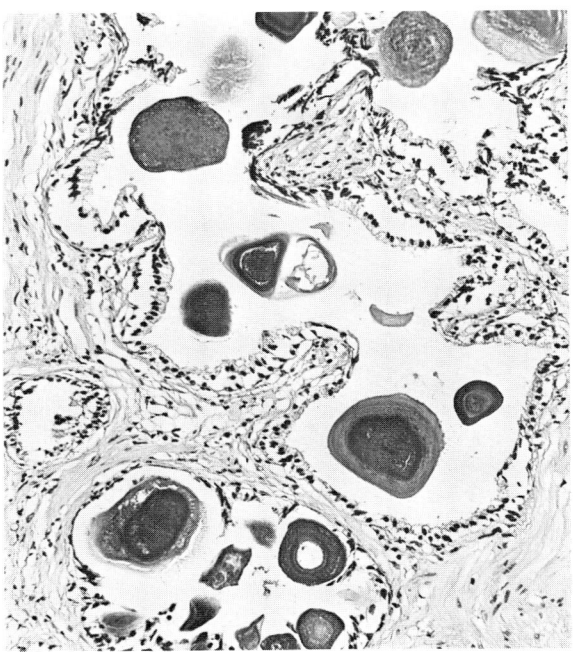

Figure 17. Corpora amylacea, prostate. (×120)

ANUCLEAR DERIVATIVES OF EPITHELIUM

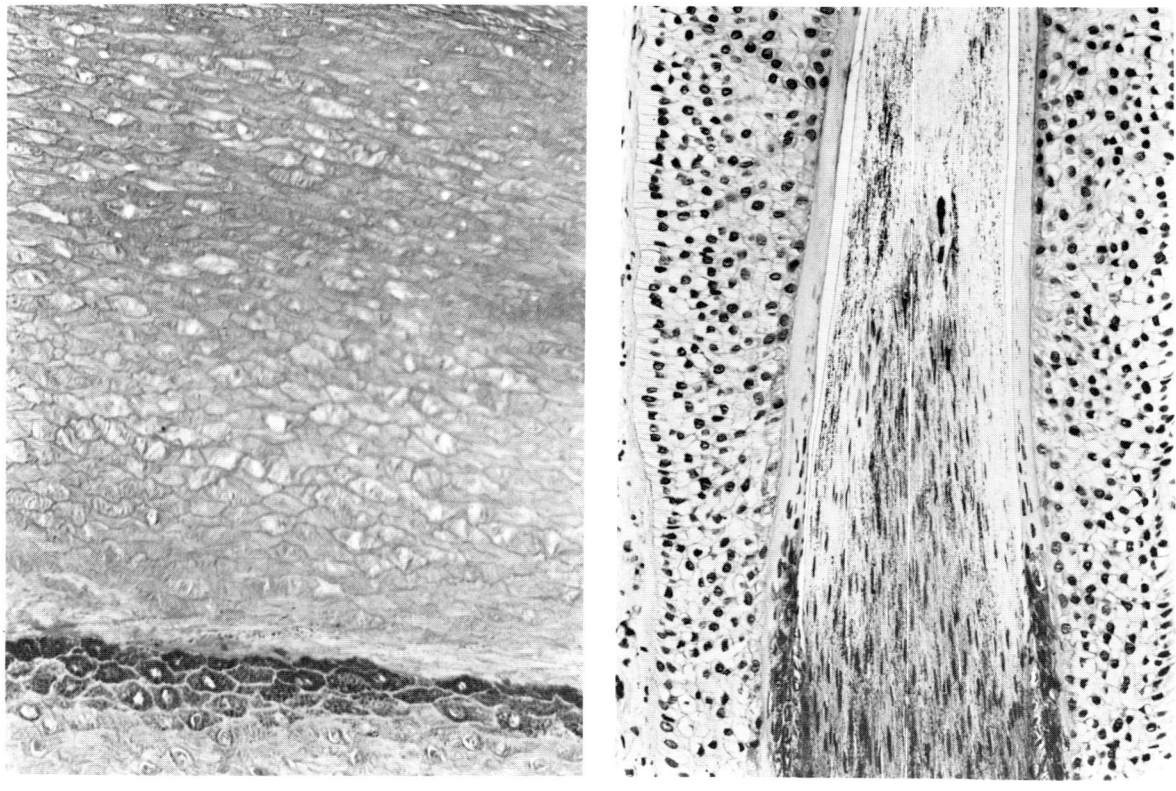

Figure 18. Keratin. (× 200)

Figure 19. Hair. (× 140)

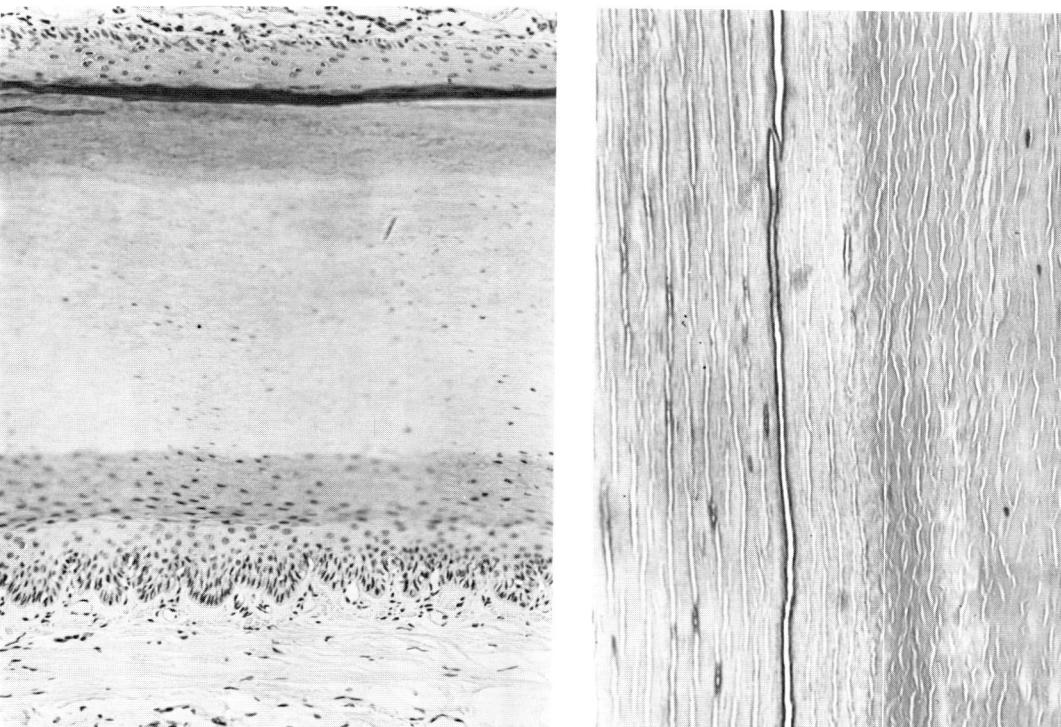

Figure 20. Nail. (× 250)

Figure 21. Lens. (× 480)

Over the skin, a fine lacy material of pale eosinophilic color, composed of degenerating epithelial cells somewhat loosely arranged and often fraying off in flakes, is keratin. A very thick layer is typical of pressure-bearing areas of skin such as the fingers, palms, and the soles of the feet. A dense compact column of keratin, slightly yellow and refractile in appearance and enclosed within a sheath is a hair shaft. Plates of bluish color, flecked with tiny linear fragments of nuclear residues arranged in parallel with the surface, are nails. A laminar arrangement of curving, almost unstained refractile plates is typical of the lens of the eye and represents modified cytoplasmic processes of the lens epithelium, which is seen in Figure 21. External to the epithelium is the thick anuclear lens capsules, which stains like collagen in a Movat preparation but lies in the position of a basement membrane.

2
CELLS

By definition, histology is the study of cells as they are organized to form tissues, rather than the isolated units of cytology. In their purest form, tissues are aggregates of cells from the same family, and cells can therefore be described in two ways: first, according to the general class of tissue to which they belong (epithelial, neural, muscle, or connective tissue cells) and then as individual members (e.g. ciliated columnar epithelial cells.) Identification of cells by morphology usually depends on a combination of features. Size by itself is not particularly important, although large cells are to be separated from small cells. Shape is much more useful, including surface modifications, as illustrated in Figures 22 through 31. Substructure includes cytoplasmic granules and vacuoles as well as nuclei of different sorts (Figs. 32 through 43).

Cytoplasmic granules may be naturally pigmented as with the black or brown granules of melanin or the brown granules of hemosiderin. The latter can be much more precisely identified and even roughly quantitated by Perls' reaction and the formation of Prussian blue precipitates. Yellow granules may be lipofuscin, which is inconstant in its chemical composition, and may stain with lysochromes or by the periodic acid-Schiff methods, and sometimes by acid fast techniques, these different reactions reflecting variable degrees of oxidation of lipids. With H & E staining, cells may contain eosinophilic, basophilic, or neutrophilic granules whose nature varies greatly. In white blood cells they reflect enzymes, and in the pituitary they represent different hormones. Pale granules may be glycogen, while gray to purple granules are usually zymogenic. After fixation in chromate, brown granules may be found in the adrenal and intestinal mucosa, so the reacting cells are termed chromaffin and enterochromaffin respectively. If formalin fixation is used, this reaction is lost. Nevertheless, the enterochromaffin cells may still be identified because they are able to reduce silver salts to metallic silver (argentaffin reaction). Other granules related to polypeptide hormones can be visualized in endocrine and paracrine (Feyrter, 1958) cells by argyrophilic methods (Fernandez Pascual, 1976). More specific identification involving immunoperoxidase techniques (Taylor, 1978) and specific antibodies rests on artificially induced precipitates.

Cytoplasmic vacuoles may be mucin, lipid, glycogen, or water, and to distinguish these possibilities, frozen sections may be needed, with appropriately chosen coloring reactions. Thus, the identification of lipids in adipose tissue and in myelin requires cryostat sections and lysochromes such as oil red O or the Sudan dyes. Glycogen is identified by positive PAS staining, removable by prior treatment with disastase. Mucin can be stained by mucicarmine or alcian blue as well as the the PAS reaction.

Nuclei are found in all cells of the body except two. The first is a mature erythrocyte, which in section appears as a small eosinophilic disc or ovoid mass, usually within a blood vessel. The second is the thrombocyte or platelet, which is an irregular particle of cytoplasm from a megakaryocyte, not seen as an individual entity in the usual histologic preparation. The size,

SOME CELLS IDENTIFIED BY SHAPE AND SURFACE MODIFICATIONS

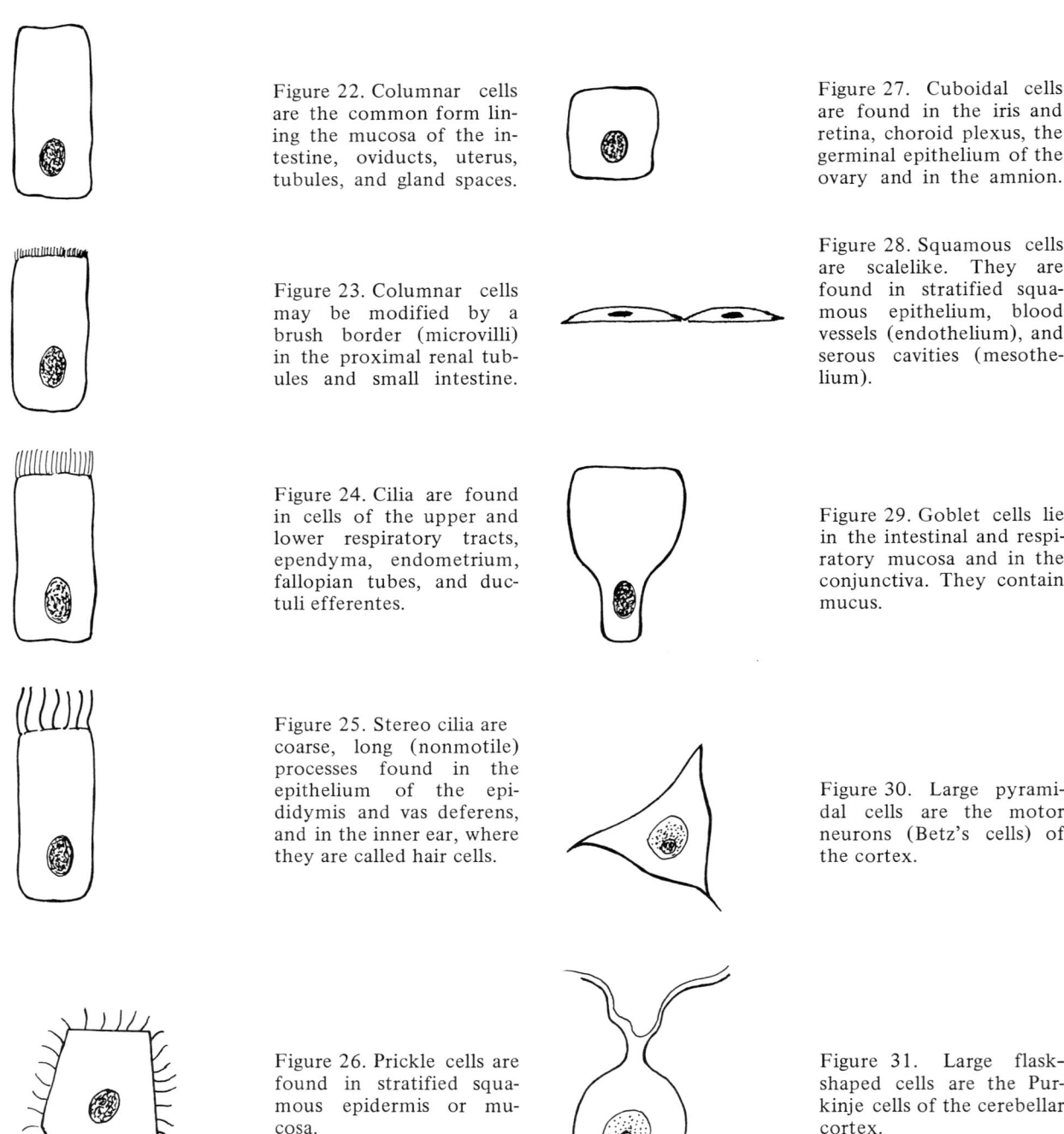

Figure 22. Columnar cells are the common form lining the mucosa of the intestine, oviducts, uterus, tubules, and gland spaces.

Figure 23. Columnar cells may be modified by a brush border (microvilli) in the proximal renal tubules and small intestine.

Figure 24. Cilia are found in cells of the upper and lower respiratory tracts, ependyma, endometrium, fallopian tubes, and ductuli efferentes.

Figure 25. Stereo cilia are coarse, long (nonmotile) processes found in the epithelium of the epididymis and vas deferens, and in the inner ear, where they are called hair cells.

Figure 26. Prickle cells are found in stratified squamous epidermis or mucosa.

Figure 27. Cuboidal cells are found in the iris and retina, choroid plexus, the germinal epithelium of the ovary and in the amnion.

Figure 28. Squamous cells are scalelike. They are found in stratified squamous epithelium, blood vessels (endothelium), and serous cavities (mesothelium).

Figure 29. Goblet cells lie in the intestinal and respiratory mucosa and in the conjunctiva. They contain mucus.

Figure 30. Large pyramidal cells are the motor neurons (Betz's cells) of the cortex.

Figure 31. Large flask-shaped cells are the Purkinje cells of the cerebellar cortex.

SOME CELLS IDENTIFIED CHIEFLY BY CYTOPLASMIC AND NUCLEAR CHARACTERISTICS

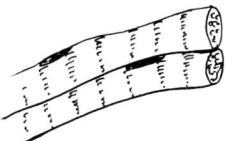

Figure 32. Transverse striation in an eosinophilic cytoplasm identifies skeletal and cardiac muscle cells.

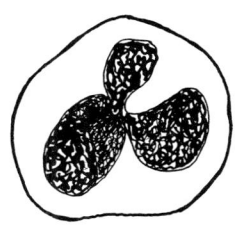

Figure 38. Very large multilobed nuclei are unique to the megakaryocyte.

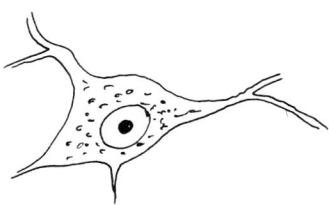

Figure 33. Dendritic cells with brown pigment are melanocytes of the skin.

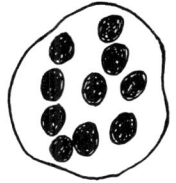

Figure 39. In bone, large cells with multiple nuclei are osteoclasts.

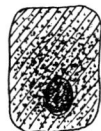

Figure 34. A finely granular, or ground glass, cytoplasm characterizes serous cells of the salivary glands.

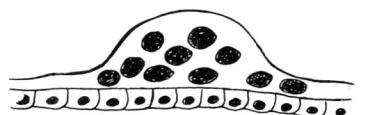

Figure 40. Multiple round nuclei in a cytoplasmic sheet identify syncytiotrophoblasts.

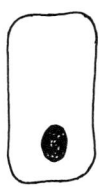

Figure 35. Clear or vacuolated cytoplasm may be due to the mucus of a mucous cell.

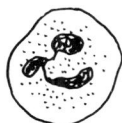

Figure 41. Small, multilobed nuclei of blood granulocytes are further distinguished by their granules — eosinophilic, basophilic, or neutrophilic.

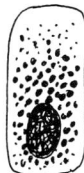

Figure 36. Bright red supranuclear granules in columnar cells identify the Paneth's cells of the intestinal crypts.

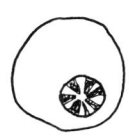

Figure 42. A small cell with basophilic cytoplasm and eccentric nucleus with clockface chromatin is a plasma cell.

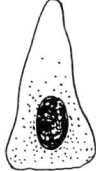

Figure 37. Faint basal granules, which can be stained black with silver reduction techniques, identify the argentaffin cells of the intestine.

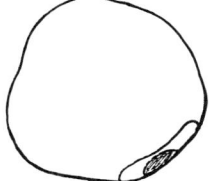

Figure 43. A large empty cytoplasmic space with eccentric nucleus identifies the fat cell.

shape, and substructure of nuclei are seldom so unique that they confer specific identification on the cell in which they are found. Exceptions are the multilobed nuclei of magakaryocytes and polymorphonuclear leukocytes. Other cells have distinctive multiple nuclei as in striated muscle cells, osteoclasts, and syncytial trophoblasts. In lymphoid tissue notched nuclei are thought to indicate a different type of lymphocyte from those with round nuclei. In bone marrow, a finely punctate chromatin distinguishes primitive red cells from the more irregularly clumped chromatin of white cells.

The identification of extracellular elements relates to the thickness and staining reactions of fibers and the refractility and texture of more amorphous material. Somewhat bluish fibers are elastin, although this may at times stain pink, particularly in the interlaminar ligaments and ligamenta flava of the spine. Very fine fibers of reticulin may be seen after the induction of silver precipitates. Dense eosinophilic material with fine parallel lines in circular or parallel arrangements, with cells in an inlaid format, identifies bone (decalcified). The matrix is hyaline cartilage is smooth and blue; similar tissue that contains elastic fibers is elastic cartilage, and if the background is more eosinophilic with visible collagen fibers, it is fibrocartilage. A pale, almost invisible material around stellate cells is mucopoly saccharide or connective tissue mucin (glycosaminoglycans) seen in the myxoid tissue of the unbilical cord and in heart valves. A thin lamina or plate of PAS positive material typically found between an epithelium and its associated connective tissue stroma is a basement membrane.

All of the parameters mentioned are used in various combinations in the identification of cells (Table 2). Sometimes weight is placed on surface characteristics, such as cilia or prickles, sometimes on shape, as in goblet cells, sometimes on cytoplasmic content, as in serous cells, and sometimes on intercellular matrix, as with cartilage cells.

The names applied to cells may also refer to their function, as in olfactory cells, which clearly refers to the sense of smell, and decidual cells, which refers to the shedding of leaves of a deciduous tree. In other situations numerical preponderance is used, so the dominant cells of the parathyroid glands, gastric glands, pineal, and pituitary may all be termed chief cells. Others are designated by letters, as in the acidophils of the pituitary, which are sometimes called A or alpha cells, or in the basophils, termed B or beta cells. The difficulty in finding a single descriptive name, particularly when there are several distinctive characteristics, each of which could be used for identification, has favored the continued use of eponyms (Table 3).

3
TISSUES

The identification of tissues begins by looking at the general format or layout, followed by detailed consideration of the types of cells and any matrix present.

Epithelium is identified by the close apposition of fairly large polyhedral cells, giving a tessellated format. Indeed, it is the arrangement of cells rather than their embryologic derivation that defines this class of tissue. However, mosaic, inlaid, fibrillary, or punctate formats occur in more than one tissue family (neural, muscle, or connective tissue). It may therefore be helpful to review the basic morphologic characteristics of these.

Neural tissues are those which contain neurones or their long cytoplasmic extensions known as axons. If neurones are supported by a dense meshwork of astrocytes, whose cytoplasmic processes are usually known as glial fibers, it is central nervous system tissue. If, on the other hand, axons are enveloped in Schwann's cells and in connective tissue, it is peripheral nervous tissue. The basic neural construction may be found in inlaid, fibrillary, or

Table 2

CELLS IDENTIFIED IN OTHER WAYS

By tissue of origin	chondrocyte	found in cartilage
	fibrocyte	found in fibrous tissue
	ganglion cell	found in a nerve ganglion
	granulosa cell	found in the granulosa of ovarian follicles
	hepatocyte	found in liver parenchyma
	islet cell	found in pancreatic islets
	lymphocyte	found in lymph and lymphatic tissue
	muscle cell	found in muscle
	olfactory cell	found in olfactory mucosa
	osteocyte	found in bone
By position in a tissue	basal cell	stratum germinativum of skin
	hilus cell	eosinophilic cells in the hilus of the ovary
	interstitial cell	eosinophilic cells between seminiferous tubules
	juxtaglomerular cell	cells in the wall of the afferent arterial and adjacent mesangium
	littoral cell	cells lining the splenic and lymph node sinuses
	parietal cell	acidophilic cells in the periphery of gastric glands
	satellite cells	found around neurones in ganglia
By dominance	chief cell	parathyroid; stomach, pineal, pituitary; paraganglia
By function	osteoclast	removal of bone
	calcitonin (c) cell	secretion of calcitonin
	olfactory cell	sensation of smell
	zymogenic cell	production of enzyme precursors
	myoepithelial cell	contractile cells around small ducts

Table 3

CELLS COMMONLY DESIGNATED BY EPONYMS OR LETTERS

By eponyms	Betz	large pyramidal cells of motor cortex
	Clara	nonciliated nonmucous cells in terminal bronchioles
	Golgi II	neurones in the granular layer of cerebellum, (larger than the small cell majority) with short axons
	Hensen	clear cells, organ of Corti
	Hoffbauer	phagocytic cells, often vacuolated, in chorionic villi
	Kulchitsky	serotonin-containing cells of gastrointestinal mucosa
	von Kupffer	phagocytic stellate cells in hepatic sinusoids
	Langerhans	clear dendritic cells in the upper epidermis
	Leydig	interstitial epithelioid cells of testis
	Paneth	eosinophilic granular cells of small intestine
	Purkinje	large flask-shaped neurones with branching broad processes in cerebellar cortex
	Schwann	myelin sheath cells of peripheral nerve
	Sertoli	supporting cells of testis
By alphabetic assignment	A or alpha	acidophils of pituitary, glucagon cells of pancreas
	B or beta	basophils of the pituitary, insulin cells of pancreas
	B cells	lymphocytes associated with immunoglobulin production
	C cells	chromophobes of pituitary, calcitonin cells of thyroid
	D cells	somatostatin cells of intestine and pancreas
	EC_1 cells	argentaffin cells producing serotonin and substance P
	EC_2 cells	argentaffin cells related to motilin
	EG cells	enteroglucagon cells of intestine
	H cells	VIP producing cells of intestine
	I cells	cholecystokinin cells of intestine
	K cells	gastric inhibitory peptide cells
	T cells	lymphokine related lymphocytes
	X cells	trophoblastic cells in placental septa and other areas of placenta

punctate formats.

Muscle is a highly specialized contractile type of tissue recognized histologically by the long eosinophilic cytoplasmic processes of its cells. When cut longitudinally, the general appearance is that of a fibrillary tissue whose fibers represent cytoplasmic cell extensions; if cut transversely, the format is more comparable to that of a mosaic. Different types of muscle are identified by the presence or absence of cross striations and by the situation and number of nuclei in each cell.

Connective tissues are of two morphologically distinct kinds. In the first, the individual cells are segregated by varying amounts of collagen, reticulin, elastin, myxoid, cartilaginous, or osseous matrix. The general format may be mosaic, inlaid, or fibrillary, and within each format, specific types of segregated connective tissue are identified by cellular characteristics and by the type of intercellular matrix present. The second kind of connective tissue includes myeloid and lymphoid tissues. Cells here are neither visibly separated by matrix nor closely joined together. The general format is punctate, and further identification depends on the types of cells present.

Tissues with Tessellated Formats

The general appearance in tessellated formats is comparable to that of floor tiles, although when cells are small they may appear overlapped, as in an imbricated arrangement (which describes fish scales or tiles on a roof). This format is synonymous with epithelium, and three major architectural arrangements are found. Some epithelia cover a reasonably flat open surface as in skin, the body cavities, and large tubes. Others line small spaces such as tubules and acini and appear in sections as rings or incomplete circular profiles of contiguous cells. In a third arrangement, which may be described as enclosed, no open surface is seen, but the epithelium forms solid confluent sheets of cells as in the liver or endocrine glands.

a. Among flat, open-surfaced epithelia, different species are identified by the contour of the surface, whether smooth or irregular, by the number of layers of cells, and by different types of cells. Although many surgical biopsy specimens consist of little more than epithelium, there are so many distinctive variants that the part from which the tissue came can usually be fairly well localized. Surface cells are frequently modified for specialized purposes. This may consist of flattening, in what is believed to be a protective mechanism associated often with keratinization. Cells with specialized external processes facilitating movement, such as cilia, or immobile processes, such as stereocilia (of unknown function), may be incorporated in the surface layer, and there are also cells that produce mucin for the lubrication of the surface.

There are, however, some technical difficulties. Due to the possibility of oblique sectioning, it may be hard to distinguish between a single row of epithelial cells as opposed to a double row and between double rows and multiple cell rows. It may also be impossible to distinguish between the true stratification of the ciliated epithelium in parts of the nasal cavity as opposed to the pseudostratified ciliated mucosa (where all cells touch the basement membrane) of most of the respiratory tract.

Multilayered epithelia are identified in different ways, often according to the nature of the most superficial layer. A surface of flat cells, identifying a stratified squamous epithelium, comes in four modifications. (1) The keratinizing stratified squamous epithelium of the epidermis; (2) the nonkeratinizing stratified squamous mucosa, which lines openings from the skin such as the mouth and esophagus, and the vaginal, urethral, and anal mucosae; (3) the stratified squamous epithelium with associated goblet cells, which is unique for parts of the conjunctiva; and (4) the thin, extremely flat layer that forms the corneal epithelium.

A stratified columnar cell mucosa in which there are ciliated surface cells, is often termed respiratory because it is virtually restricted to that tract. There are also stratified columnar epithelia without cilia, and there are stratified epithelia in which the cells remain polyhedral, e.g. transitional epithelium.

An epithelium consisting of a single layer of columnar cells is found in the lining of the stomach and intestines, the gallbladder, and the fallopian tubes and uterus. Uniformly tall columnar cells with clear mucous-secreting cytoplasm are found in the fovea of the stomach and in the gallbladder and endocervical mucosa, and small fragments of this kind of epithelium cannot be distinguished. However, if deeper areas of mucosa are included, there are likely to be more distinctive cells enabling specific identification, as with the acid-secreting cells of the stomach, or Paneth's cells of the intestine.

A single layer of flattened squamous epithelium lines the serous cavities (mesothelium) and blood-containing spaces, both heart and vessels (endothelium). By themselves, mesothelium and endothelium cannot be localized to any particular anatomic area, although their origin may be deduced from the nature of subjacent tissues. There is the added difficulty that this kind of epithelium is extremely thin and often fails to survive processing so that the artifactual appearance of a bare open surface is presented.

b. The epithelium that forms the tubules, acini, and follicles of exocrine glands and other microcavitary parts is usually seen as rings around spaces. Serous cells, mucous cells, bichromic and sometimes mixtures of serous and mucous cells may be found, but identification depends heavily on the whole micropart unit — the size and contour of the space, the nature of secretions, and supporting stroma. This is dealt with later, under the heading of microcavitary sections.

c. Deep, enclosed epithelial tissues do not form a natural open surface, despite the sheet-like breadth of the tissue and the numerous cells present. Their identification depends in part on tissue arrangement but also on the size, shape, and other characteristics of individual cells. Single plates or laminae in a radiating arrangement are seen in the liver; double parallel plates are found in the fasciculata of the adrenal glands. A whorling arrangement is seen in the zona glomerulosa of the outer adrenal cortex. Large cells come from the liver; adrenal cortex and medulla; the corpus luteum; and the sebaceous glands. Small enclosed epithelial cell groups come from the parathyroid, while combinations of large and small cells come from the anterior pituitary. Cell shape is not particularly useful, since all are polyhedral, but cytoplasmic staining can be most valuable, as when acidophil or basophil granules are included, identifying the anterior pituitary. Small collections of large oxyphilic cells are found in the parathyroid after puberty. Cells of the liver contain pale granules of glycogen, while finely vacuolated cells with lipid indicate adrenal cortex, corpus luteum, or sebaceous glands. In the adrenal medulla, adrenalin-containing cells are believed to react more darkly on fixation with chromates than those containing nonadrenaline.

Mosaic Formats (Epithelioid)

Among the mosaic formats are found tissues from neural, muscle, and connective tissue families. Moderately large epitheloid cells in a glial background identify the pineal gland. Muscle tissue may also resemble a mosaic if the fibers are cut transversely. An epithelioid appearance, in which there is a relatively scanty collagen-elastin-reticulin-acid mucopolysaccharide matrix, is found with the carotid body, the interstitial cells of the testis, decidua, and brown fat.

Tissues with an Inlaid Format

These may be neural or connective tissues.

A finely granular light pink inlaid format in which there are scattered neurones and more numerous astrocytes, oligodendroglial, and microglial cells is gray matter. The granularity is chiefly due to the innumerable fine branching processes of the astrocytes and to the relative absence of myelin close to the nerve bodies or somata. Here and there visible fibers may be found. The general background is often described as neuropil. The further identification of gray matter depends largely on its position but to some extent on the neurones. These come in two chief sizes, large and small. The former have prominent nuclei and conspicuous nucleoli, while the cytoplasm contains dark granules or bodies known as Nissl substance. In general, large triangular neurones have a motor function, and large spherical neurones are sensory. Some have distinctive shapes or cytoplasmic features such as pigment and so can be more precisely identified.

An inlaid tissue where there is collagen or acid mucopolysaccharide falls into the connective tissue family. Abundant hyalinized eosinophilic collagen with scattered spindle-shaped fibroblasts is seen in the corpus albicans of the ovary, and calcified collagen (also eosinophilic after decalcification) is the matrix of bone. An amorphous light pink or blue matrix with small polyhedral cells isolated by ones or twos in lacunae is chondroid and may be seen in three forms — hyaline, elastic, and fibrocartilage. An abundant pale mucoid or myxoid material with stellate cells is present in the umbilical cord.

Fibrillary Formats (Neural, Muscle, and Connective Tissues)

These are dominated by threads or fibers of large or small diameter, in a variety of arrangements. When they lie in parallel, the general appearance can be described as streaming; in one form, the bundles appear to be interwoven. Other fibers appear to be tangled, to be whorled, or to form an open network.

Fibrillary tissues of neural type include white matter and peripheral nerves. The former is identified by very fine fibers, representing innumerable axons, with associated supporting glial cells, chiefly astrocytes. No collagen is found except in the connective tissue septa of the optic nerve and in the fibers associated with perivascular connective tissue. White matter with a streaming format identifies a fiber tract. In some areas, tracts pass between small masses of gray matter and variations in their relative amounts may be distinctive enough to allow reasonably specific localization. In other white matter, the fibers form irregular tangles.

Peripheral nerve fibers, which also have axons in a streaming arrangement, are coarser in texture, and the cell population includes Schwann's cells with short indented nuclei, as well as fibroblasts with collagen. The Schwann's cells are related to the formation of the lamellated myelin sheaths. Nerves may include, throughout their course, scattered neurone cell bodies, but these are best recognized in the well-defined nodular aggregates known as ganglia on the dorsal roots of the spinal cord and in the sympathetic chain. Neurone somata are also found among peripheral nerve fibers in Auerbach's myenteric and in Meissner's submucosal plexuses of the intestinal wall.

In muscle, the format is unusually coarse because the fibers are the cytoplasmic extensions of myocytes, which are very large eosinophilic cells. Skeletal, cardiac, and smooth types of muscle are identified according to the size of the fiber, their arrangement, presence or absence of striations, and the situation of the nuclei, whether peripherally or centrally placed. In two situations, a woven interdigitating appearance is found — in the tongue and in the uterine wall.

Fibrillary forms of connective tissue include a streaming arrangement in tendons and ligaments, and a tangled format in the umbilical cord and loose areolar connective tissue. A network is found in adipose tissue and in the chorionic villi. In the former, the cells are actually arranged in a mosaic, but preparation of the section for histology dissolves out of fat, leaving only a meshwork of cell walls with intervening collagen, reticulin, and capillaries. In the immature chorionic villi, the reticulate appearance is due to the loss of cytoplasmic contents of more watery mucopolysaccharide nature.

Punctate Formats (Neural and Connective Tissues)

Small, densely staining, round naked nuclei, closely packed together, are found in the developing ganglia of the embryo, in the dentate gyrus of the hippocampus, in the cerebellar cortex, and in the retina. They are most easily identified as neurones by their anatomic location, while in the hippocampus and cerebellar cortex, a glial background may be seen. Apart from the ganglia, there is also a distinctive bandlike arrangement.

A punctate format is also found in the myeloid and lymphoreticular subclass of connective tissues, identified chiefly by cytologic characteristics. Myeloid tissue, however, is enclosed within bones and closely associated with adipose tissue. The individual cells show all grades of differentiation from primitive to mature white and red cells, with associated megakaryocytes. A more homogeneous, less variegated appearance is seen in lymphoid tissue, but there are still large and small cell types, as well as plasma cells and histiocytes, to enable identification.

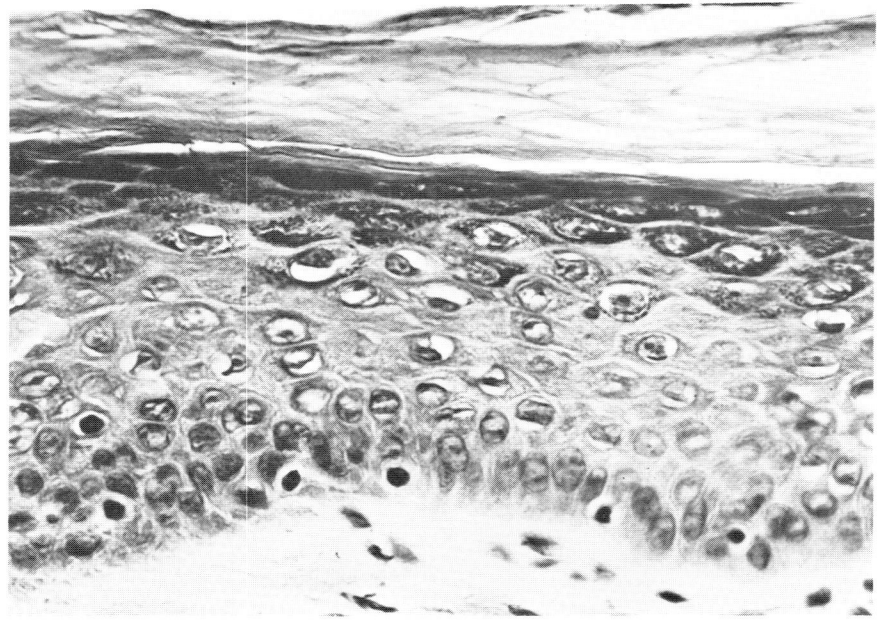

Figure 44. Epithelium with large cells in a tessellated format and with a natural open surface. The upper layer is composed of anuclear keratin. Immediately beneath are three or four rows of darkly staining cells containing keratohyalin (the granular layer) followed by approximately five rows of prickle cells, or acanthocytes, (the stratum Malpighi), and below these, a row of basal columnar cells (stratum germinativum). Among the latter are scattered clear cells with dark nuclei, which are melanocytes. High level clear cells (Langerhans) have histiocytic affinities. *Epidermis* (×480)

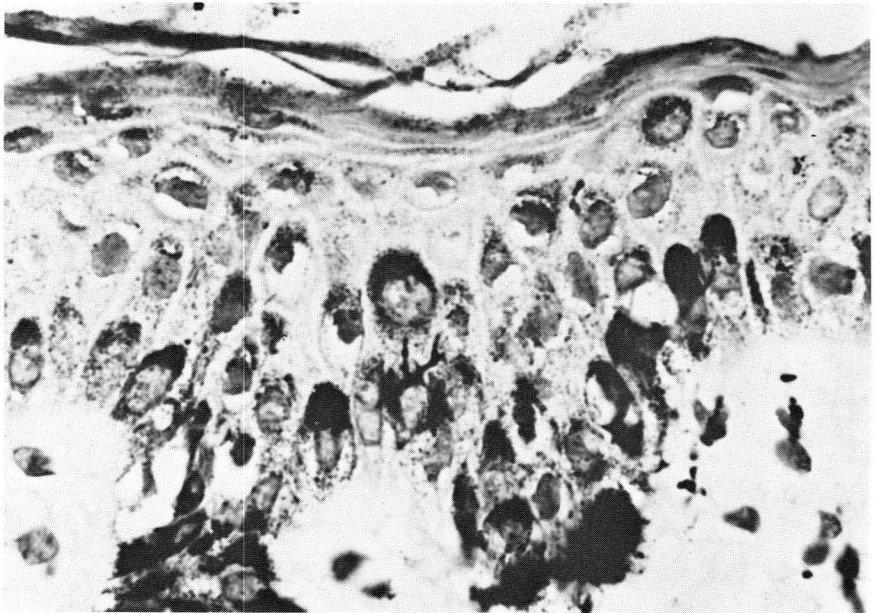

Figure 45. Melanocytes made visible by inducing silver precipitates on them. The cell in the center of the basal row has arborizing, dendritic processes shown in black. Melanin granules are frequently dense enough to obscure many of the melanocytes. They are also found in small numbers in the acanthocytes, or prickle cells, of the stratum Malpighi and in the desquamating keratin. *Epidermis with melanocytes,* Masson-Fontana silver reaction (×720)

A stratified squamous epithelium with keratinization is found only in the skin.

TESSELLATED FORMATS: SURFACE EPITHELIA

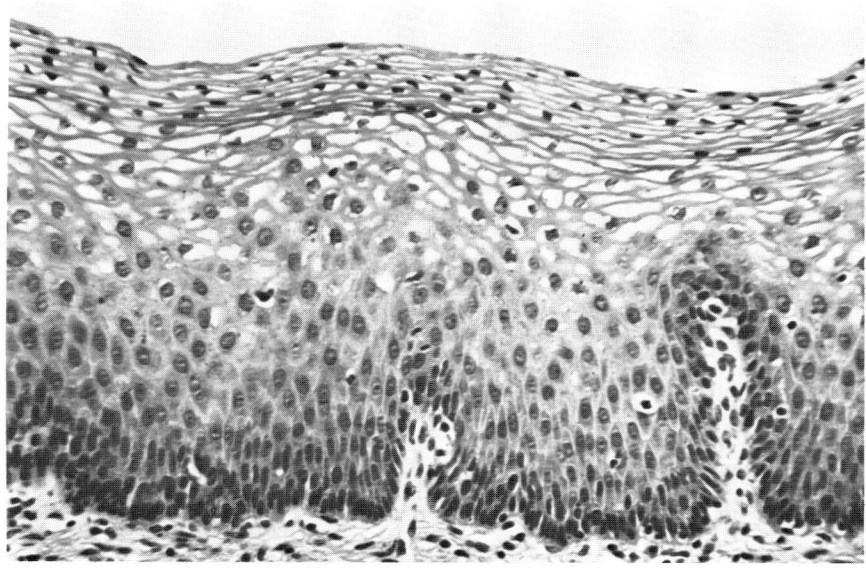

Figure 46. Also a stratified squamous mucosa, but the epithelial cells show empty spaces, representing glycogen lost in processing. Glycogenated mucosa may be found in the lower esophagus, vagina, and ectocervix. *Ectocervix* (×200)

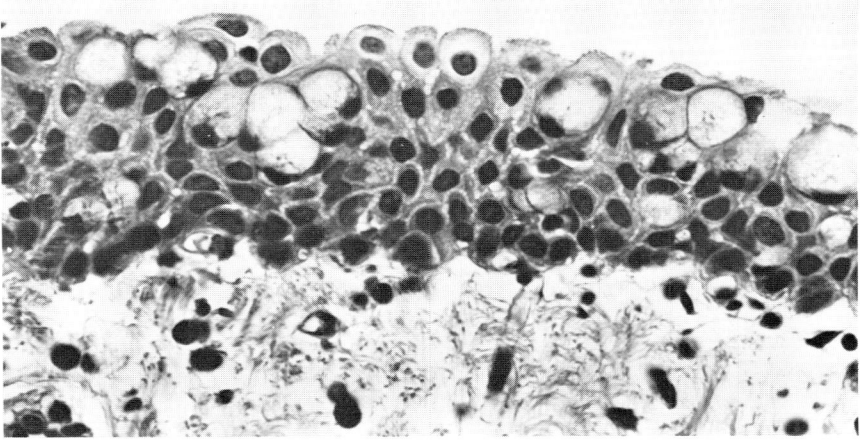

Figure 47. Round empty goblet cells, with eccentric nuclei, interspersed among cells of a stratified columnar epithelium (or in a stratified epithelium with prickle cells as shown here), identify the *conjunctiva* (×480)

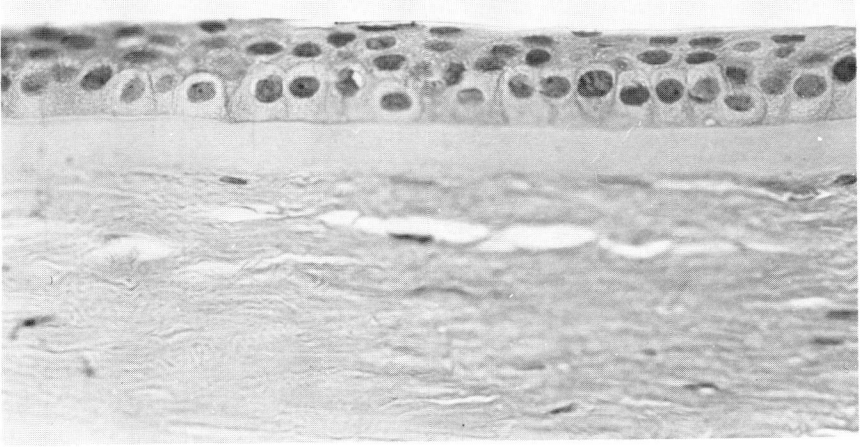

Figure 48. A stratified squamous layer only three or four cells deep with unusually plump basal cells and a completely flat lower surface, which lies on a thick basal lamina (Bowman's membrane), identifies the *cornea* (×480)

A stratified squamous epithelium that lacks a granular layer and is non-keratinizing comes from a mucosal surface that is in continuity with the skin or from the esophagus.

TESSELLATED FORMATS: SURFACE EPITHELIA

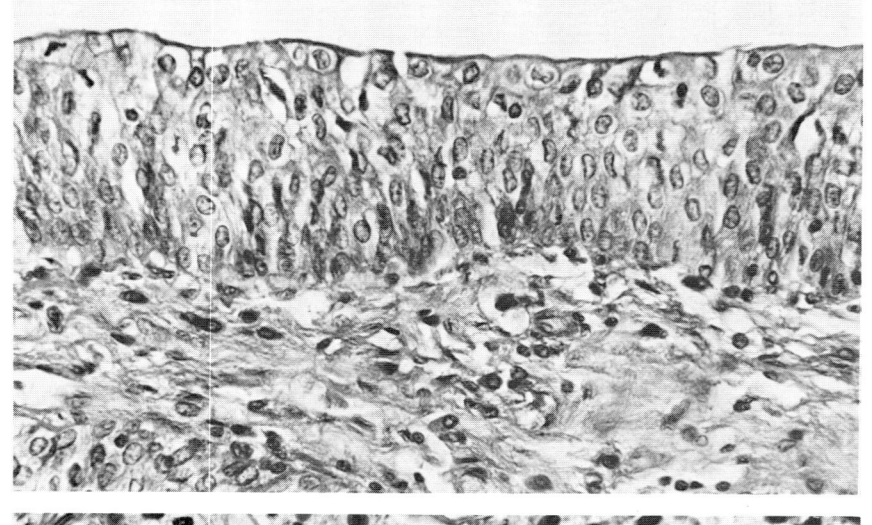

Figure 49. This stratified polygonal epithelium shows no particular differentiation, and the surface cells have a slightly hobnail, or bulging, appearance. Such epithelium identifies the urinary tract. *Ureter* (× 480)

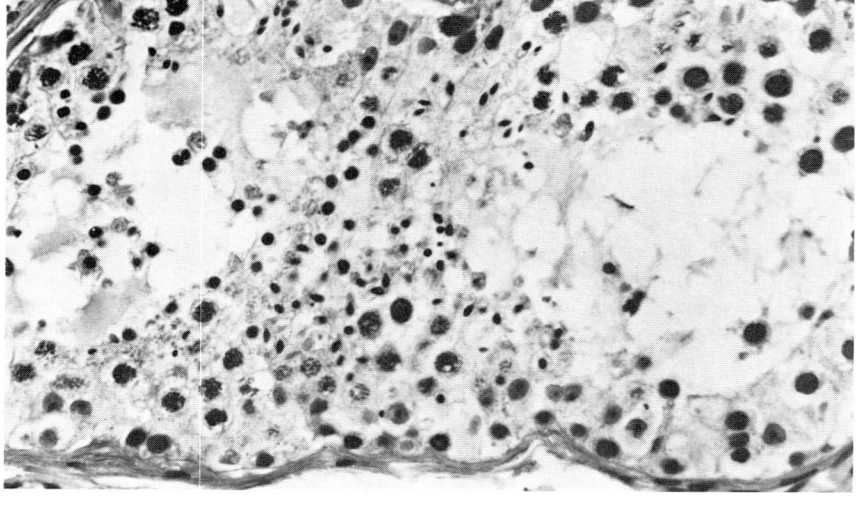

Figure 50. Here the cells are stratified but varied in size with large peripheral cells giving rise to smaller cells, which finally show the spearhead and tail typical of spermatozoa. *Seminiferous tubules* (× 300)

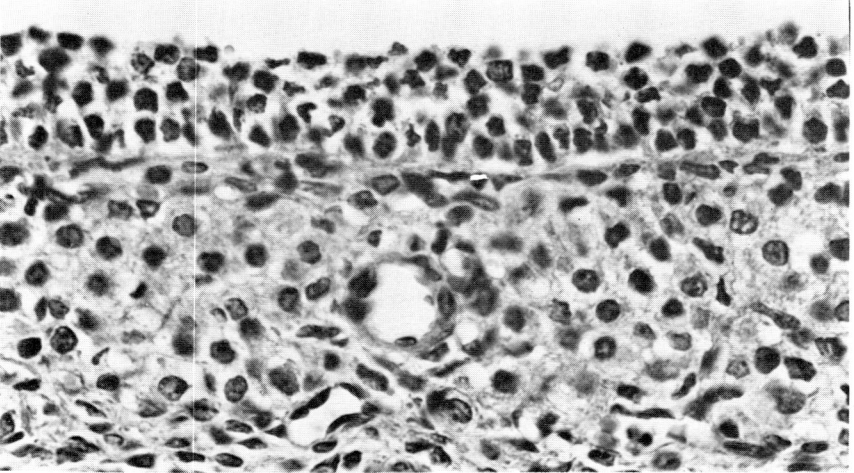

Figure 51. This epithelium has smaller, less regularly arranged cells with a less sharply demarcated surface. They overlie a second layer of epithelioid nature (the cells of the theca interna) a combination unique for the ovary. *Granulosa cell layer* (× 480)

Stratified epithelium with polygonal cells but showing no flattening of the surface, no mucin, keratin, or prickle cell differentiation is found in a restricted number of locations.

TESSELLATED FORMATS: SURFACE EPITHELIA

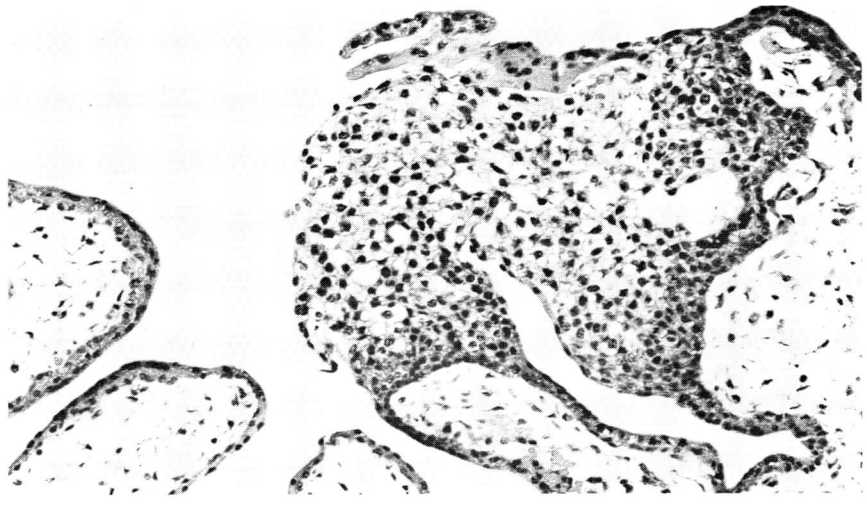

Figure 52. Small masses of polyhedral cells (cytotrophoblasts) associated with syncytial giant cells (upper margin) and appearing intermittently within a double row of epithelium (syncytiotrophoblasts on the surface and cytotrophoblasts beneath) over a myxoid stroma, are unique to the chorionic villi. *Trophoblast* (×135)

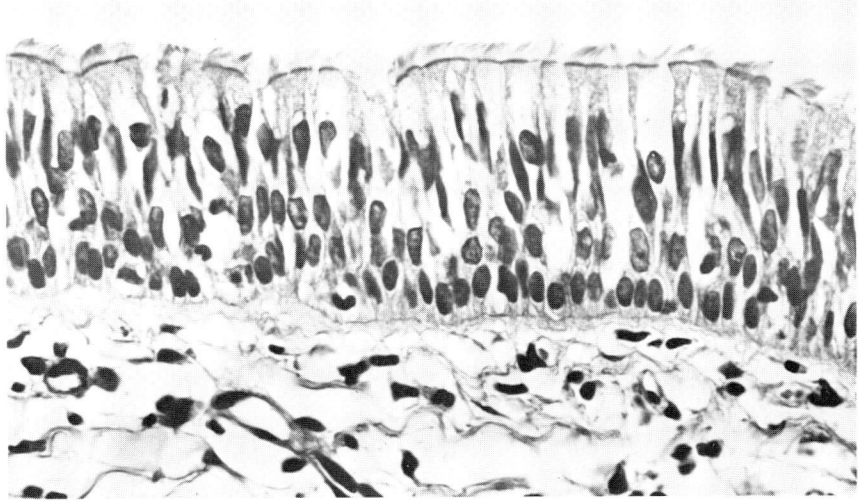

Figure 53. A pseudostratified columnar cell epithelium with cilia visible as fine hairs on the free surface comes from the upper or lower respiratory tract — nasal passages, trachea, and bronchi. *Trachea* (×480)

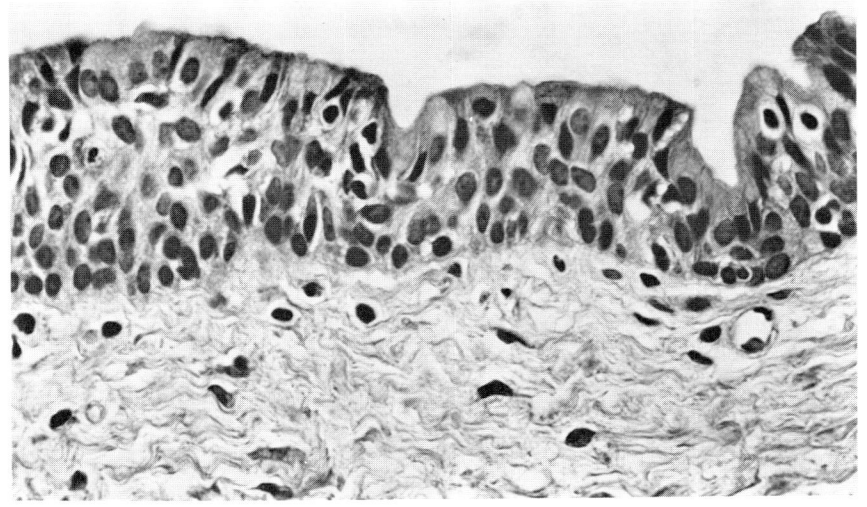

Figure 54. This stratified epithelium has a surface layer of columnar cells, an arrangement seen in ducts of exocrine glands and at the junction of stratified squamous and columnar mucosae. It is thus found in the larynx, the anus, and the mid part of the urethra. *Duct, Bartholin's gland* (×480)

TESSELLATED FORMATS: SURFACE EPITHELIA

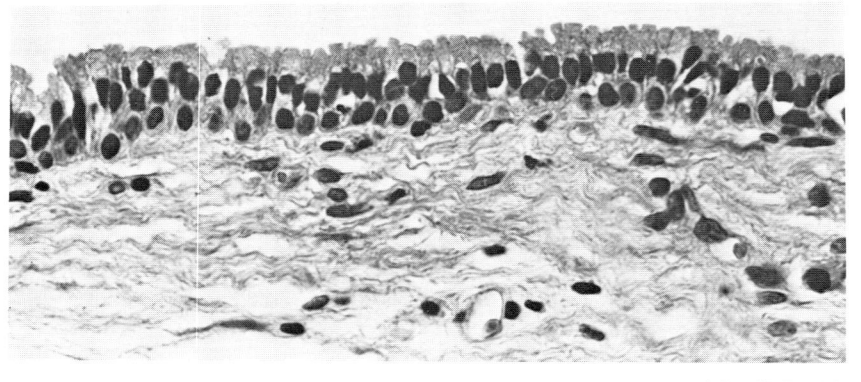

Figure 55. A double cell layer with surface of columnar cells is also common in the larger ducts of many exocrine glands. The peripheral layer may have flattened nuclei and myoepithelial characteristics. *Duct, Bartholin's gland* (× 480)

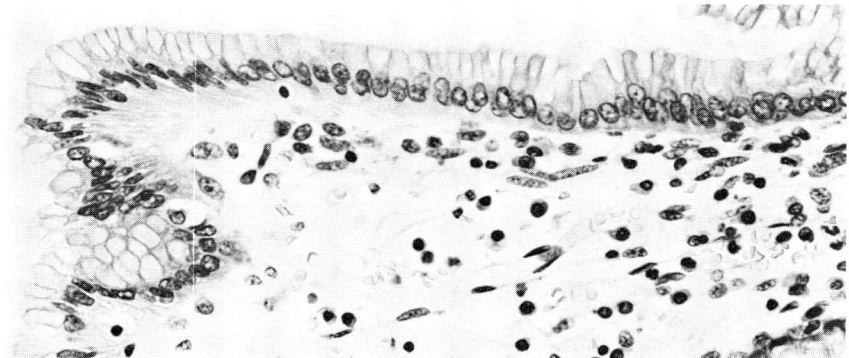

Figure 56. A single layer of tall columnar cells with clear or sometimes opalescent cytoplasm is found in the fovea of the stomach, the gallbladder, and the cervix uteri. These are individually distinguishable only if their deeper parts and supporting stroma are visible. *Foveal epithelium, stomach* (× 480)

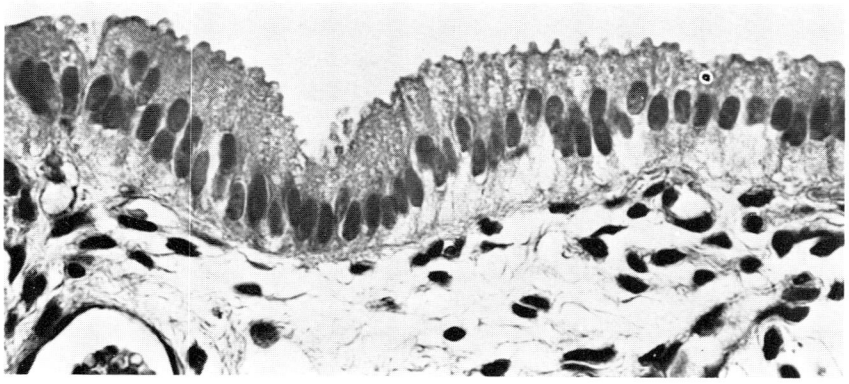

Figure 57. This is also a simple columnar epithelium but comes from the gallbladder. Sometimes it may be recognized because of brown pigment, which may be seen in the cytoplasm. *Gallbladder* (× 480)

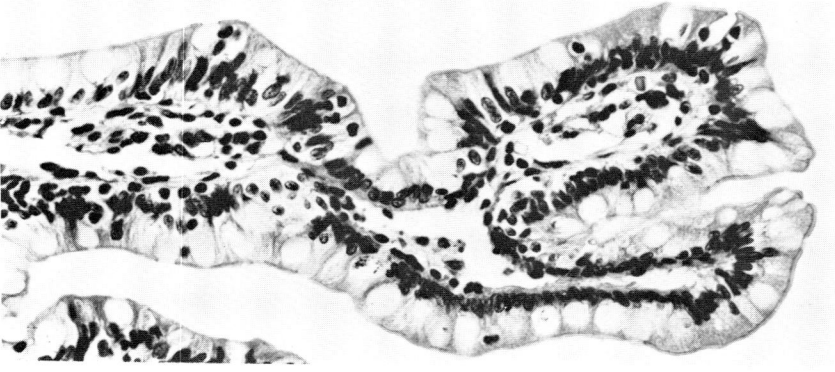

Figure 58. A simple columnar epithelium with interspersed goblet cells identifies the intestinal mucosal epithelium. The goblet cells become increasingly numerous in more distal parts and in the terminal large bowel are so numerous that they may dominate the picture. *Small intestine* (× 480)

TESSELLATED FORMATS: SURFACE EPITHELIA

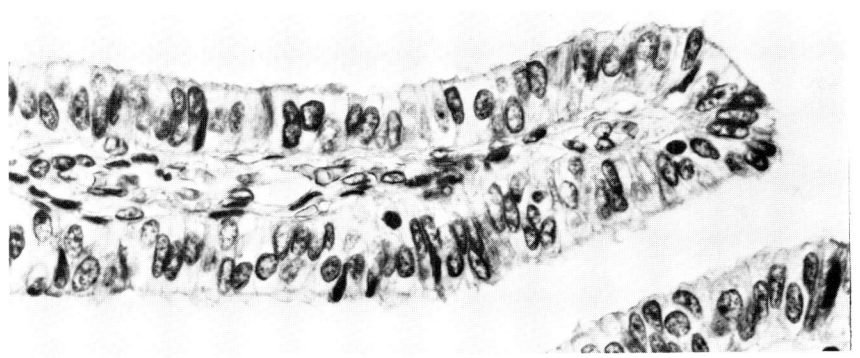

Figure 59. A single layer of columnar epithelium, which includes ciliated cells, comes from the fallopian tube or endometrium. If the ciliated cells are combined with narrow peg cells and with columnar cells with surface cupolae of cytoplasm, whose nuclei project above the general surface layer, the resultant variegated appearance is characteristic of *fallopian tube.* (×480)

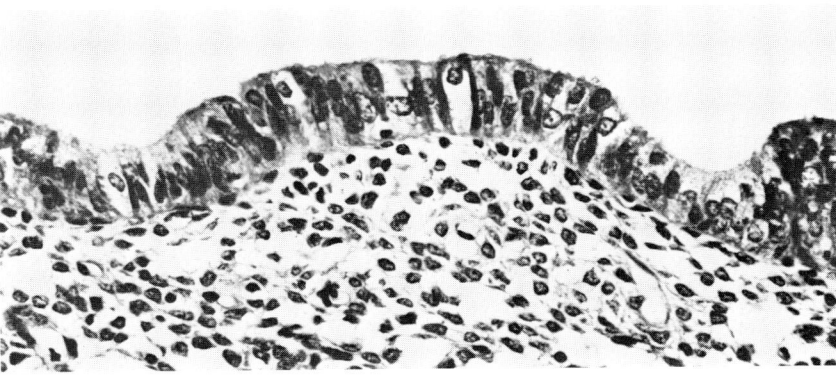

Figure 60. A more regular arrangement of columnar cells, a few ciliated, others with dark cytoplasm, is typical of the endometrium. Here there is likely to be some attached stromal tissue with rather scattered cells having oval nuclei in a loose arrangement with myxoid or fibrillary characteristics. *Endometrium* (×480)

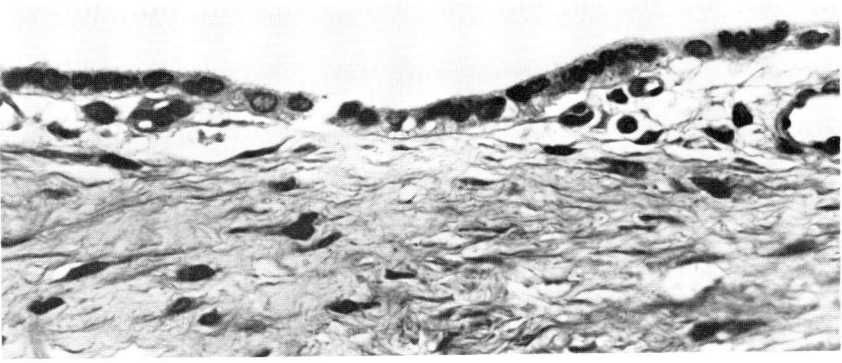

Figure 61. A cuboidal epithelium lines the amnion, thyroid follicles, posterior iris, and anterior lens of the eye. *Amnion* (×480)

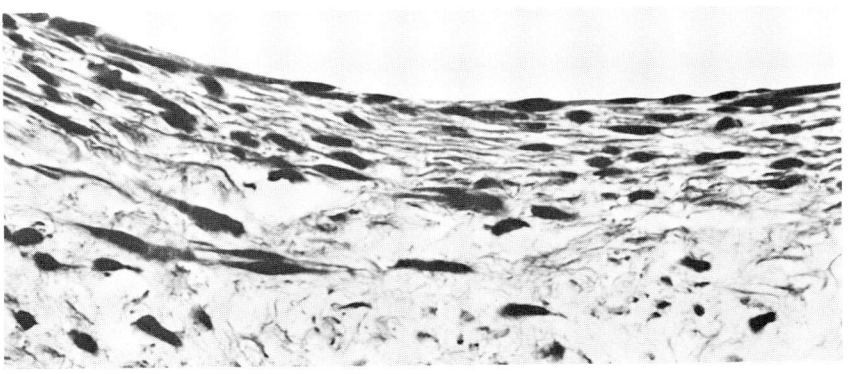

Figure 62. A single layer of very flat epithelial cells lines the serosal cavities and blood vessels as mesothelium and endothelium respectively. *Vein* (×480)

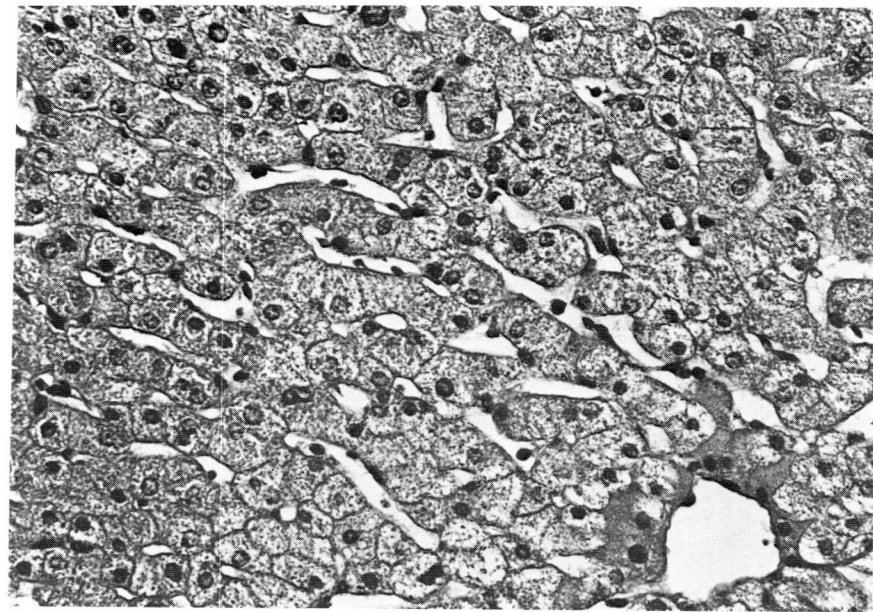

Figure 63. Large epithelial cells in single rows or plates, some parallel, but others diverging. In H & E sections, the cytoplasm is pale with tiny granules. *Liver* (×300)

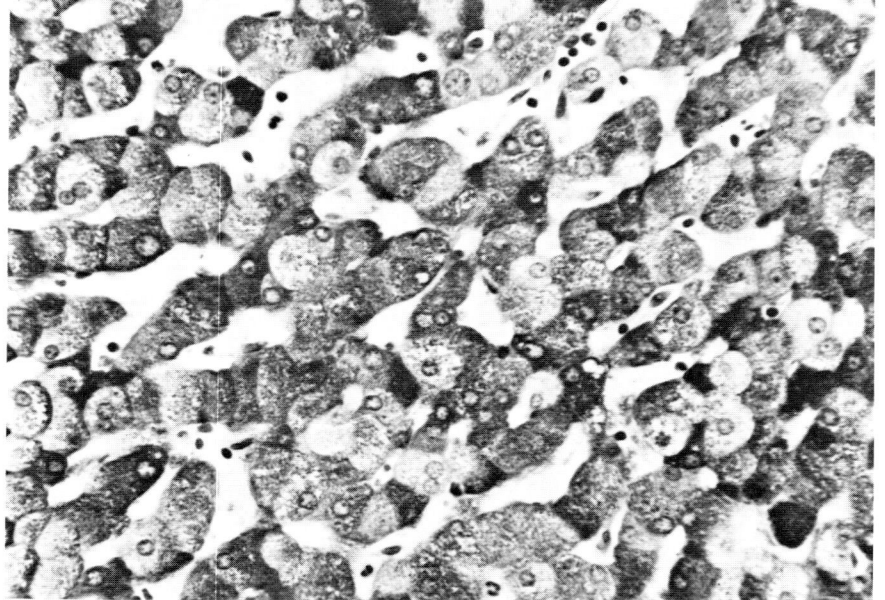

Figure 64. Periodic acid-Schiff (PAS) staining (with resultant magenta color) indicates some cytoplasmic substance, which can be reduced to an aldehyde group, and the presumption is that it may be a sugar. If preliminary treatment with diastase abolishes this reaction, the material is glycogen. *Liver*, PAS (×300)

Deep epithelia are identified by the arrangement, size, shape, and differentiation of cells. Large cells are found in the liver, adrenal cortex, corpus luteum, and sebaceous glands; small epithelial cells in the parathyroid; and a combination of large and small cells in the anterior pituitary.

ENCLOSED EPITHELIA

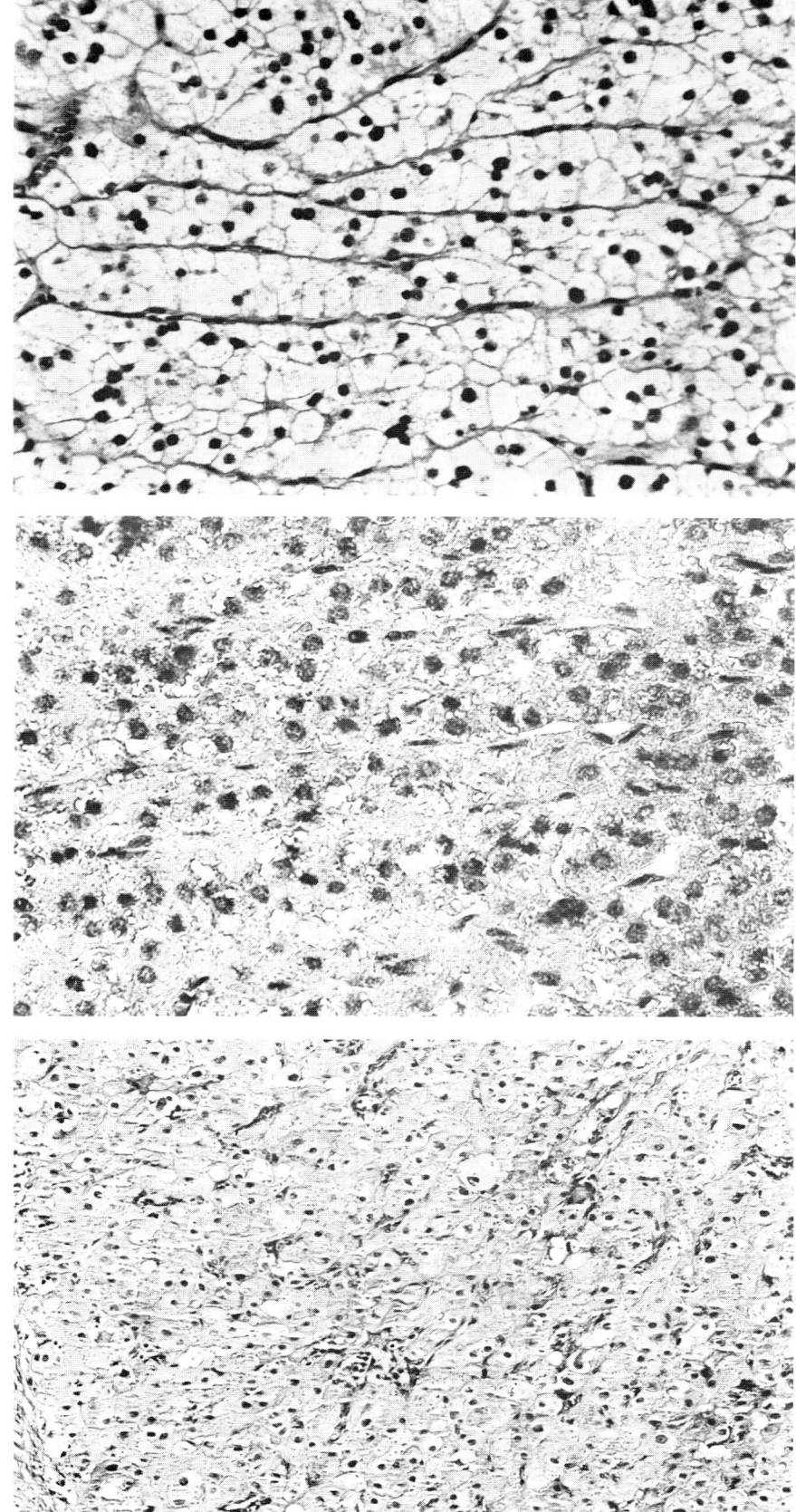

Figure 65. Relatively large cells in regular rows, often double, and separated by a scanty but highly vascular stroma. The cytoplasm is extremely pale and vacuolated. *Adrenal* (× 250)

Figure 66. Lysochrome coloring of the same gland prepared through Carbowax® shows that the pale vacuolated appearance of the cells was due to lipid; this is largely cholesterol ester. *Adrenal,* oil red O (× 250)

Figure 67. Again, large pale cells containing lipid, but there is no particular architectural arrangement. Specific identification depends on the surrounding tissues. *Corpus luteum, ovary* (× 120)

ENCLOSED EPITHELIA

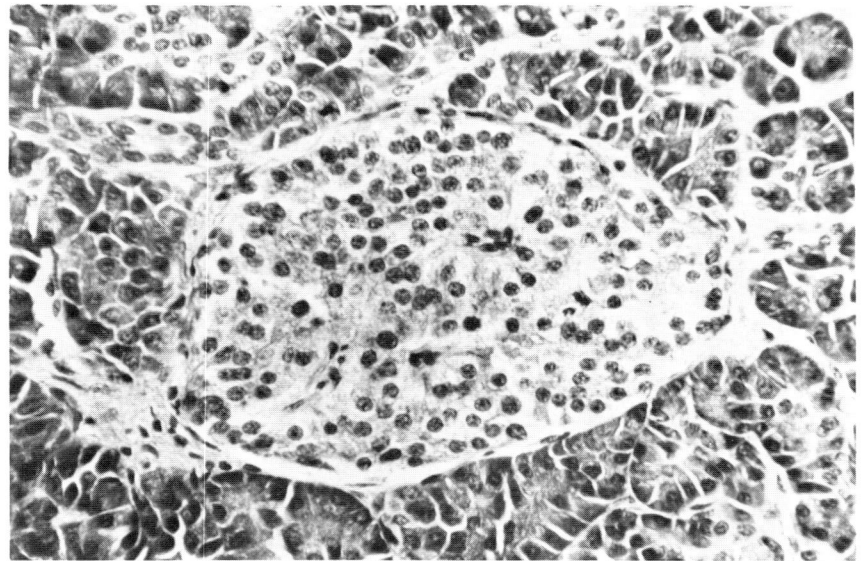

Figure 68. Small epithelial cells in spheroidal islands are typical of the *islets of Langerhans* of the pancreas. (× 320)

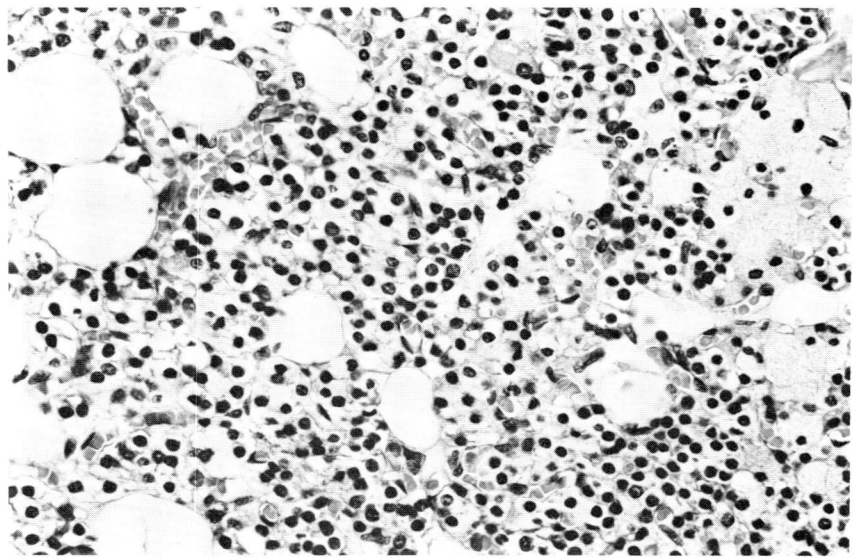

Figure 69. Small epithelial cells without organized pattern but in adults associated with fat cells are found in the parathyroid. On the right are large (oxyphilic) cells, which are a normal component after puberty. *Parathyroid* (× 480)

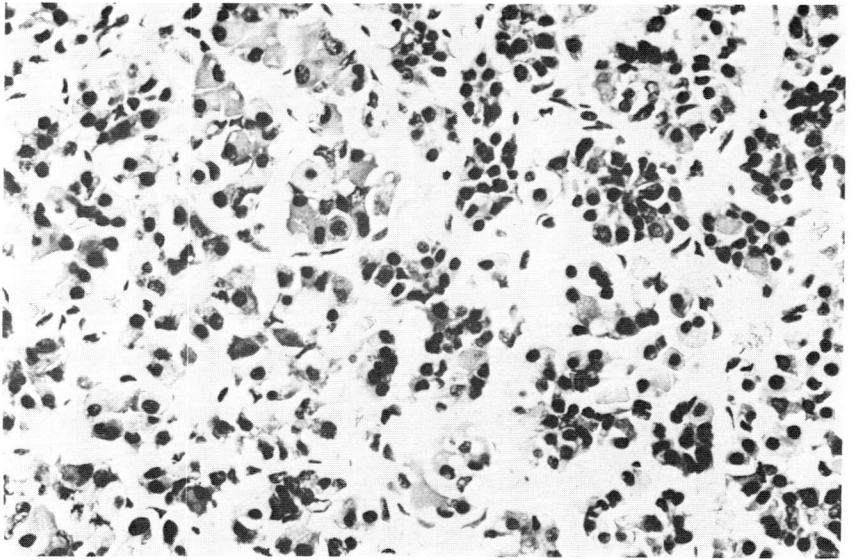

Figure 70. A combination of small and large cells in a highly vascularized stroma is typical of the pituitary. Distinctive basophilic, eosinophilic, and unstained cytoplasm can be seen in different cells in H & E sections, although difficult to appreciate here. *Pituitary* (× 480)

MOSAIC (EPITHELIOID) FORMATS: CONNECTIVE TISSUES

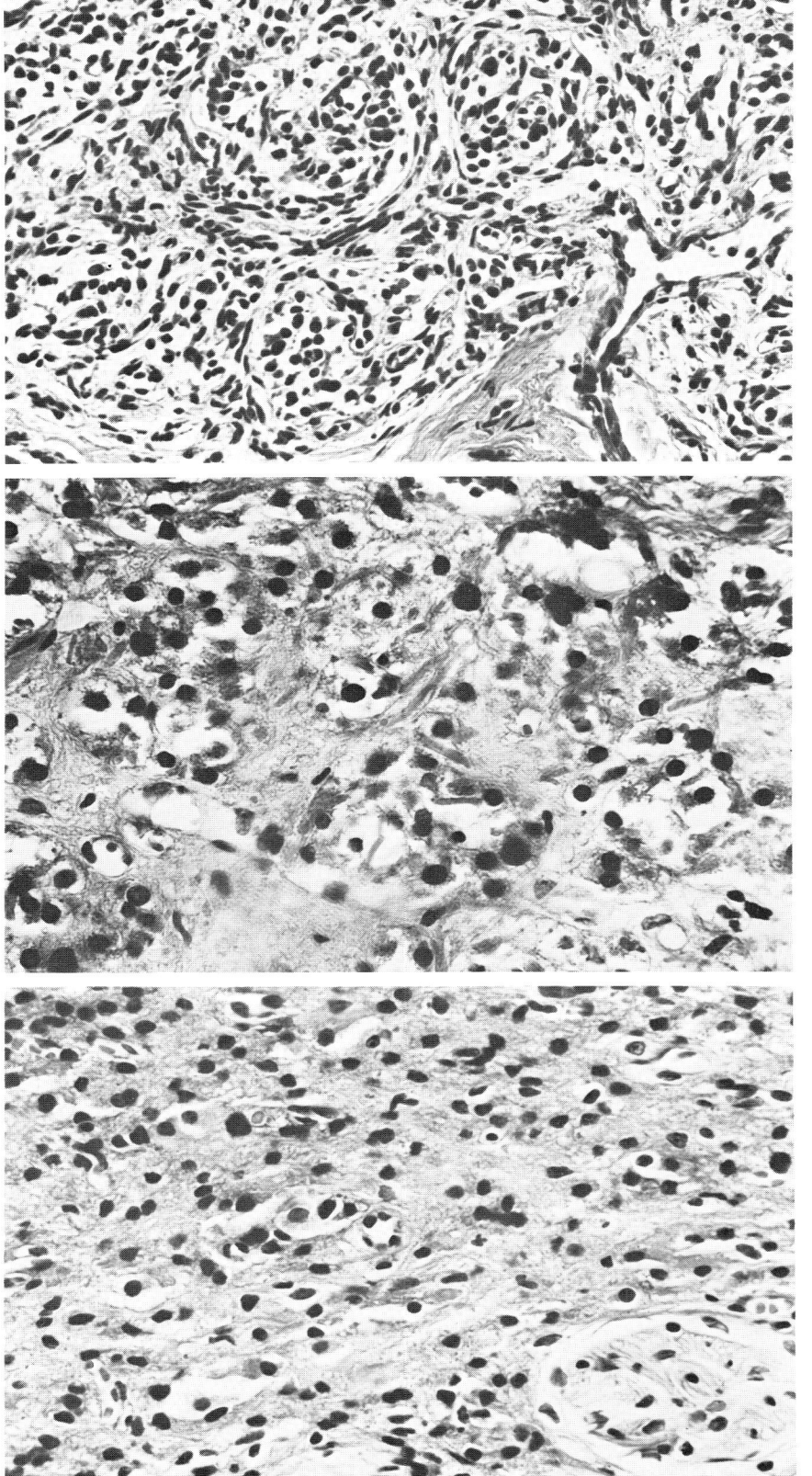

Figure 71. A mosaic format, which has epithelioid cells in a mesenchymal background and which has some thicker septa of fibrous tissue, is seen in paraganglia. *Carotid body* (×250)

Figure 72. These epithelioid cells with a loose connective tissue matrix come from the testis and are associated with small rodlike crystals (Reinke). Several are seen here in the center of the figure. Similar crystals may be found in the hilus cells of the ovary. *Leydig cells* (×320)

Figure 73. This mosaic of epithelioid cells is associated with small nerves and vessels and comes from the hilus of the ovary. *Interstitial or hilus cells* (×320)

Tissues with a mosaic format in which the cells are segregated by collagen, elastin, reticulin, or acid mucopolysaccharide belong to the family of connective tissues.

MOSAIC (EPITHELIOID) FORMATS: CONNECTIVE TISSUES

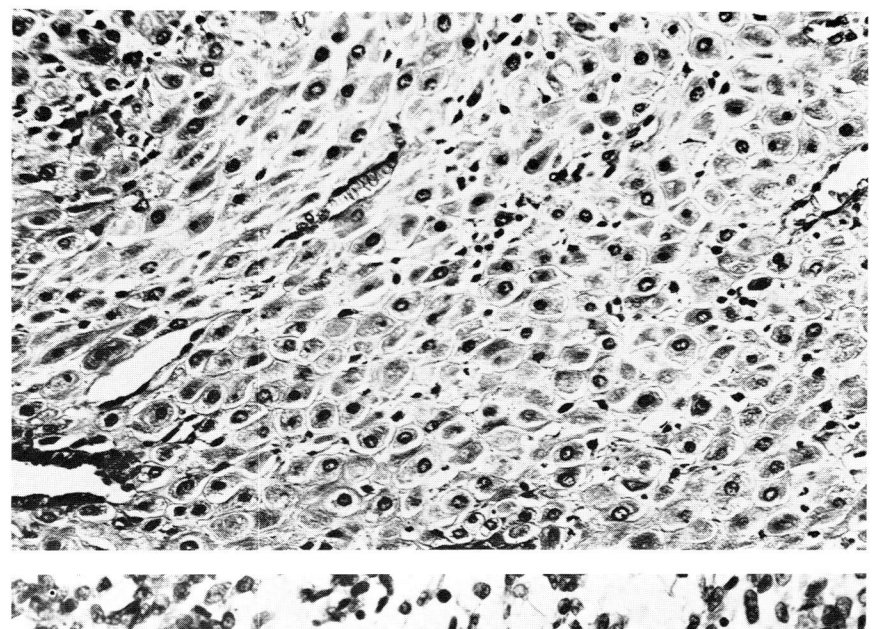

Figure 74. Large epithelioid cells separated by small clefts representing acid mucopolysaccharide. This is the altered endometrial stroma seen in pregnancy. *Uterine decidua* (× 200)

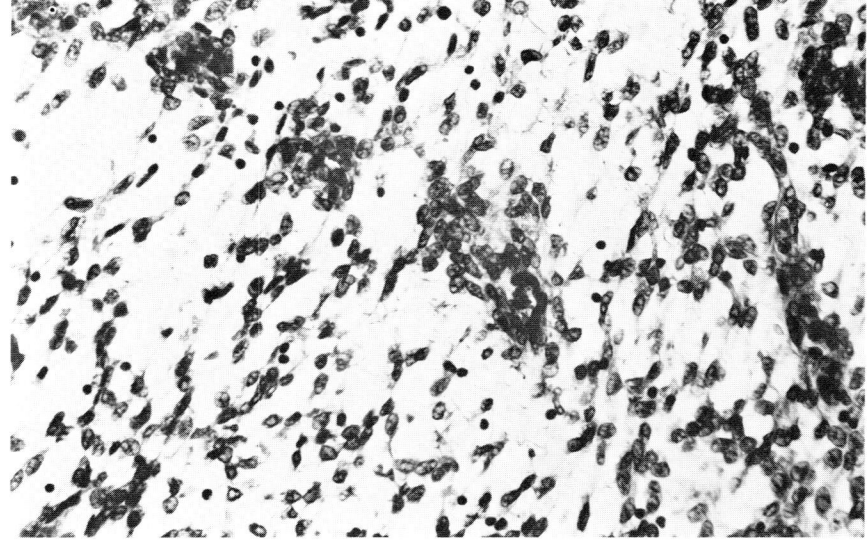

Figure 75. The format here is not strictly a mosaic but more comparable to a fibrillary tangle, but the figure is placed here for contrast with the decidua above. The cytoplasm of the cells is inconspicuous, and there is much ground substance. This is *endometrial stroma* as seen in the proliferative phase of the cycle. (× 250)

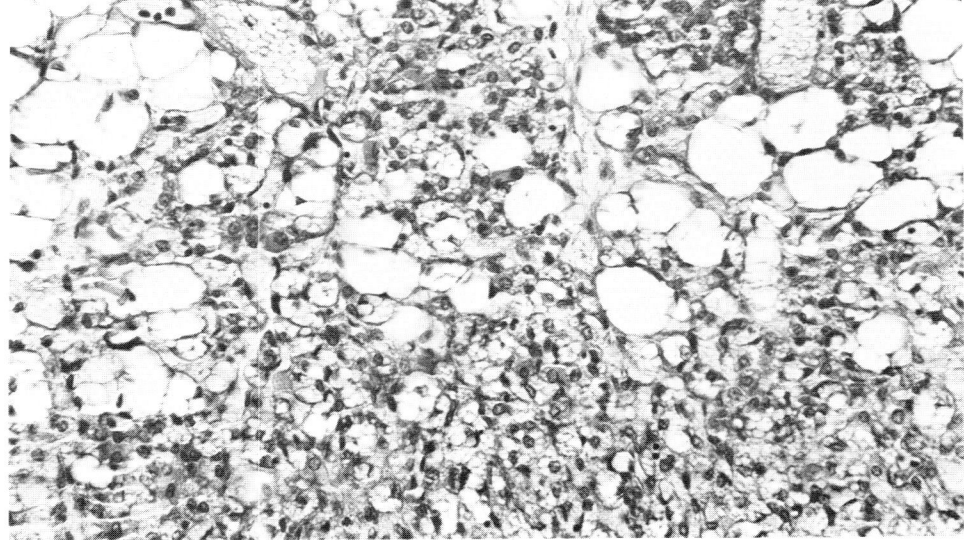

Figure 76. Along the lower margin are closely packed, finely vacuolated epithelioid cells, merging with easily recognized fat cells of adult type. *Brown fat* (× 200)

INLAID FORMATS: NEURAL TISSUES

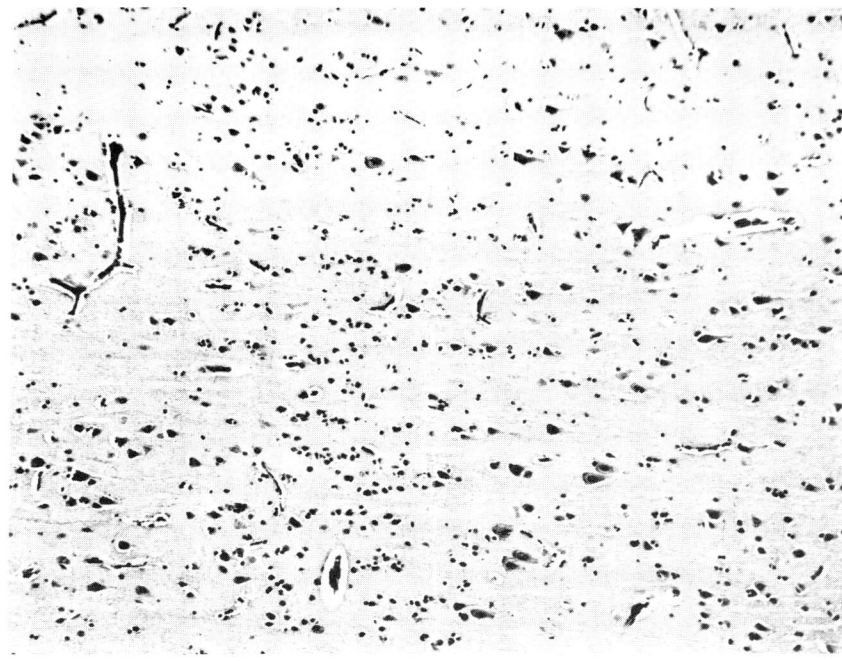

Figure 77. The format here is inlaid, with a finely granular, slightly linear background in which are scattered neurones, astrocytes, oligodendrocytes, and microglia. The larger triangular cells that appear to be arranged in rows with their apices pointing (towards the meninges) are pyramidal neurones. *Brain cortex*, gray matter (×80)

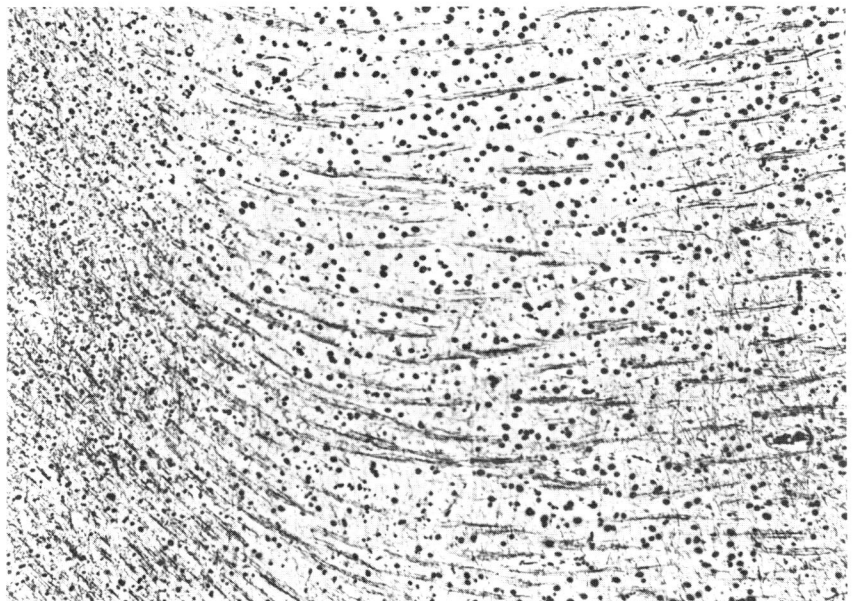

Figure 78. An area comparable to that shown in Figure 77, when subjected to Bodian's silver reaction, shows numerous axons running horizontally through the gray matter (in the right two-thirds) and curving to enter the dense fibrillary white matter in the left margin of the field. *Cerebral cortex* (×80)

DISTINCTIVE NEURONES

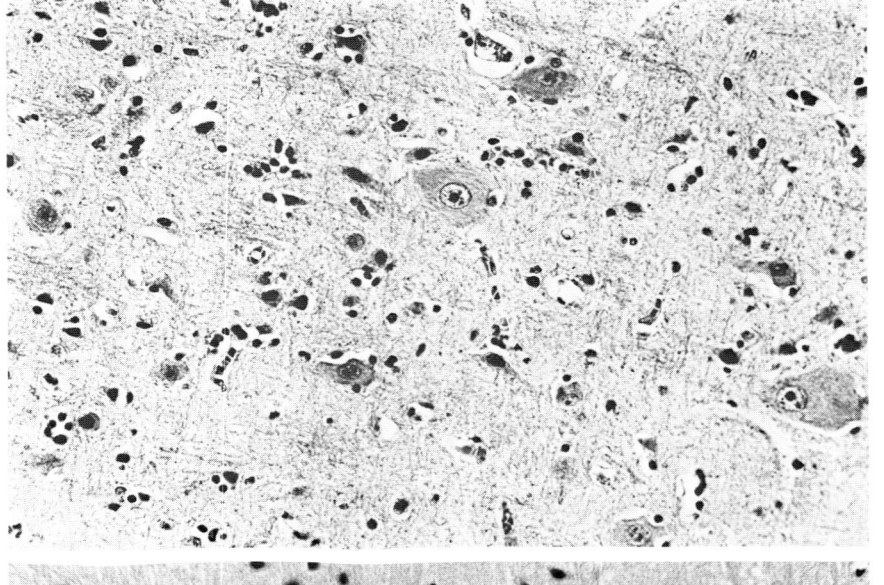

Figure 79. The very large pyramidal cells with prominent nuclei and nucleoli are the Betz's cells from the motor cortex; the small round haloed nuclei come from oligodendroglia, the oval nuclei from microglia, and the larger round nuclei from astrocytes. The dark granules in the cytoplasm of Betz's cells are Nissl bodies. *Cerebral cortex* (× 200)

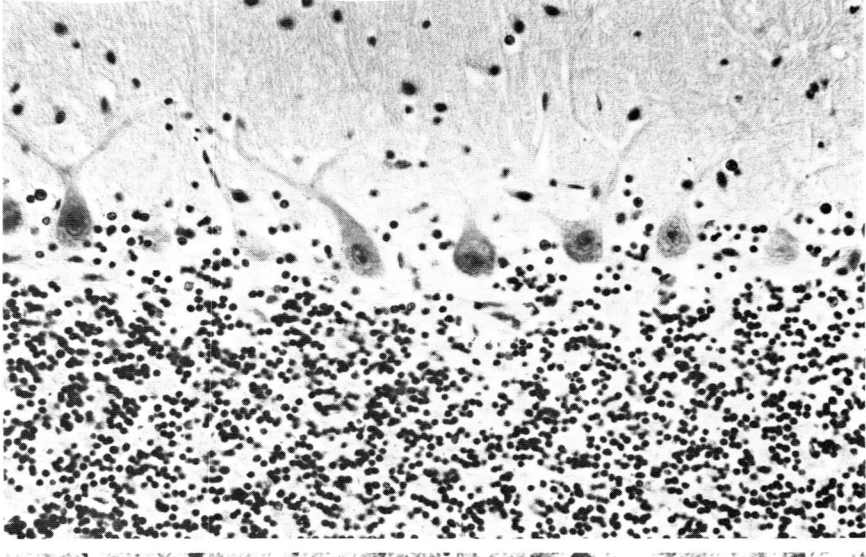

Figure 80. These large flask-shaped neurones with coarse dendritic processes, some showing obvious branching, are Purkinje cells. The upper gray matter contains astrocytes; the lower half shows small neurones of the granular layer of the cerebellum, interrupted by small clear areas known as islands or glomeruli, largely formed from dendrites. *Cerebellar cortex* (× 200)

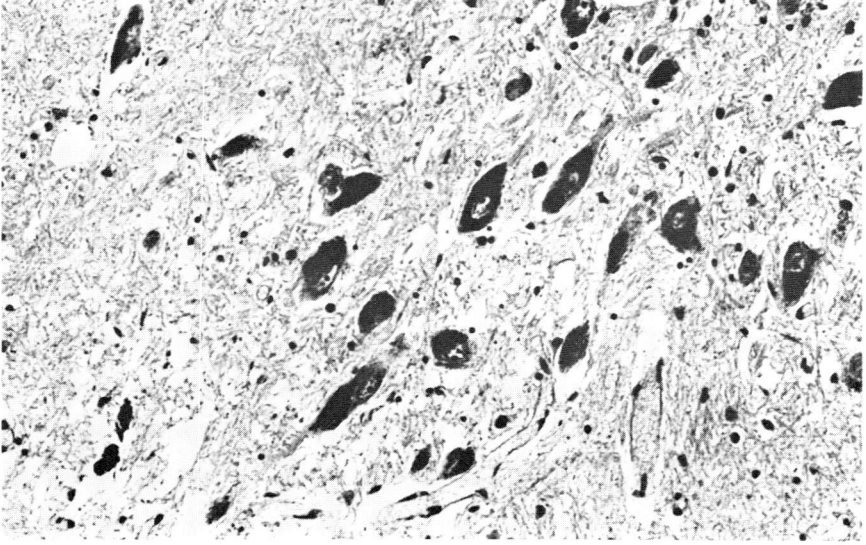

Figure 81. These are also large neurones, but their cytoplasm is obscured by black pigment (melanin), which may be seen in the substantia nigra, locus ceruleus, dorsal nucleus of the vagus, and occasionally in other neurones, including dorsal root ganglia. *Substantia nigra* (× 150)

Some large neurones can be distinguished by their size, shape, and cytoplasm differentiation.

INLAID AND FIBRILLARY FORMATS: NEURAL TISSUES

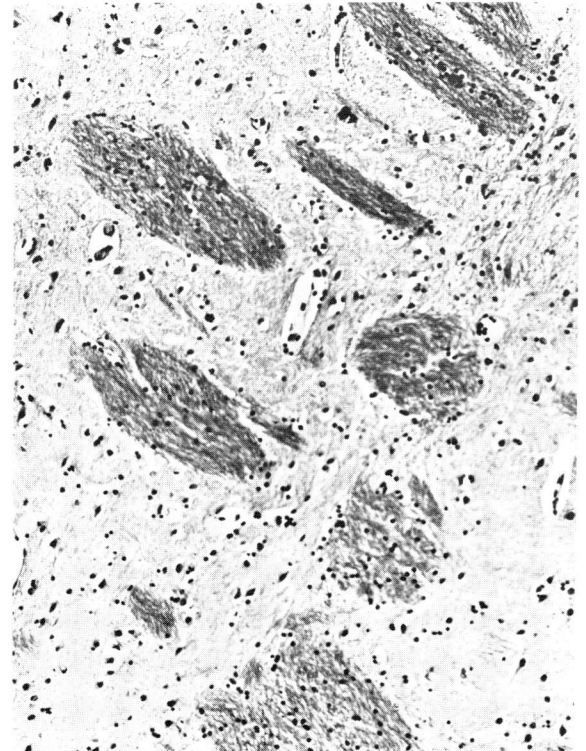

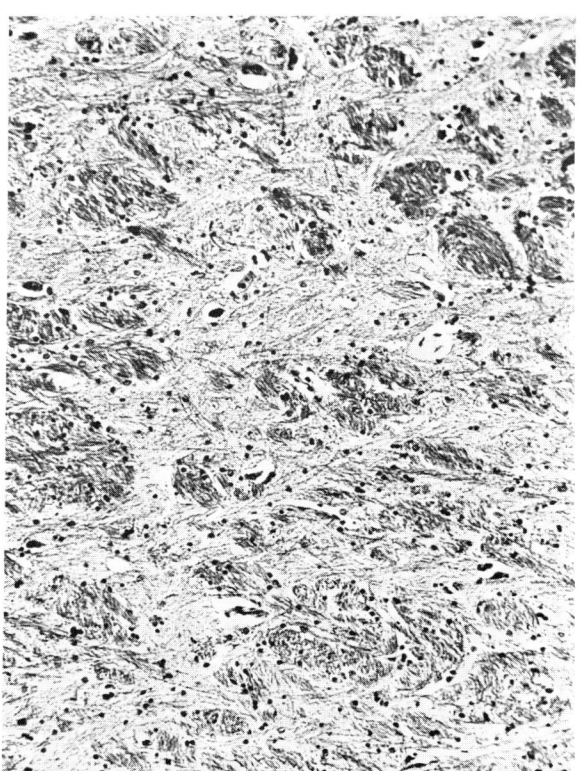

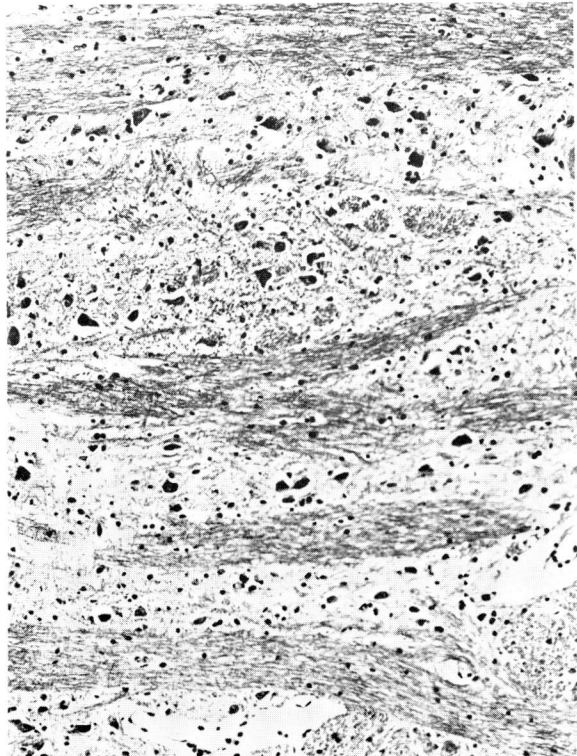

Figure 82. (Upper left) Relatively large, widely separated bundles of fibers running through gray matter identify the *putamen*. (×80)

Figure 83. (Upper right) Here there are more closely grouped fiber bundles in gray matter, an arrangement that identifies the *globus pallidus*. (×80)

Figure 84. (Lower left) Where fiber bundles run in an almost regular parallel fashion, dividing off large areas of gray matter (nuclei), the structure is the *pons*, cut transversely. (×80)

Certain areas where fiber tracts and gray matter intermingle can be recognized by the arrangement and relative proportions of the two elements.

INLAID FORMATS: CONNECTIVE TISSUES

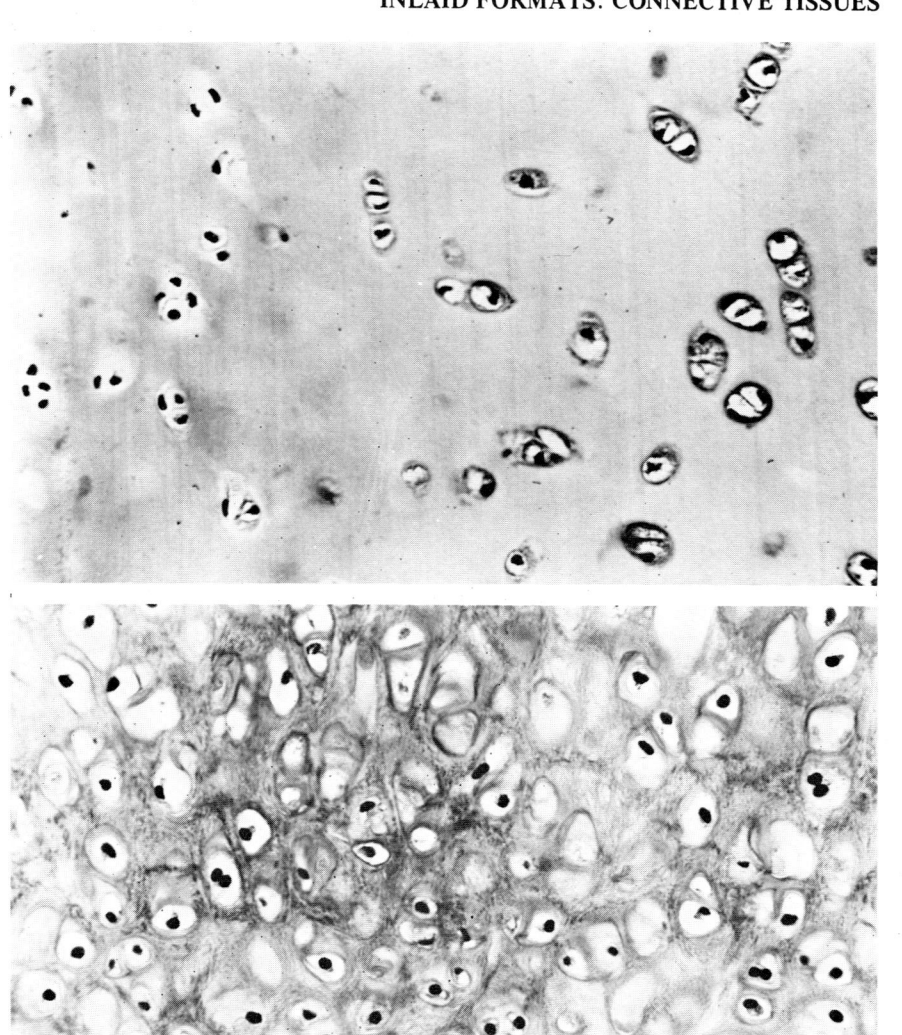

Figure 85. Round or oval cells, in small clusters of two or three, widely separated and embedded in a sea of matrix material, identify cartilage. Different varieties are recognized by the intercellular material. A large amount of proteoglycan, staining with a bluish color and smooth in texture, identifies hyaline cartilage. The densely staining zone immediately around the cartilage cells is known as the capsule. Hyaline cartilage is seen in the embryonic skeleton, the cartilages of the nose and the respiratory tract, the epiphyseal plates, and the articular cartilages. *Hyaline cartilage* (× 200)

Figure 86. Cells of similar appearance, but more distinctly encapsulated and associated with fibers that can be seen in the matrix, identify elastic cartilage. The nature of the fibers can be confirmed by appropriate connective tissue stains. Elastic cartilage is found in the external ear, epiglottis, and some laryngeal cartilages. *Pinna* (× 250)

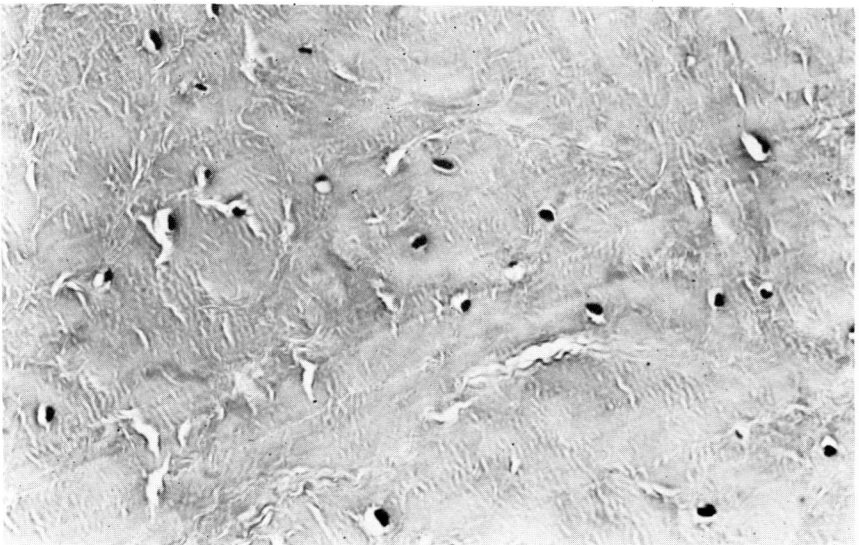

Figure 87. Here the matrix is distinctly fibrillary, and a large amount of collagen can be demonstrated. Cells are smaller, and usually the lacunae contain only one chondrocyte. This is fibrocartilage, found in the menisci — at the insertion of tendons, the symphysis pubis, and the periphery of the intervertebral discs. *Semilunar cartilage* (× 250)

Connective tissues having an inlaid format are classified by the nature of the matrix, which may be chondroid, osseous, or fibrous.

INLAID FORMATS: CONNECTIVE TISSUES

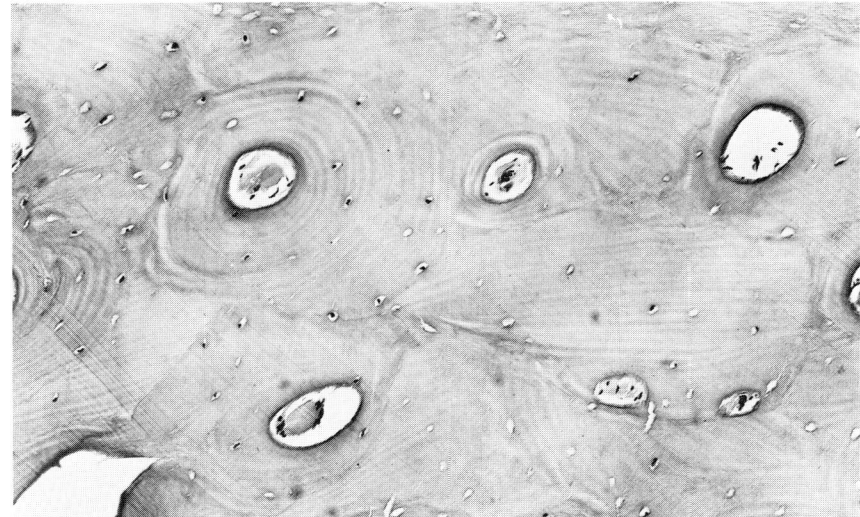

Figure 88. An inlaid format with small single cells in a dense eosinophilic matrix with faintly fibrillary characteristics is decalcified bone. The cells are osteocytes, and here they are arranged in rings, centered on canals that carry blood vessels, to form haversian systems, or osteons. Canals with larger vessels communicating with the bone surface, and without concentric lamellae, are Volkmann's canals. *Cortical bone* (×80)

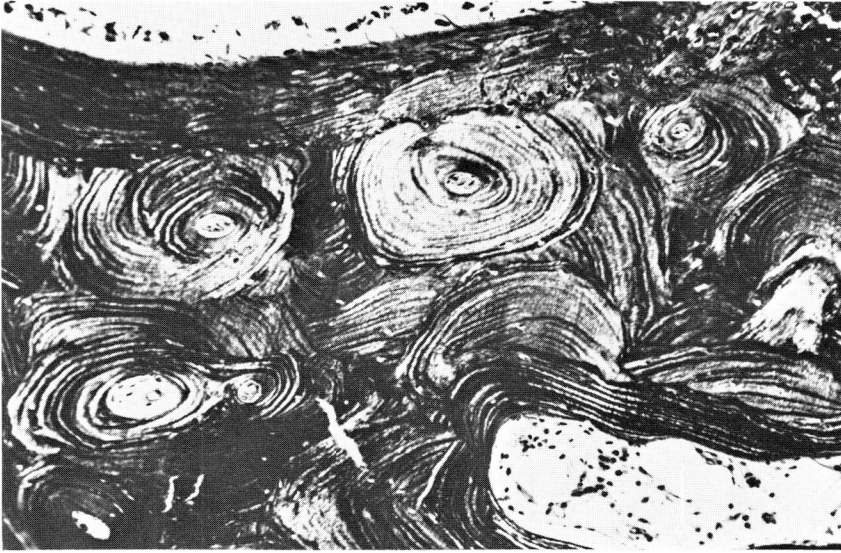

Figure 89. A similar preparation when examined by polarized light shows the concentric haversion lamellae of the osteons, as well as the parallel bands of subperiosteal circumferential lamellae (upper margin) and the small interstitial lamellae, between the osteons. *Bone*, polarized light (×100)

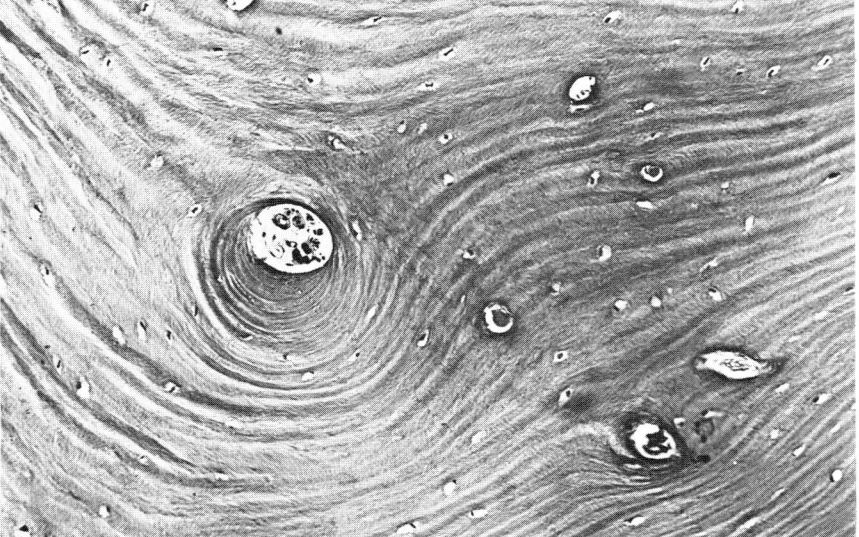

Figure 90. Special stains for collagen reveal something of the underlying nature of bone, which is essentially composed of collagen fibers seen here, which are impregnated with hydroxyapatite crystals, which have been removed by decalcification. Larger collagen fibers passing irregularly into bone from the periosteum are Sharpey's fibers. *Cortical bone*, Movat pentachrome (×120)

In the inlaid format of bone, the diagnostic characteristic of the matrix is its dense calcification. The preparation of sections requires preliminary decalcification. In adults, bone is usually lamellar in construction, with the lamellae arranged in concentric rings to form osteons or in flat plates to form trabeculae.

INLAID FORMATS: CONNECTIVE TISSUES

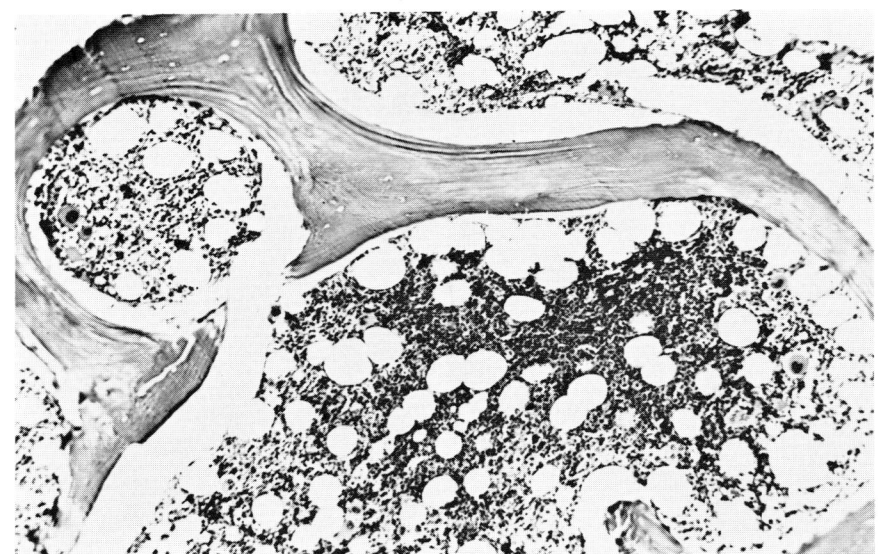

Figure 91. Parallel lamellae of bone, packed together to form flat narrow anastomosing trabeculae, or beams, are found beneath the denser osteons of cortical bone. In infants and in the flat bones and vertebrae of adults, the spaces between the trabeculae contain adipose and myeloid tissues. *Trabecular bone* (×80)

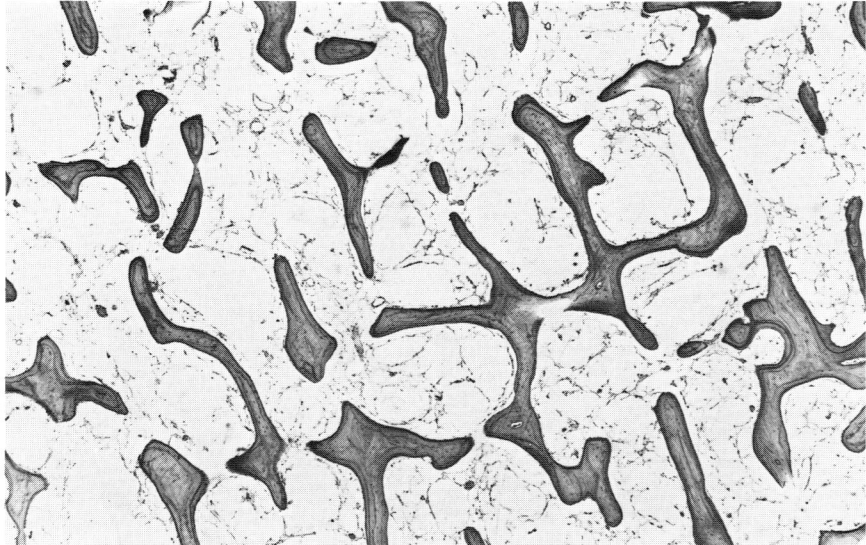

Figure 92. Here the trabeculae are separated by fatty tissue only, with prominent vessels. This is typical of the spongy or medullary bone of the long bones in adults. This comes from an elderly man. *Femur, trabecular bone* (×20)

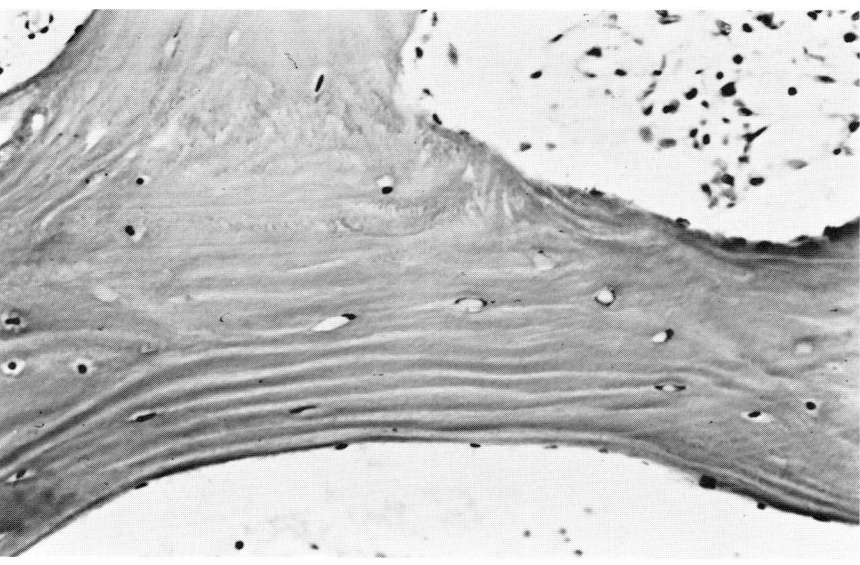

Figure 93. At higher magnification the lamellar structure is easily seen. The single cells between lamellae contain the mature osteocytes while lined along the periphery of the trabeculae are the bone-forming osteoblasts. *Trabecular bone* (×200)

INLAID FORMATS: CONNECTIVE TISSUES

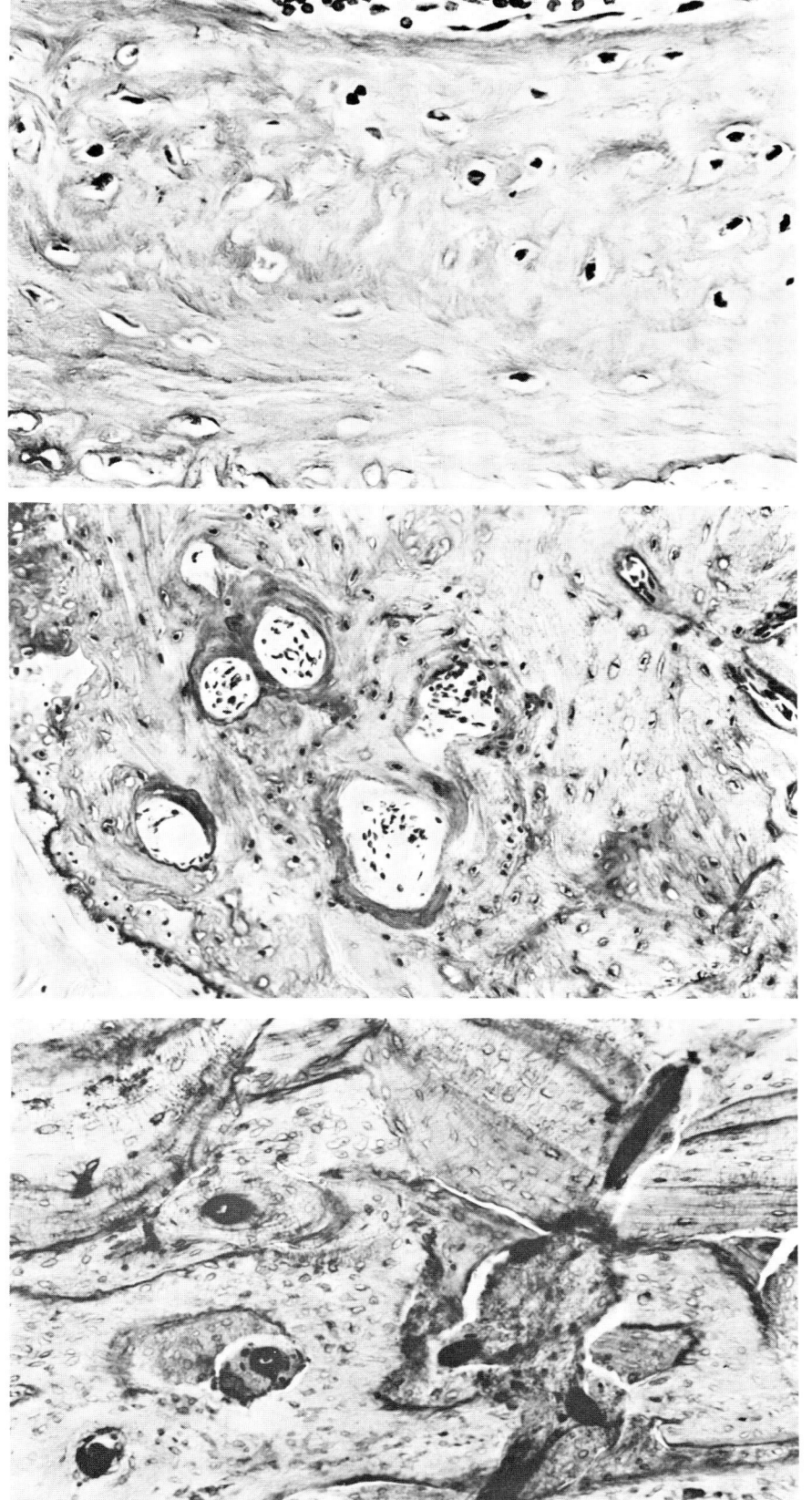

Figure 94. This section also has been decalcified (if not, the calcium salts would have resulted in an intense granular blue-staining reaction). Lamellae are not seen, but the matrix has a fibrous appearance, which is variously described as woven bone, new bone, or fibrillary bone. This comes from the cortex of the femur from a fetus. *Woven bone* (× 275)

Figure 95. The woven bone normal to the fetus is almost entirely replaced by lamellar bone in adults but persists in the ossicles, the petrous temporal bone, and the cementum of a tooth. Here the spaces contain connective tissue but no marrow. *Stapes* (× 120)

Figure 96. The densest bone in the body is said to be the temporal bone, and this can be recognized by a rather mosaic pattern, chiefly of fiber bone but showing some lamellae, both straight and circular. *Petrous temporal bone* (× 120)

INLAID FORMATS: CONNECTIVE TISSUES

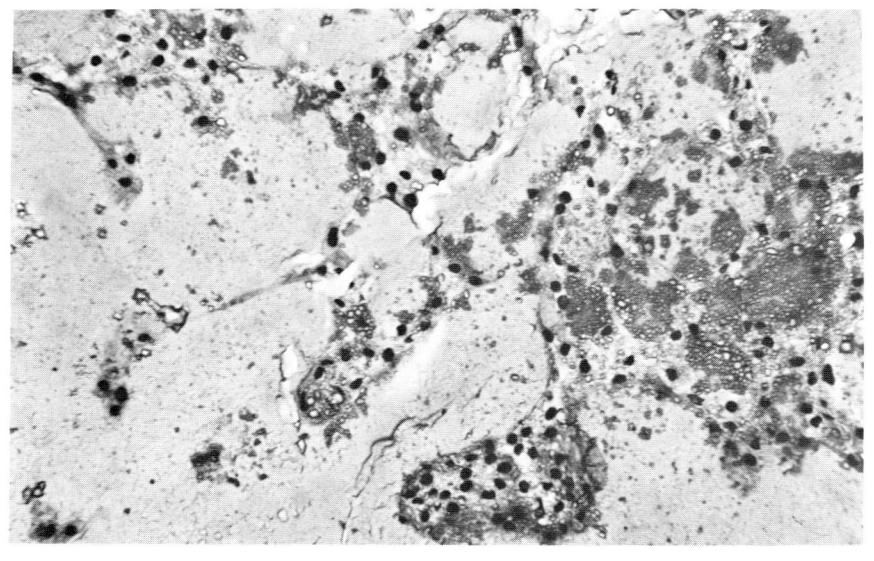

Figure 97. This shows a large amount of amorphous mucoid matrix in which there are clusters of epithelioid cells, with a somewhat vacuolated cytoplasm. This appearance is typical of the *nucleus pulposus* of the fetus. Movat × 200

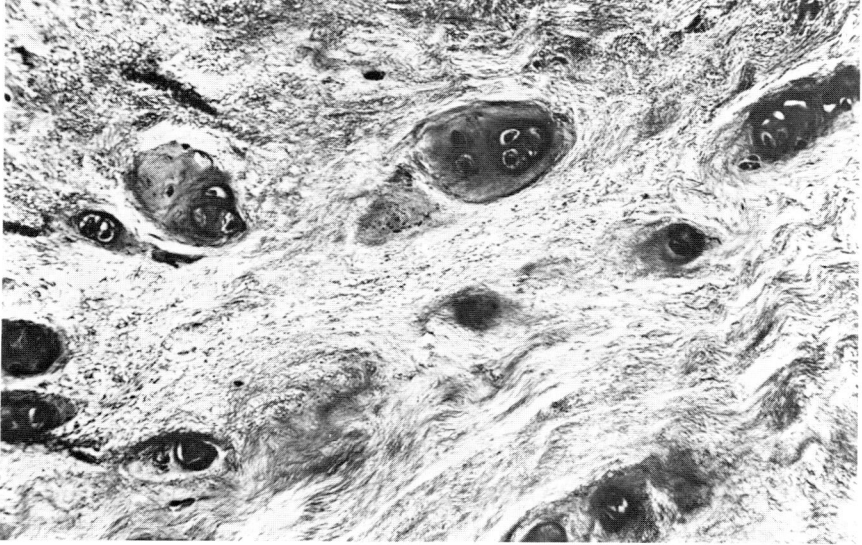

Figure 98. Here the cells are in small clusters and strongly resemble ordinary chondrocytes, each cell in its own lacuna. There is, however, a large amount of intercellular proteoglycans (acid mucopolysaccharide). The fibrillary background so evident here is barely discernible in H & E sections. This is from a fifteen-year-old girl. *Nucleus pulposus,* Movat × 200.

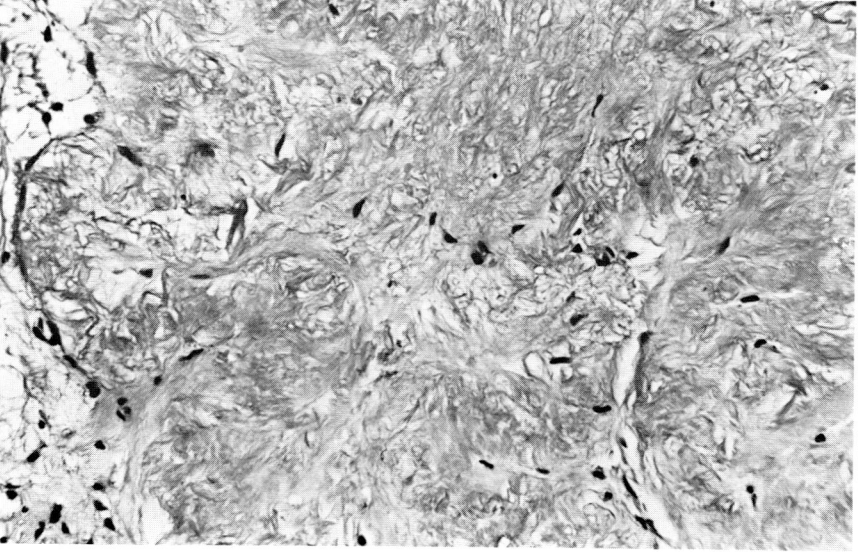

Figure 99. Here there is an abundant matrix with the staining characteristics of collagen, although the general appearance is not fibrillary as with ordinary fibrous tissue but is smooth and hyaline and only occasionally threadlike. *Corpus albicans* (× 200)

FIBRILLARY FORMATS: NEURAL TISSUES

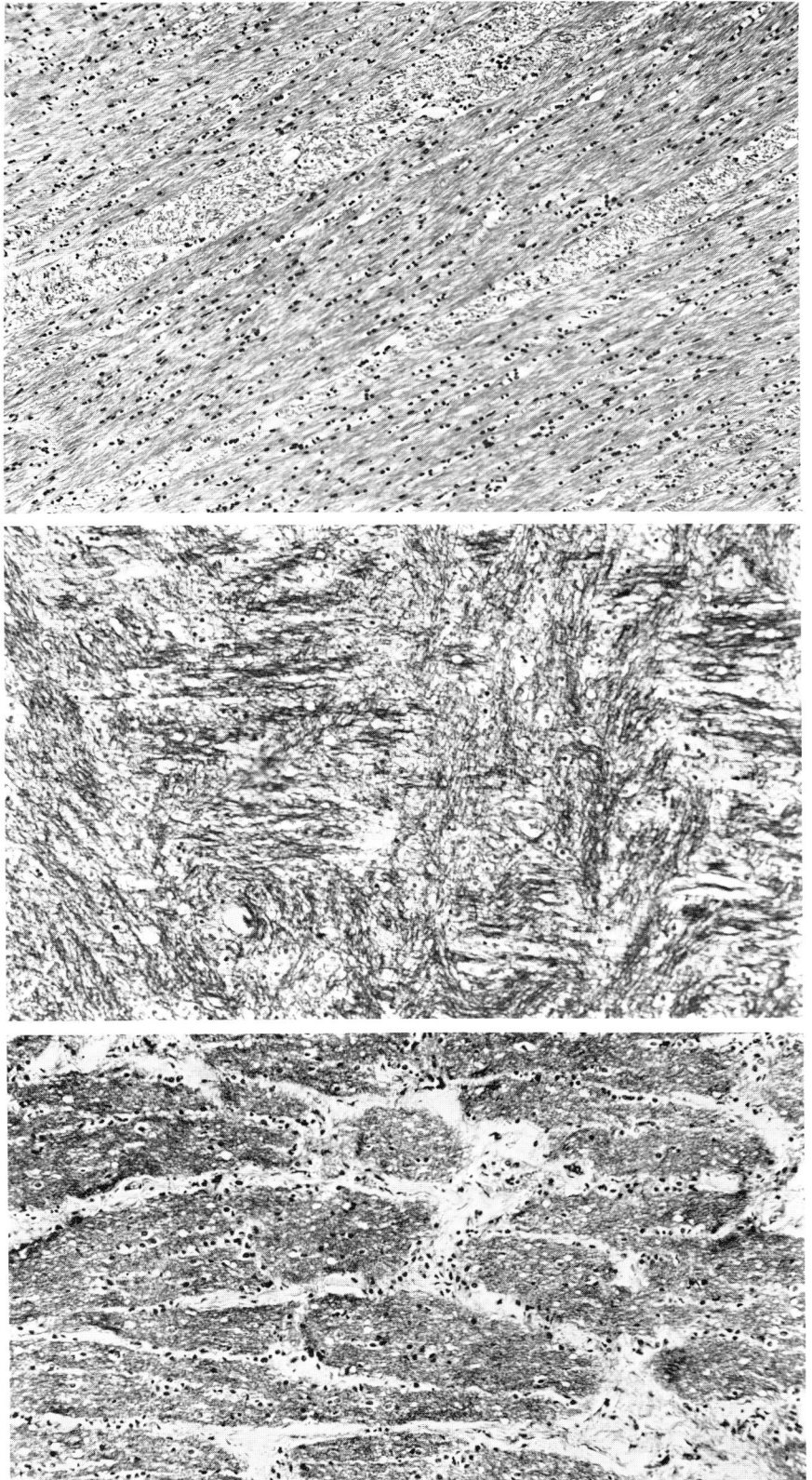

Figure 100. Fine parallel fibers arranged in broad bands, which include the small round nuclei of oligodendroglia and larger round nuclei of astrocytes, identify fiber tracts. The two narrower bands with a punctate appearance have been cut transversely. A section of this size could come only from one of the larger fiber tracts. *Internal capsule* (×80)

Figure 101. Similar fine fibers showing an interwoven pattern can be found at the angle where the internal capsule and corpus callosum interdigitate. (×120)

Figure 102. Fine streaming fibers, again with astrocytes and a glial matrix, but this time including septa of collagenous tissue, which here appear pale, are unique to the *optic nerve*. (×100)

A streaming arrangement of very fine fibers, which are found to be myelinated axons supported by the glial fibers of astrocytes, identifies the fiber tracts of the white matter of the central nervous system.

FIBRILLARY FORMATS: NEURAL TISSUES

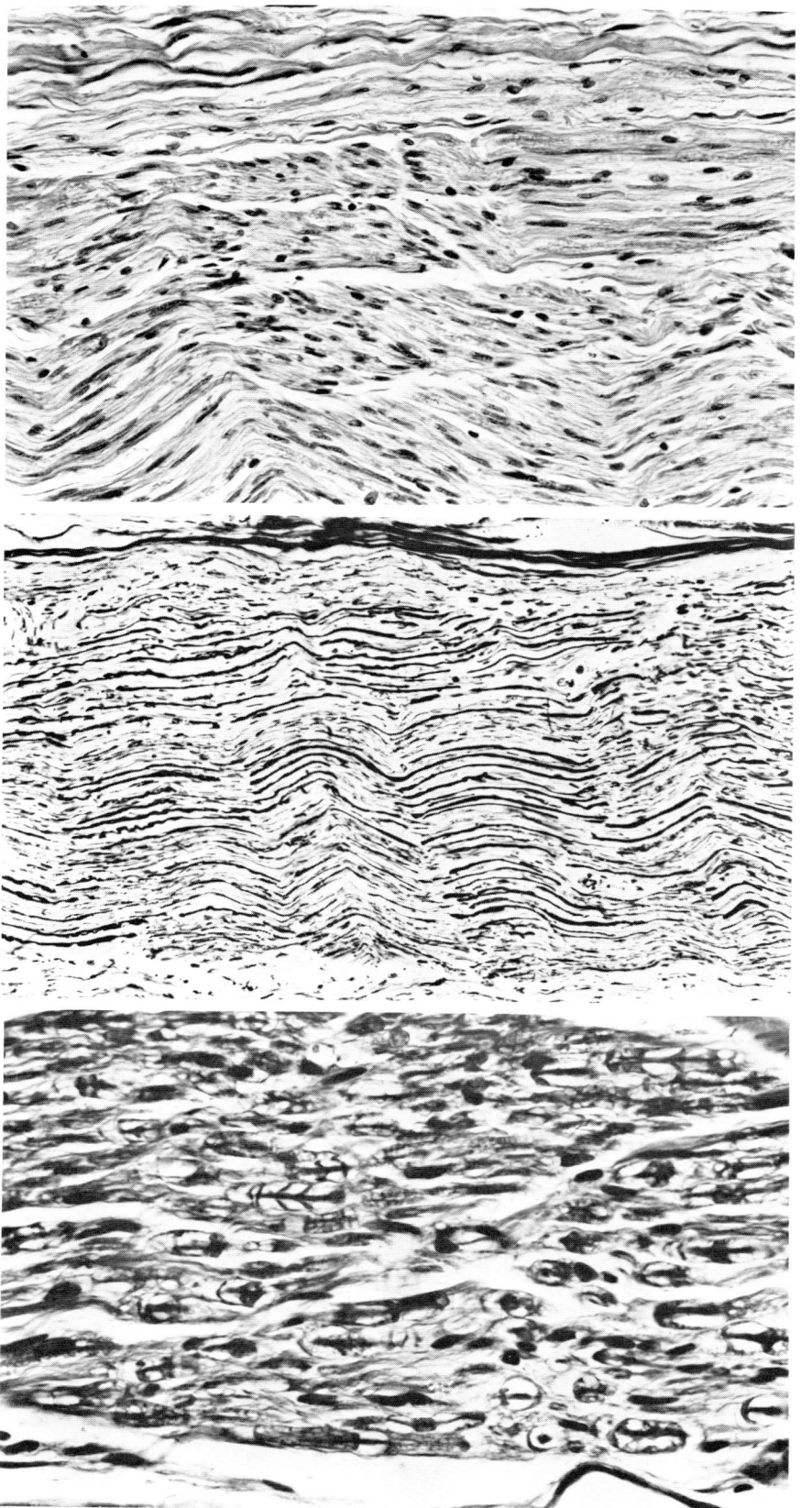

Figure 103. A coarser fibrillary tissue with a streamlined undulating appearance. It also contains myelinated axons, but among them are also collagen and reticulin fibers as well as Schwann's cells, identified by their short, slightly bent nuclei. This combination identifies peripheral nerve. The upper margin of this plate shows ordinary fibrous connective tissue. Schwann's cell nuclei are often arranged in register and thus have a palisaded appearance. *Peripheral nerve, longitudinal section* (×120)

Figure 104. Here silver stains have been employed to outline the axons, or long cytoplasmic processes, of the nerve cells. They appear in parallel rows and again an undulating appearance is seen. *Peripheral nerve,* Bodian (×120)

Figure 105. In H & E sections, axons are identified as dark lines, and the myelin that surrounds them has been dissolved out and is represented by the pale areas. The lateral dark extensions, which give the appearance of airplane wings or arrowheads, represent condensations of the schwannian membranes of the myelin sheath; they are responsible for the Schmidt-Lanterman clefts in a fat-stained preparation where they form clear spaces interrupting the heavily colored myelin lipid. *Nerve* (×220)

A coarse fibrillary streaming format with axons that are supported by Schwann's cells and interspersed with collagen fibers identifies peripheral nerve.

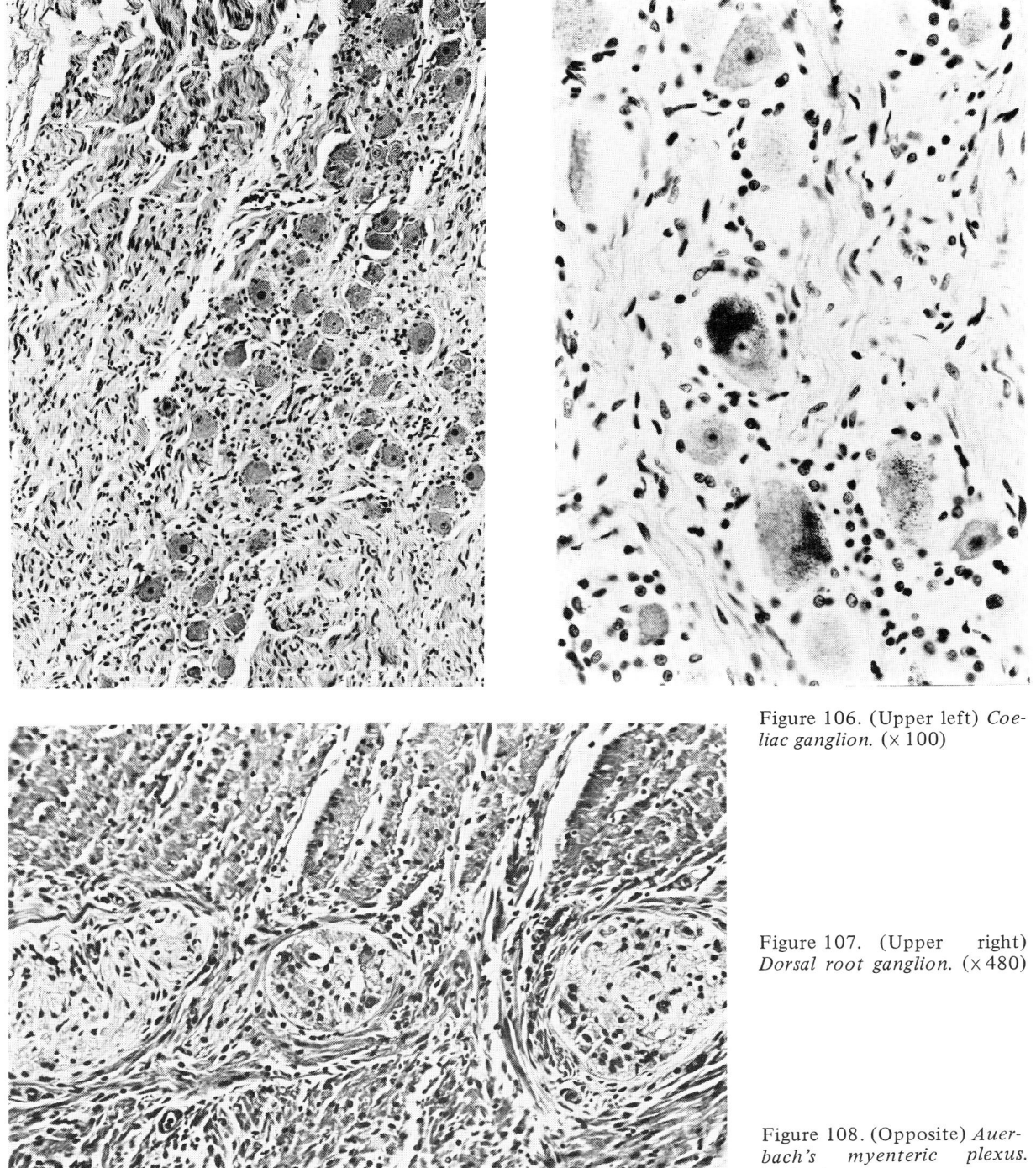

Figure 106. (Upper left) *Coeliac ganglion.* (×100)

Figure 107. (Upper right) *Dorsal root ganglion.* (×480)

Figure 108. (Opposite) *Auerbach's myenteric plexus.* (×125)

A close intermingling of neurones and peripheral nerve fibers is found in the peripheral ganglia of the dorsal nerve roots, in the ganglia of the sympathetic chain, and in peripheral plexuses. The cells immediately around the neurone cell bodies are satellite cells; these form a more complete ring in sympathetic than in dorsal ganglia. Plexuses in the intestinal wall are recognized by their association with visceral muscle. Note the pigment in the dorsal root ganglion cells.

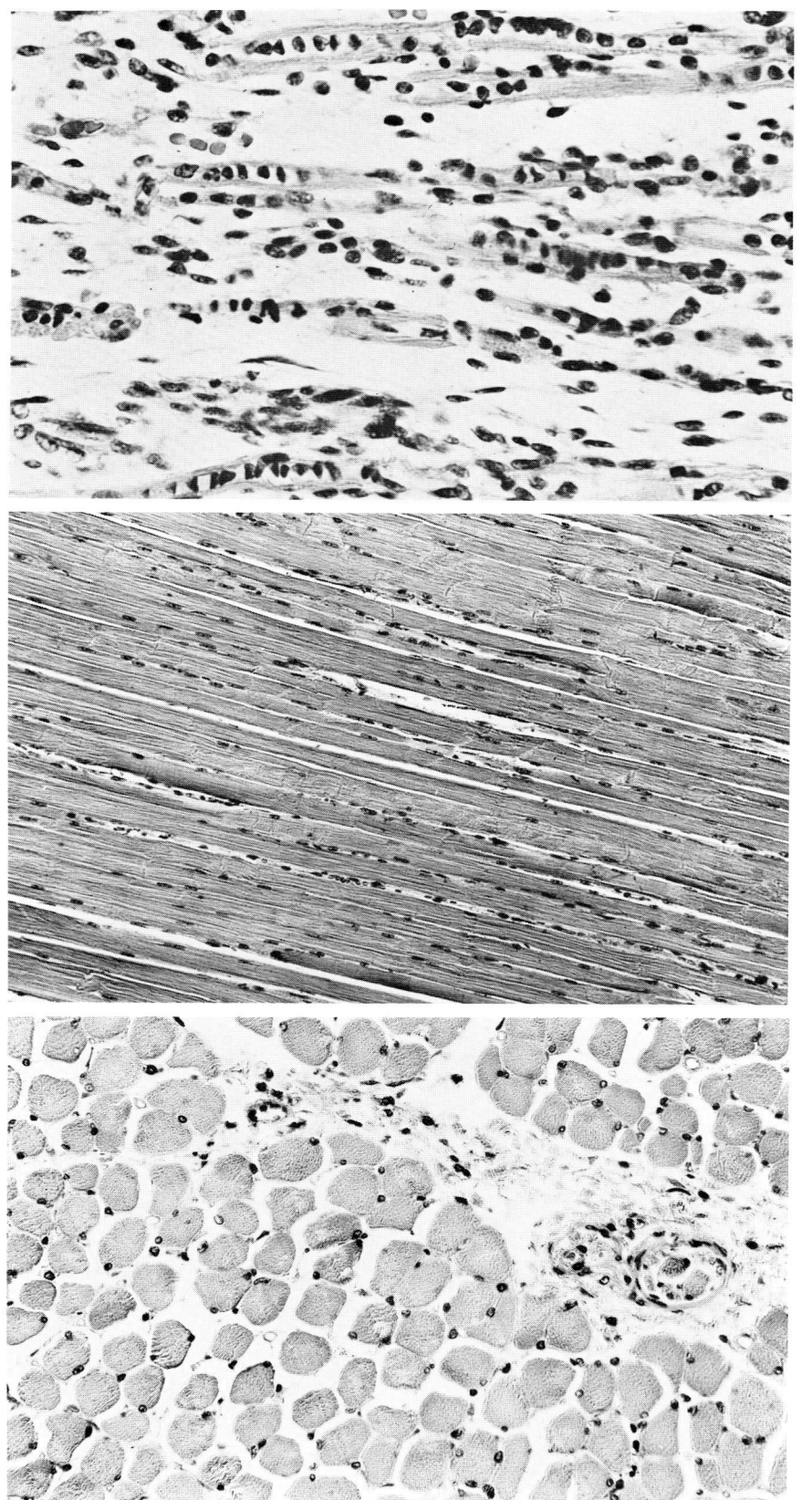

Figure 109. These fibers are very coarse and have a brightly eosinophilic cytoplasm. Several appear as hollow tubes with central rows of nuclei. Cross striations are easily seen. This is typical of *fetal striated muscle.* (×400)

Figure 110. Here the fibers are even broader and appear as darkly staining eosinophilic bands. The nuclei are now seen beneath the cell membranes at the periphery of each cell and are relatively small and oval or rectangular in shape. *Skeletal muscle,* thirteen years old (×100)

Figure 111. When cut transversely, skeletal muscle has a mosaic appearance. The peripheral position of the nuclei is more easily appreciated, and intervening connective tissue and blood vessels are more obvious. In the right center is a muscle spindle. *Skeletal muscle* (×200)

Skeletal muscle is identified as coarsely fibrillary tissue in which the fibers are formed by the elongated cytoplasm of the cells. Each cell has multiple nuclei, central in the fetus but situated beneath the sarcolemma or cell membrane in adults. The cytoplasm has cross striations.

FIBRILLARY FORMATS: MUSCLE TISSUES

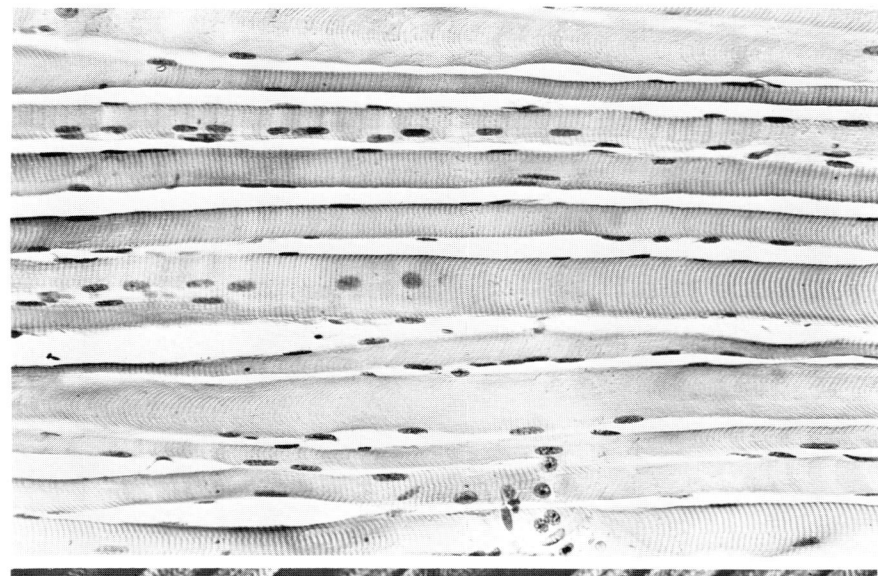

Figure 112. High power examination with racking down of the condenser may show the distinctive cross striations that identify *skeletal muscle*. (× 240)

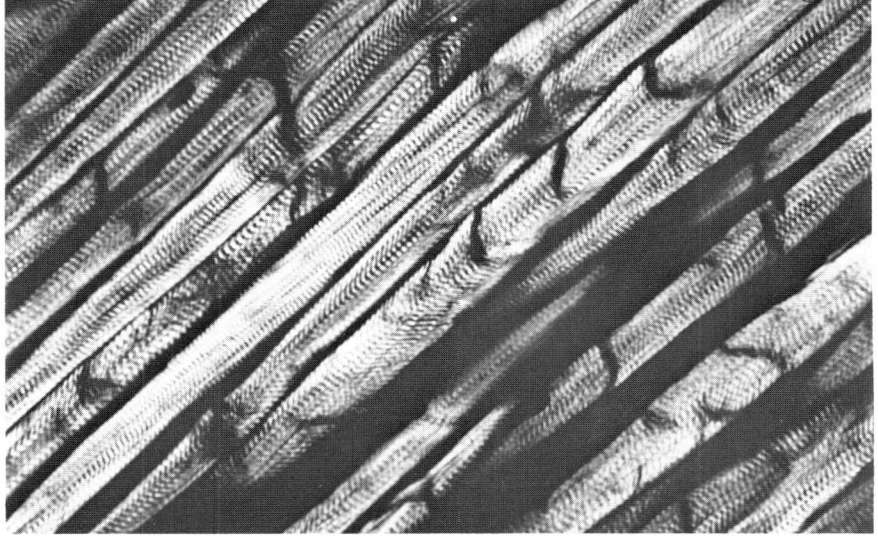

Figure 113. These cross striations are much more distinctly seen by semipolarization, as here. (× 400)

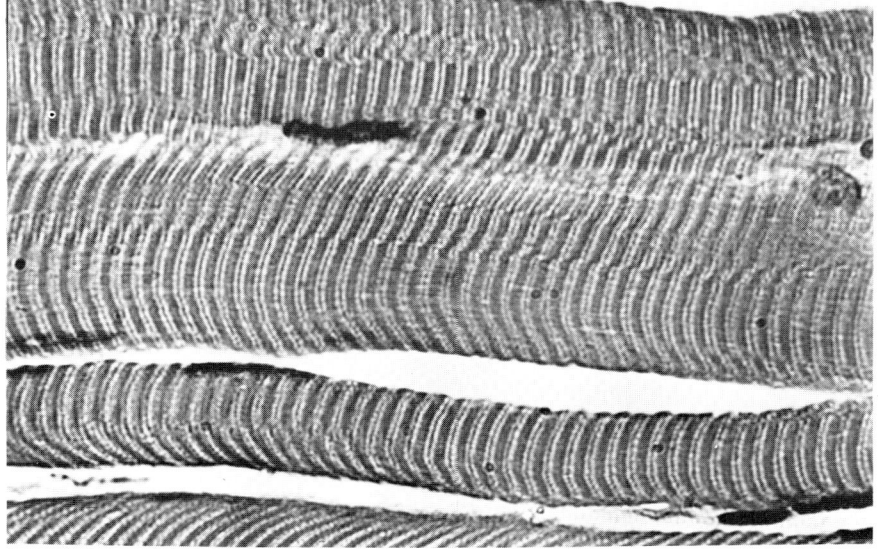

Figure 114. At very high magnification, the dark A (anisotropic) bands include central clear H (helle) lines or bands, while the light I (isotropic) bands are transected by thin, dark, but easily seen Z (Zwischen) bands. *Skeletal muscle* (× 756)

FIBRILLARY FORMATS: MUSCLE TISSUES

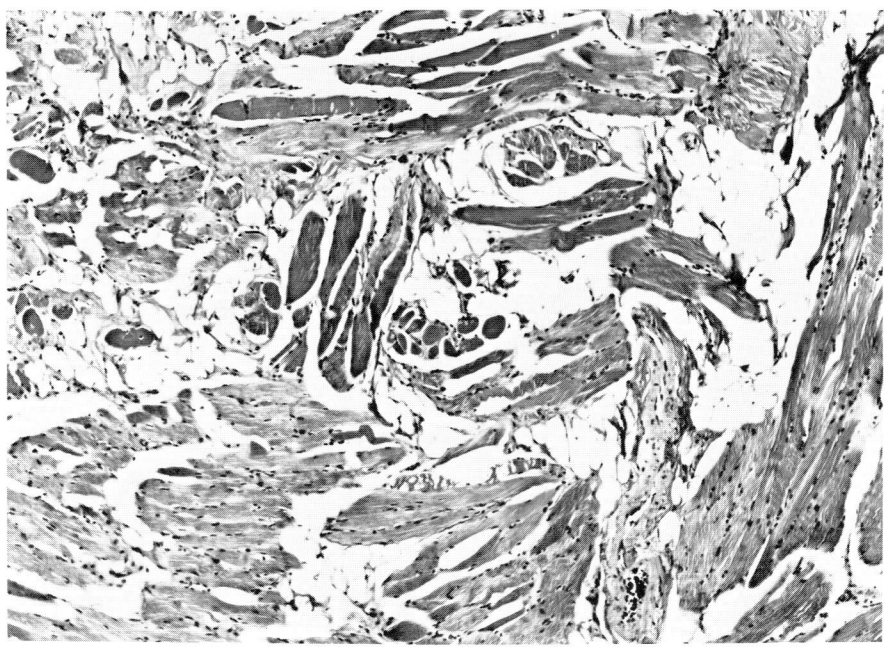

Figure 115. This arrangement is distinctive because it shows mucle fibers cut transversely and also longitudinally so that the bundles appear to be running in every direction. This arrangement is unique for the tongue, the only skeletal muscle that can be individually identified. Minor salivary glands might well be expected (as shown in Figure 160 of fetal tongue). *Tongue* (×65)

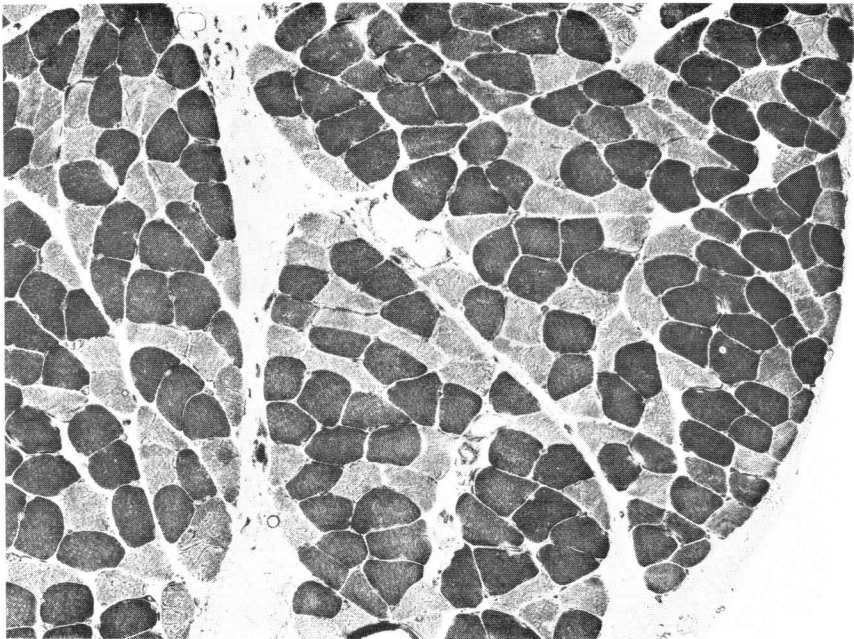

Figure 116. This mosaic format, with rectangular, triangular, and polyhedral cell profiles, represents skeletal muscle that has been cut transversely and then reacted with NADH (nicotinamide-adenine dinucleotide, reduced) to demonstrate different types of muscle fiber. Type I slow-acting red muscle fibers can be identified by their content of succinic dehydrogenase or, as here, by their NADH-tetrazolium reductase, a less specific reaction. This has resulted in the precipitation of formazan pigment from Nitroblue tetrazolium (NBT) to produce the dark-colored fibers. Type II fast-acting white fibers, which use glycogen as their source of energy, appear gray in this type of preparation. Frozen section, NADH, *skeletal striated muscle* (×100)

FIBRILLARY FORMATS: MUSCLE TISSUES

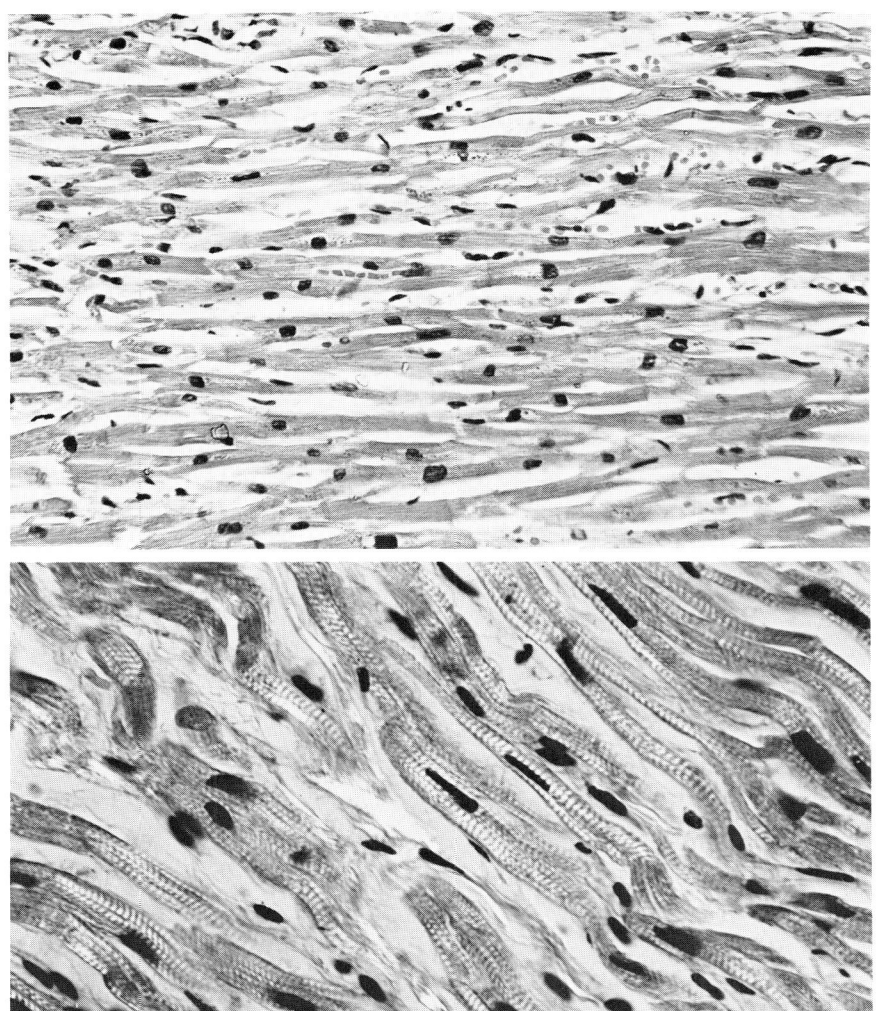

Figure 117. Striated muscle fibers that have their nuclei placed centrally and that show anastamoses, or junctions, come from the heart. Cardiac fibers vary in their thickness with the age of the patient and with the particular part or chamber of the heart. They are smallest in the conducting system, larger in the auricles, larger again in the right ventricle, and largest in the left ventricle. *Cardiac muscle* (× 240)

Figure 118. Semipolarization clearly reveals the striated nature of these fibers, their central nuclei, and their intercommunications. *Cardiac muscle* (× 400)

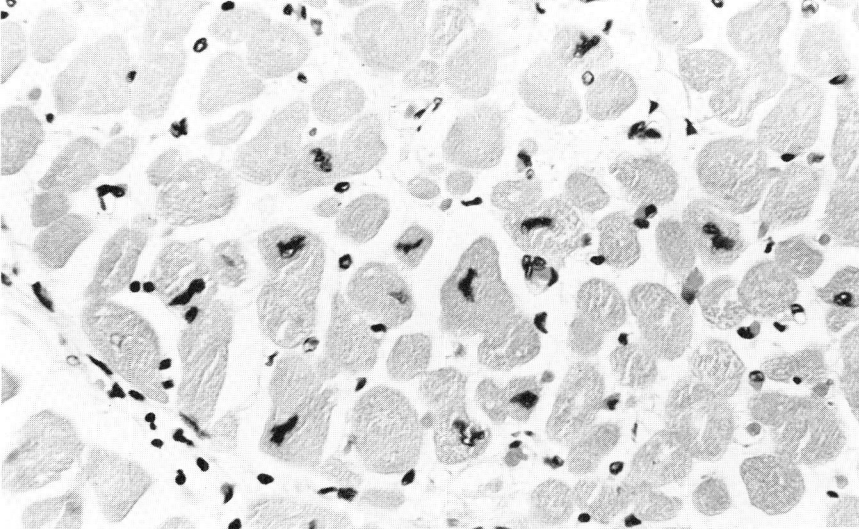

Figure 119. In transverse section, a mosaic format appears with small amounts of connective tissue between cells. The central position of nuclei in a brightly eosinophilic cytoplasm is apparent. *Cardiac muscle* (× 360)

When cut in longitudinal section, striated muscle fibers that show anastomoses and that have large oval centrally placed nuclei are identifiable as cardiac. The ends of the nuclei are frequently squared off, and yellow brown lipochrome pigment is commonly found in a perinuclear situation. This is sometimes described as wear-and-tear pigment and is almost universal in older age groups.

FIBRILLARY FORMATS: MUSCLE TISSUES

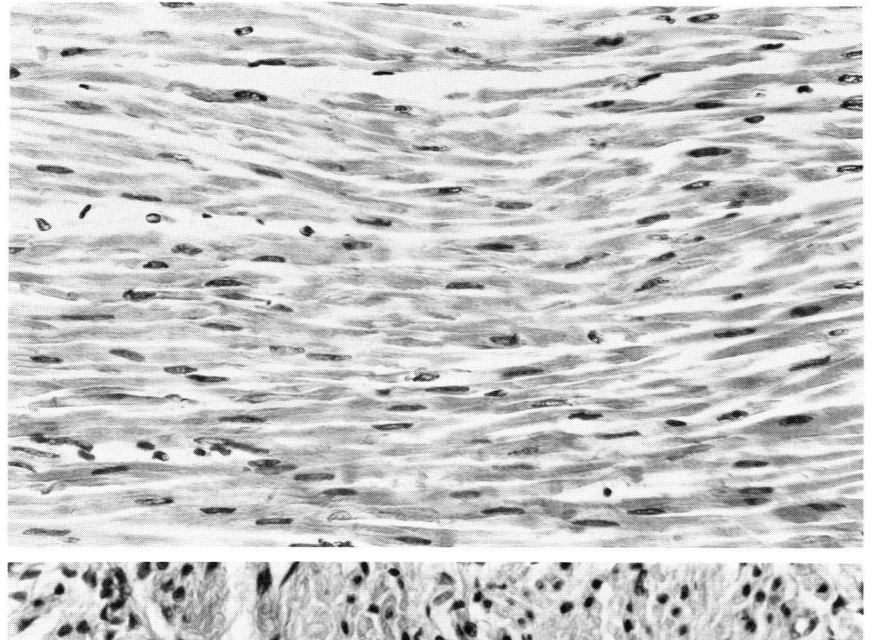

Figure 120. A tissue with a fibrillary streaming appearance composed of spindle cells, which have the eosinophilic staining of muscle fibers, without striations and with central nuclei, is nonstriated muscle. *Bladder* (× 250)

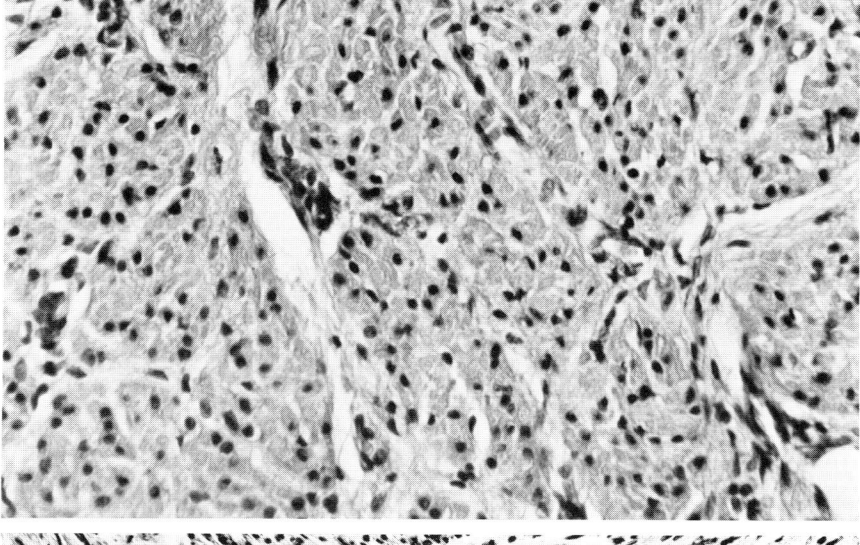

Figure 121. When cut transversely, the cells appear as a compact mosaic with central nuclei. Because of their length, many fibers are cut through a part that does not include the nucleus. *Nonstriated muscle* (× 250)

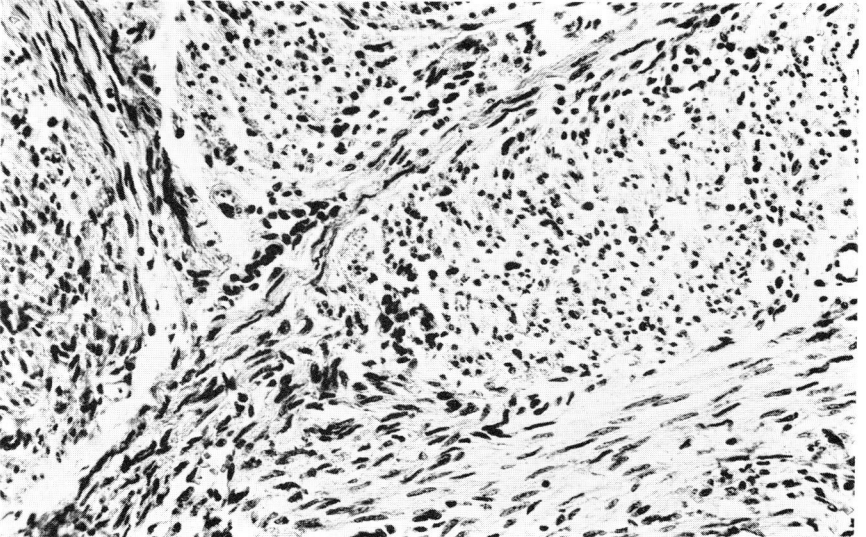

Figure 122. Nonstriated muscle bundles that run in various directions (shown here in both longitudinal and transverse cuts) are typical of the myometrium of the uterine wall. More widely separated bundles with loose connective tissue, but again irregularly arranged, may be seen in the wall of the gallbladder and the urinary bladder (as opposed to the thick sheets of intestinal muscle). *Uterine wall* (× 200)

Long spindle (as opposed to strap) cells, with eosinophilic cytoplasm suggesting muscle but having no cross striations and having straight rod-shaped central nuclei with rounded ends, identify nonstriated muscle, also known as smooth or visceral muscle.

FIBRILLARY FORMATS: CONNECTIVE TISSUES

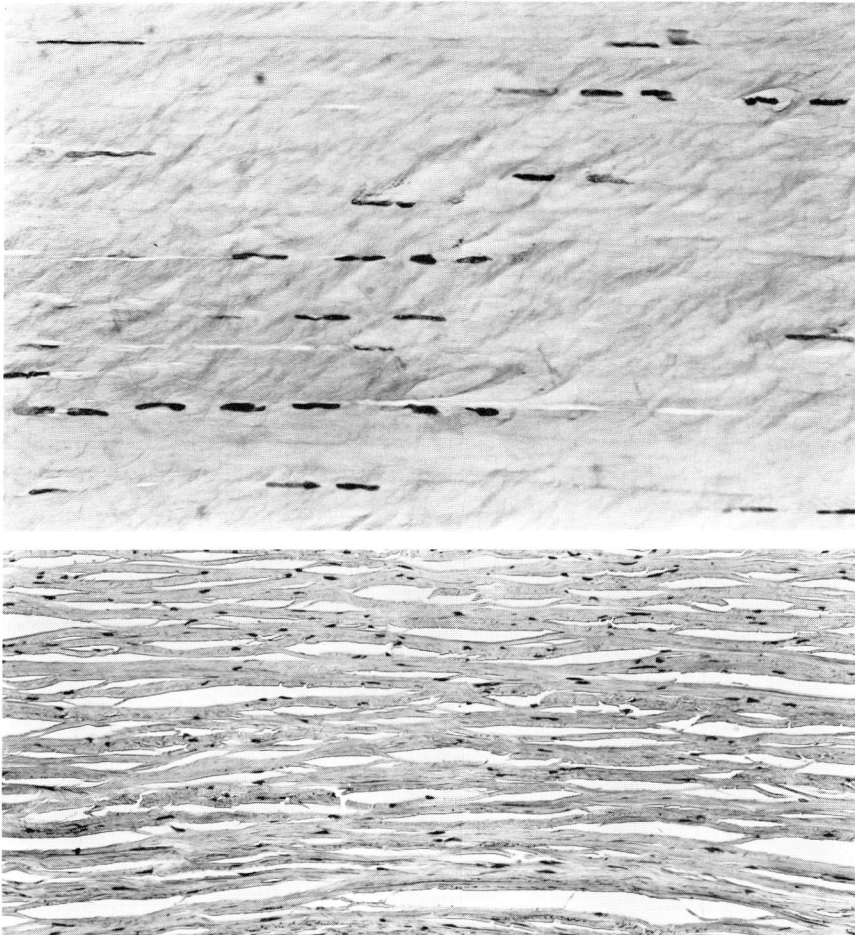

Figure 123. Very coarse, broad fibers of refractile eosinophilic collagen, between which are found the rather serpentine, sharp-pointed nuclei of fibrocytes, identify tendon or ligament. The collagenous nature of the fibers can be demonstrated by appropriate special connective tissue stains. *Tendon* (× 200)

Figure 124. Thinner bands of collagen with smaller, less regularly arranged fibers are seen in the *sclera*. (× 100)

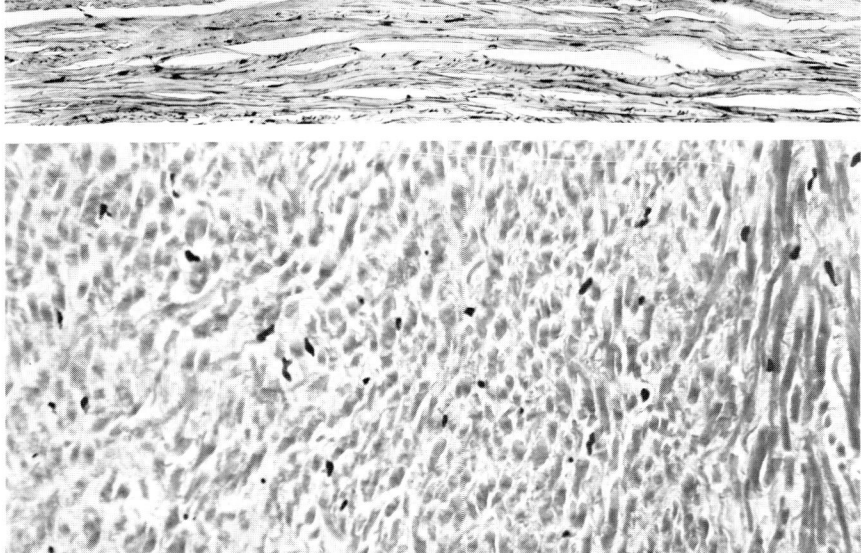

Figure 125. Fibers with a dull pink or slightly bluish color are elastic fibers. This section has been cut to show a streaming appearance on the right and a mosaic due to transverse sectioning on the left. *Elastic tissue*, ligamentum nuchae (× 250)

A fibrillary format with a streaming arrangement of coarse fibers of collagenous nature is seen in tendons and ligaments, cornea, and sclera; with coarse elastic fibers in the yellow ligaments is associated with the spines and laminae of the vertebral column.

FIBRILLARY FORMATS: CONNECTIVE TISSUES

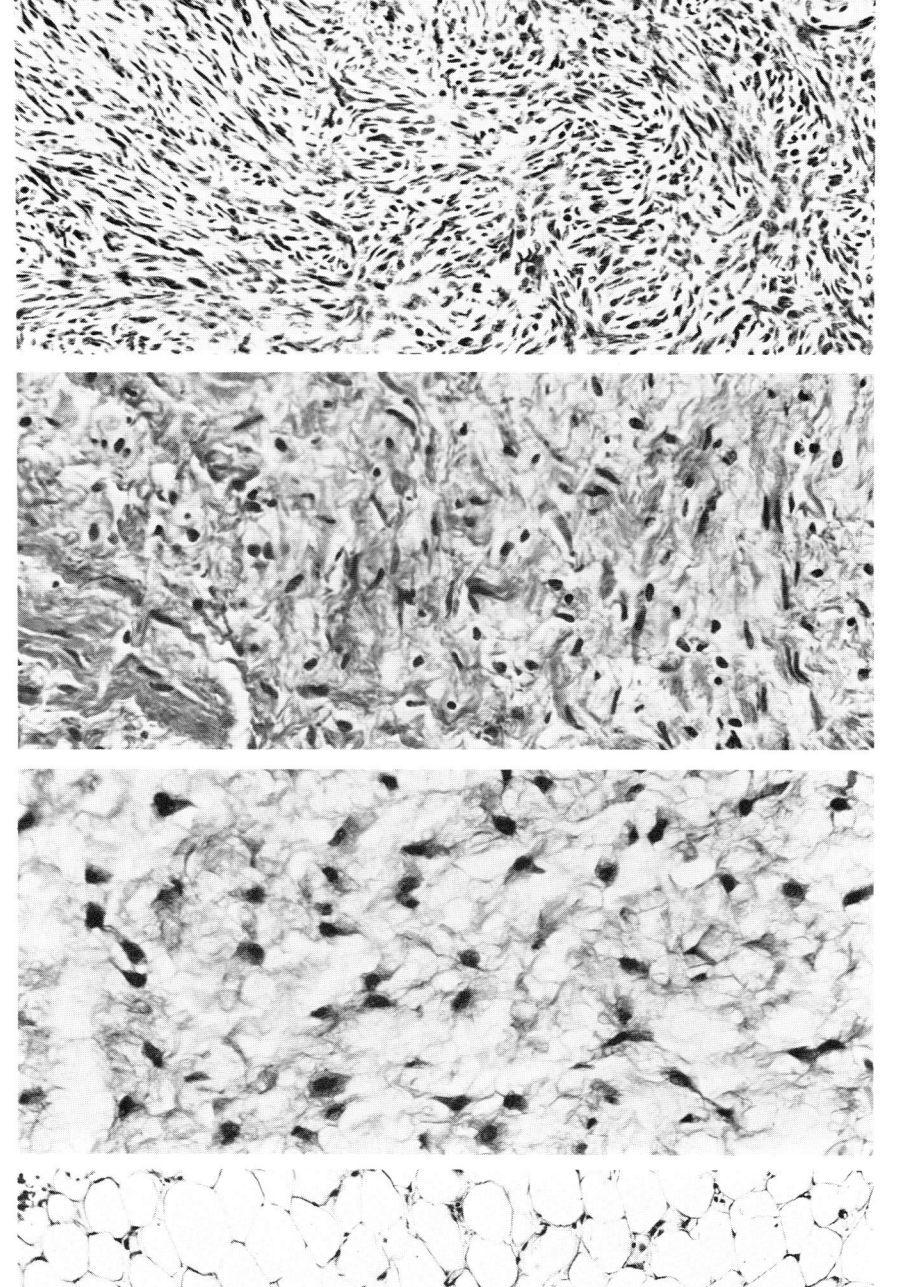

Figure 126. This fibrillary format is not streaming but shows a curlicue swirling arrangement of fibrocytes. The cell population is unusually dense, a combination that is unique to the *ovarian cortical stroma*. (× 200)

Figure 127. Irregular unpatterned tangles of collagen fibers with interspersed nuclei of fibrocytes, constitute loose or *areolar connective tissue*. (× 220)

Figure 128. A loose tangle of collagen fibers embedded in abundant mucinous (proteoglycan) background and having cells of stellate or triangular appearance identify myxoid tissue. This is seen in heart valves, the pulp of the tooth, and the *umbilical cord*. (× 300)

Figure 129. The appearance here is that of a network, an artefactual result of dissolving out the fat contained within the cells. The only remaining visible structures are the cell membranes with a few capillaries, which produce the darker thick bands. *Adipose tissue* (× 100)

PUNCTATE FORMATS: NEURAL TISSUES

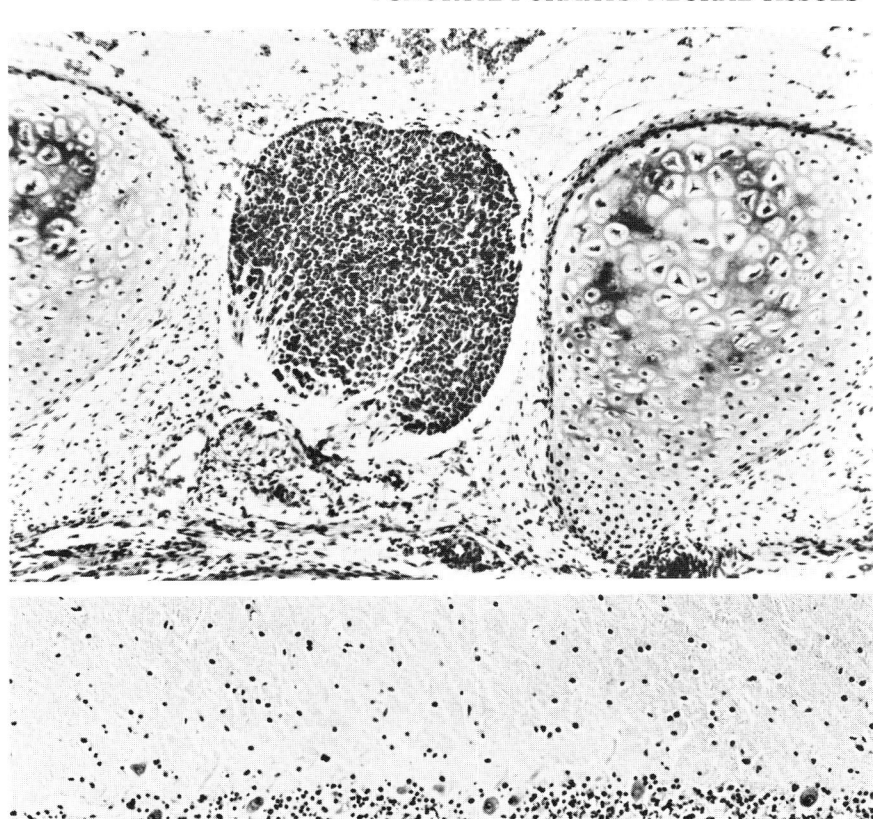

Figure 130. In the center of this figure is a fairly well circumscribed mass with a punctate format. It lies between the developing hyaline cartilages of the pedicles of the vertebra, and the combination of situation and appearance identifies this as the *dorsal root ganglion* from a fetus. (× 80)

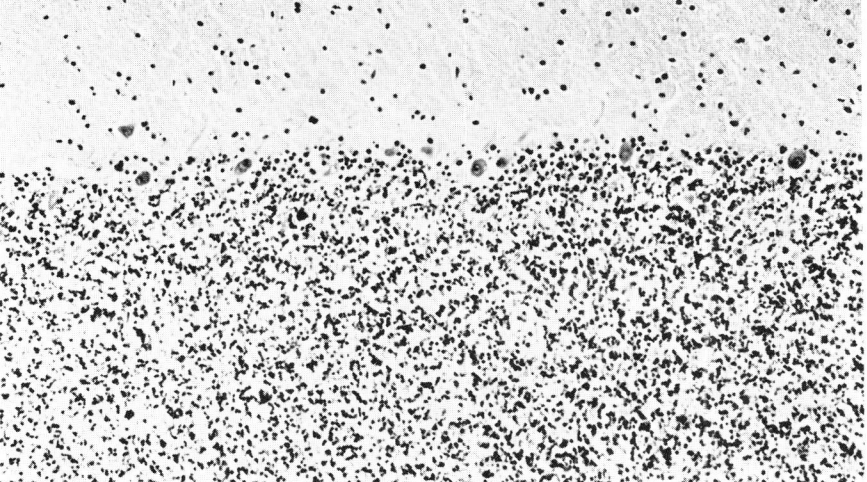

Figure 131. Another punctate format (lower two-thirds), the cells having a rather dappled arrangement and the nuclei lying on a light pink glial background. These are the small neurones of the adult *cerebellar cortex.* (× 80)

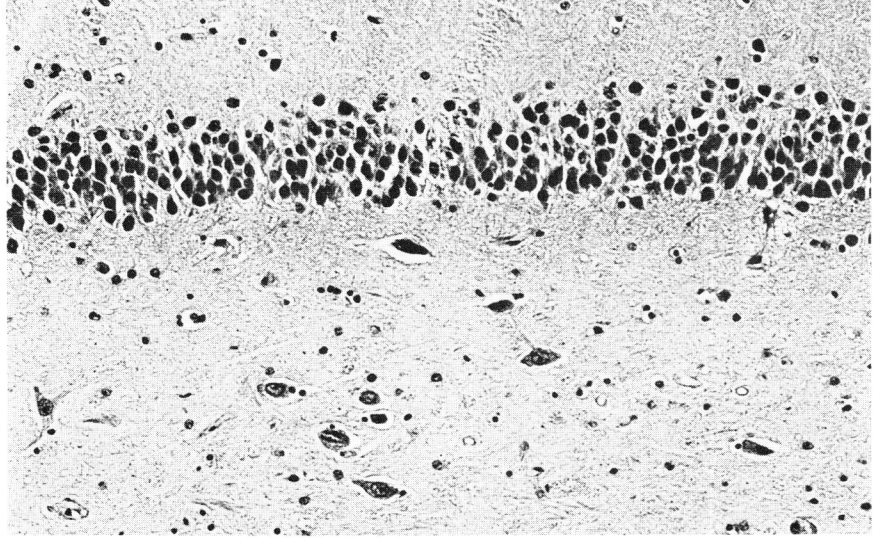

Figure 132. A narrow band of punctate tissue, running through gray matter, is identifiable as small neurones from the granular layer of the *dentate gyrus* in the hippocampus. (× 120)

A punctate arrangement in which there are small cells in a light pink glial background identifies small neurones. These occur in a limited number of locations, as illustrated. (*See also* retina)

PUNCTATE FORMATS: CONNECTIVE TISSUES (MYELOID)

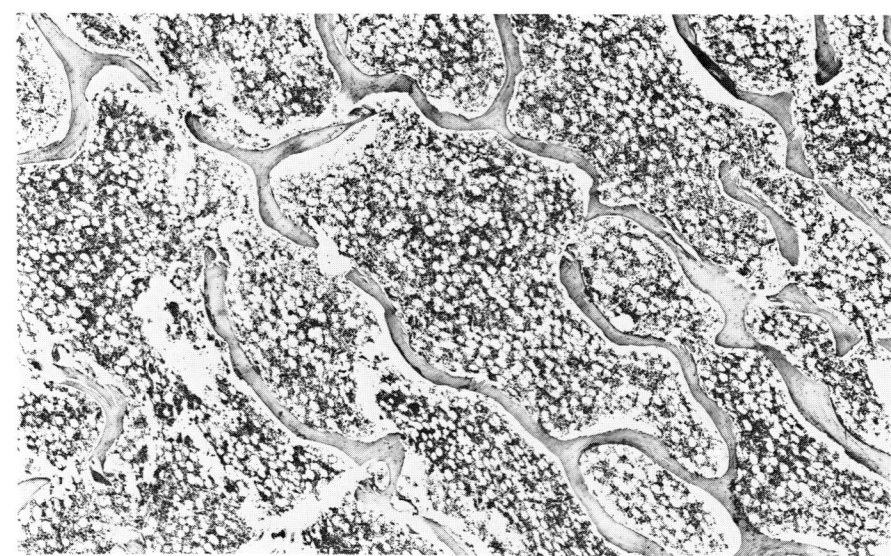

Figure 133. This plate shows three types of tissue — trabeculae of bone, a fibrillary network of fat, and punctate myeloid tissue. Normally, adipose and myeloid tissues are present in equal proportions, although in the adult this combination is restricted to the vertebra and flat bones of the rib cage, pelvis, and skull. *Bone marrow* (×20)

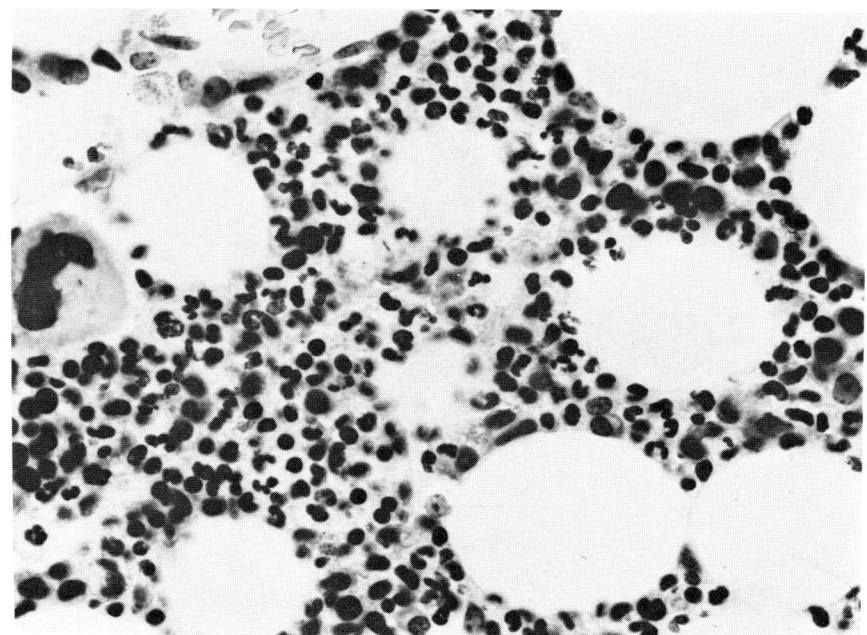

Figure 134. At the left margin of this figure is a large cell with lobed, hyperchromatic nucleus and abundant cytoplasm; it is a megakaryocyte. Below is a cluster of large, round darkly staining nuclei that identify erythroblasts. Later stages of the developing erythroblasts are smaller in size but retain their dark round nuclei. Some of these are seen towards the left lower center. The granulocytic series is readily recognized by the characteristic multilobed nuclei in the polymorphonuclear and band stages, although the latter may be difficult to distinguish from monocytes. Cells with indented round or oval vesicular nuclei are myelocytes and myeloblasts. In sections, primitive granulocytes may be difficult to separate from erythroblasts, although the nuclear chromatin of the latter is finer than that of the myeloblast, which is more likely to have an oval or indented nucleus and a more lightly staining cytoplasm. *Bone marrow* (×480)

PUNCTATE FORMATS: CONNECTIVE TISSUES (MYELOID)

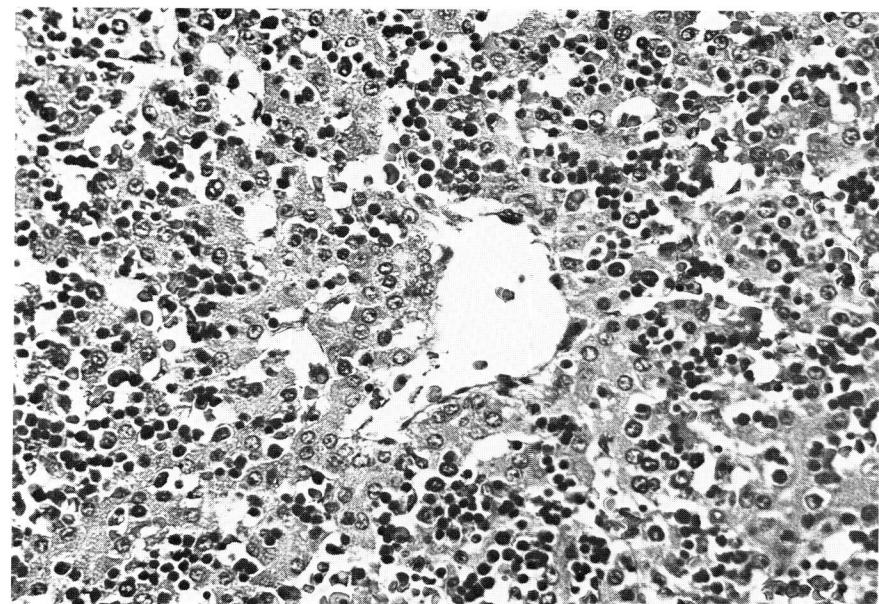

Figure 135. In the fetus, red cells are produced in the liver, spleen, and other tissues, persisting in the liver until birth. Here the section shows hepatic plates, but these are largely obscured by small groups of cells within the sinusoids, most cells having small dense round nuclei and therefore belonging to the red cell series. Developing granulocytes with irregular nuclei are also present. *Fetal liver with erythropoesis* (× 250)

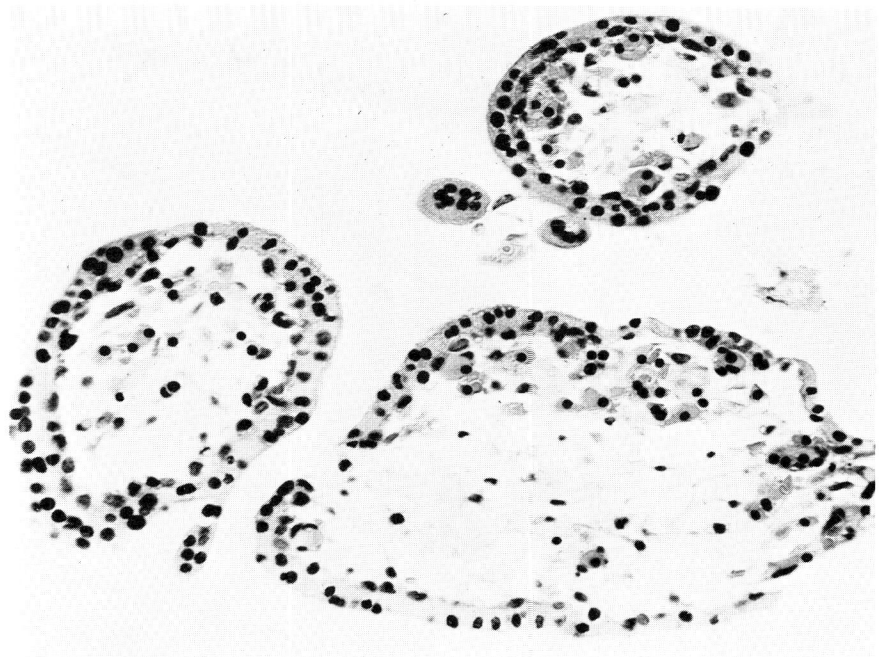

Figure 136. These structures have a myxoid connective tissue core with Hofbauer cells and are covered by a double layer of epithelial cells (trophoblasts) among which there are one or two syncytial giant cells. This identifies immature villi. In the placental vessels there are also developing red cells, identified by small round densely staining nuclei and by rather copious brightly eosinophilic cytoplasm appearing gray in the photograph. *Immature chorionic villi with nucleated red cells* (× 300)

PUNCTATE FORMATS: CONNECTIVE TISSUES (LYMPHATIC)

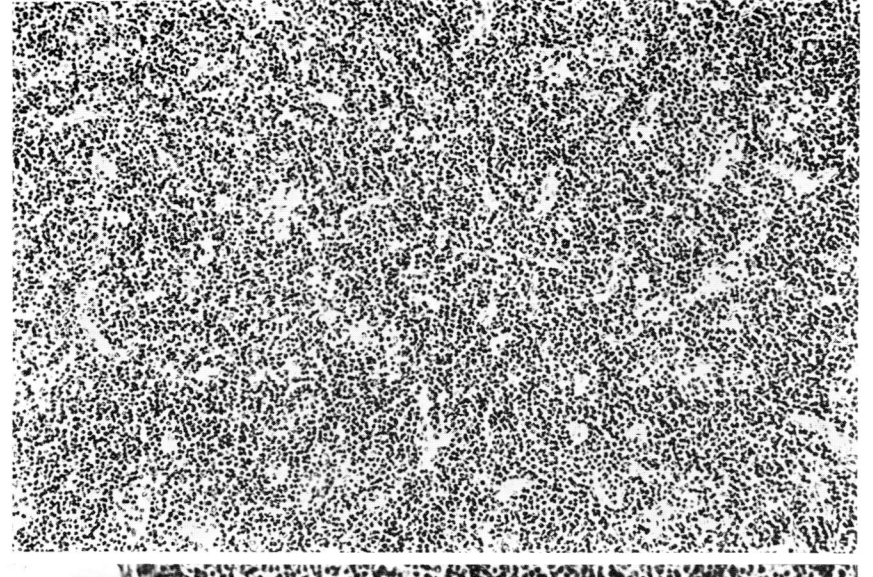

Figure 137. This tissue has a punctate format and is dominated by the small round nuclei of lymphocytes, among which are scattered larger cells, generally termed histiocytes, which are most obvious by their clear cytoplasm, giving the effect of holes. *Lymphatic tissue,* lymph node (× 120)

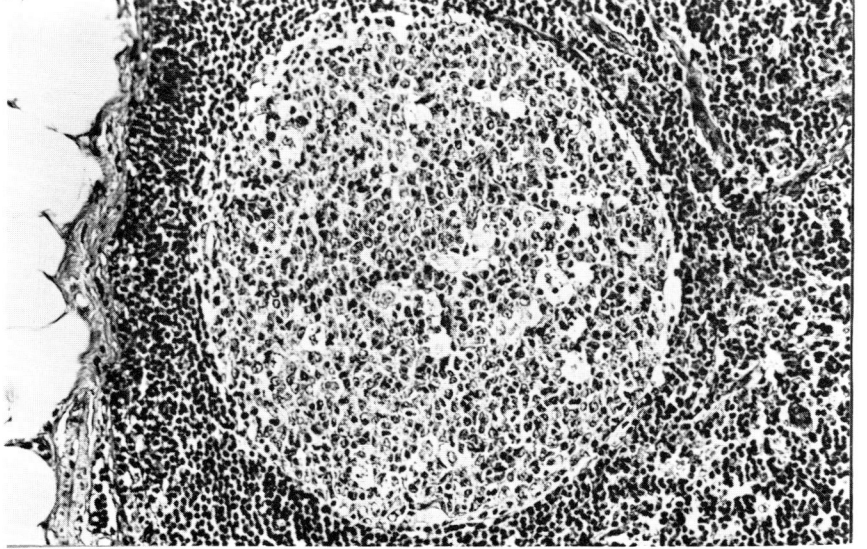

Figure 138. In this figure the peripheral small lymphocytes are condensed around a central collection of larger cells, the secondary nodule, or germinal center in a lymph node. In the germinal center, cells belong to the B series, while those in the interfollicular zones are T, or thymus-dependent, cells. *Lymph node* (× 160)

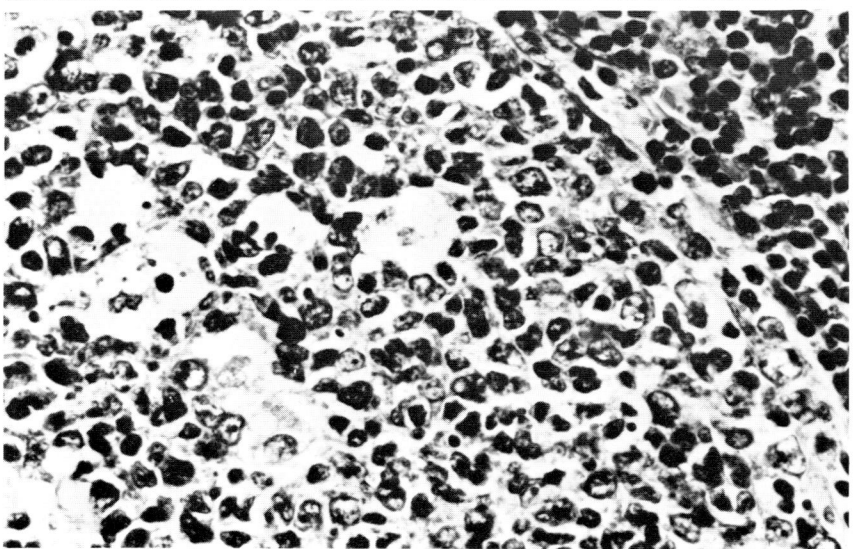

Figure 139. Higher power examination of the germinal center shows histiocytes with abundant pale cytoplasm containing nuclear debris, sometimes known as tingible bodies. Other large nuclei with prominent nucleoli, which sometimes touch the nuclear membrane and which are associated with scanty methyl green pyronin (MGP) positive cytoplasm, are immunoblasts. Cells of large or intermediate size with indented or cleaved nuclei are presently regarded as activated B cells. Typical small lymphocytes are seen in the upper right corner. *Germinal center* (× 480)

Practical Identification

4
PARTS

The most complete identification of any part would require description of its size, shape, position, and the nature of its subunits. However, the first three of these parameters may not be discernable in the histologic section, sometimes because the part has been too big and sometimes because the biopsy has been too small, as after needle, punch, or curette sampling. Fortunately, substructure by itself is usually enough to enable identification.

It has been found in practice that a useful approach is to begin with the general appearance of the section itself, making four categories, which are admittedly empirical. Two groups are based primarily on the contour of the section, while two relate to substructure (Figs. 140 through 143).

Lineate Sections

A flat natural open surface indicates that the section has come from the wall of a large cavity or from the external body wall. If slightly curved, it may suggest derivation from a large, hollow viscus or tube. Because of a surface line of epithelium, and (usually) parallel underlying striations due to the layered arrangement of the subepithelial tissues, the general appearance is lineate. Sometimes there are two parallel epithelial surfaces, which indicate a full thickness section of some thin wall, fold, or partition, such as the diaphragm or stomach wall. A section taken through the free edge of a fold results in a conoid section, an appearance seen in preparations from the margin of the eyelid, nares, and lips; from the edge of skin folds such as the pinna, prepuce, or labia; or from plates such as the turbinates, the soft palate, the epiglottis, or the margin of the tongue.

Annulate Sections

An annulate section indicates origin from some hollow cylinder, which since the section fits the slide, is less than 2.5 cm in diameter. The substructure is again laminar so that the appearance is both circular and striated. (Sometimes tubular structures are deliberately cut lengthwise, when they acquire the appearance of a flat lineate section and must be approached as such.)

Multiperforate Sections

In multiperforate sections the most striking feature is a multiplicity of small cavities, indicating origin from some structure that has a microcavitary construction, usually of modular unit type. It is true that some multiperforate parts retain a recognizable size and shape in the section, as with the ovary and possibly certain others, but by far the most constant and reliable feature is internal structure, which is therefore used as the basis for identification.

Solid Sections

Solid sections are characterized by confluent sheets of cells, usually from a single tissue family, but sometimes combining tissues from different families. In making this a distinct category, some liberties have been taken with parts to be included and excluded. For example, the walls of body cavities and some large hollow viscera are essentially solid in section, but they have already been treated as lineates because of their free open surface and laminar construction. On the other hand, the liver contains blood vessels (as in all solids) but also scattered bile ducts. It is treated as a solid because the dominant appearance remains such. The spleen has innumerable blood-filled sinusoids and could legitimately be discussed as a multicavitary structure. However, these are not so conspicuous as the solid lymphoid aggregates of the white pulp, which gives a strong resemblance to other lymphoid parts, with which it is therefore considered.

Quite a number of small solids can be cut across so that their size and shape can be described. Indeed, configuration may be diagnostic by itself, as with the tricorne appearance of the adrenal and the cleft of the spinal cord. However, it is common to receive only small fragments of tissue when such observations cannot be made, and the most important and generally applicable consideration remains substructure. Tissue characteristics are therefore adopted as the basis for analyzing this group.

TYPES OF MICROSCOPIC SECTION

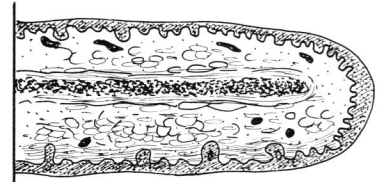 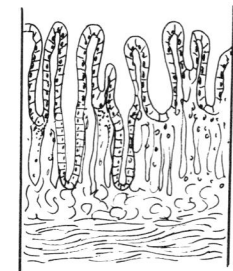 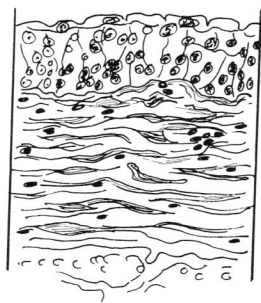

Figure 140. Lineates. Sections from large, flat, or slightly curved surfaces give microscopic preparations with a striated appearance having one or possibly two epithelial surfaces — sometimes smooth and sometimes irregular. Both the epithelia and supporting tissues differ in their nature, and particular combinations enable specific identifications.

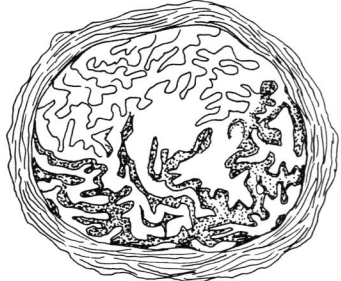 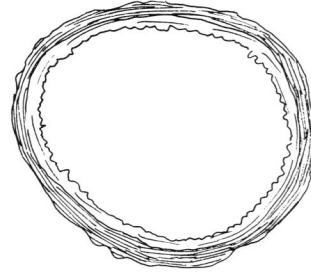 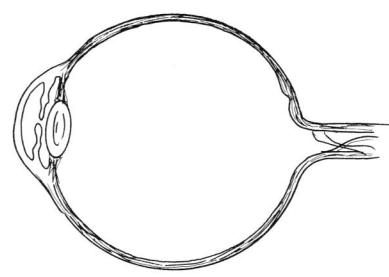

Figure 141. Annulates. Transverse cuts from hollow tubes or spheroids give ringlike sections identified again by the type of epithelium and the tissues making up the wall.

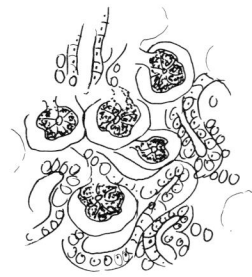 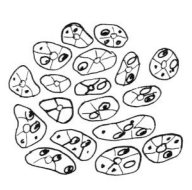 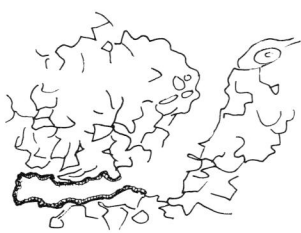

Figure 142. Multiperforates. Although some may have a definable contour, the dominant feature here is a colanderlike multiperforated appearance, and identification is most reliably made from the size and contour of spaces, the different types of epithelium, the content of spaces, and the supporting tissue.

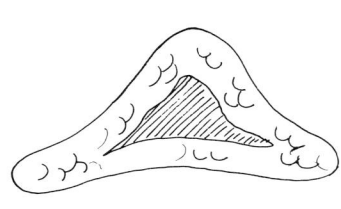 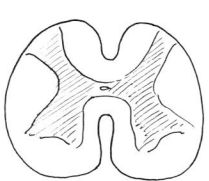 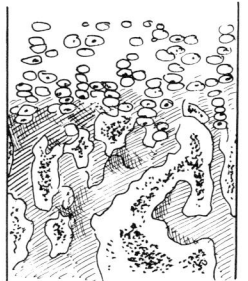 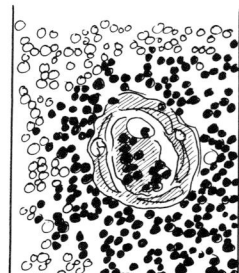

Figure 143. Solids. Smaller solids may be seen as islands with recognizable configuration, but because many specimens are too small to be identified in this way, diagnosis often depends on the types of tissue present. One family may dominate — epithelial, neural, muscular, or connective tissue — or there may be distinctive combinations.

IDENTIFICATION OF PARTS

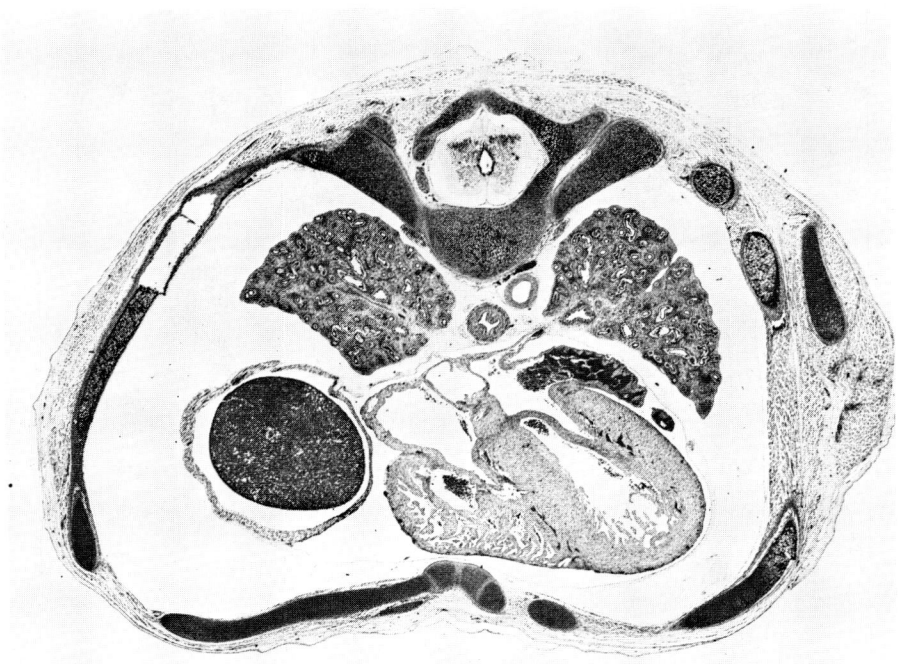

Figure 144. This section comes from a fetus of ten weeks gestation and illustrates the normal histologic appearances at this age, with unicavitary, multicavitary, and solid structures seen in miniature. It can be appreciated how samples cut from the laminated walls of cavities will appear as lineate sections, while transverse cuts of tubules will appear as annulates. Sections from modular hollow unit parts will retain a multiperforate appearance, and similarly, sections from large solids will appear as homogeneous solid sheets of cells.

This figure also allows the principles of identification to be illustrated. The thorax contains a number of cavities within an outer ringlike body wall. Internally, various organs and parts are identified by their size, shape, position, and construction. The developing vertebrae are seen above, still in the stage of cartilage and enclosing the spinal cord with its central canal. In front of the vertebrae are two small tubes seen as rings. The one on the right is the aorta, running down the left side of the vertebral column; the one on the center is the esophagus. On each side of these are rather triangular parts with multiple perforations; these are fetal lungs. On the left, the dark round solid is the liver, and the ring that surrounds it is part of the dome of the diaphragm cut obliquely. In the center at the front is the heart with its individual chambers and thick walls. *Fetus, transverse section of thorax* (× 10)

Lineate Sections

Lineate sections have a flat open surface, and any of the possible types of epithelium may be encountered. A useful division can be made between those where the margin of the section is perfectly smooth and those where it is irregular, ruffled, or fringed because of folds or indentations or, in some cases, indentations accompanied by acini giving a surface of microcavitary appearance. Smooth-surfaced, keratinizing, stratified, squamous epithelia are found in the skin, and nonkeratinizing stratified squamous mucosae in the openings from the body surface, as well as down the esophagus. Transitional epithelium lines the renal pelvis and bladder, and respiratory epithelium is found in the nasal cavities, larynx, and trachea. A flat cuboidal layer is seen in the amnion and over the peritoneal surface of the ovary, while a flat layer of squamous cells lines the serous cavity.

Surfaces of corrugated appearance with folds, villi, or tubular invaginations are all covered with a single layer of columnar cells. However, these may contain distinctive cell types, such as ciliated cells, goblet cells, and argentaffin cells, which enable more specific localization. Cytoplasmic mucus may also vary in its component acid mucopolysaccharides, giving different staining reactions according to neutral or acid composition. However, the surface columnar cells of the fovea of the stomach, the folds of the gallbladder, and the endocervix are so uniform in appearance that small fragments may not be individually recognizable.

Identification is further assisted by the nature of the supporting elements, such as muscle, which may be found in specific locations only. For example, a thin muscularis mucosae is unique to the alimentary tract (in the trachea, a similar layer of muscle is incomplete). Cartilage is a supporting tissue found in the ear, nares, nasal septum, epiglottis, larynx, or trachea. Bone is seen beneath the surface of the turbinates in the nose, the nasal septum, and possibly the larynx. An unusually dense fibrous tissue is found in the tarsal plates of the eyelids.

In many lineate sections, accessory glands may be found beneath the surface. In the skin, these are the sweat and sebaceous glands, while in the nose, oral cavity, pharynx, esophagus, and respiratory tract, there are minor glands of salivary type, providing the lubricant mucus that identifies a structure as a mucous membrane.

LINEATES WITH SMOOTH SURFACES

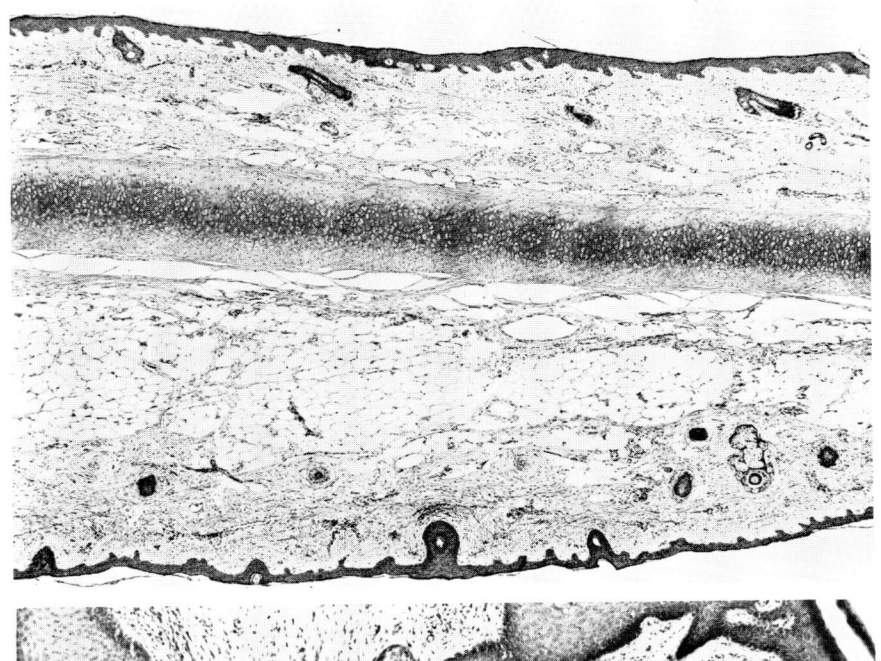

Figure 145. Between two epidermal surfaces is loose connective tissue containing skin appendages and a central narrow band of elastic cartilage. This combination is unique for the pinna. (The lobe of the ear has only adipose tissue in its core.) The posterior surface is identified by having the thicker layer of connective tissue. A similar picture is given by the skin of the alae nasi and lower nasal septum, but these are associated with hyaline cartilage. *Pinna* (×20)

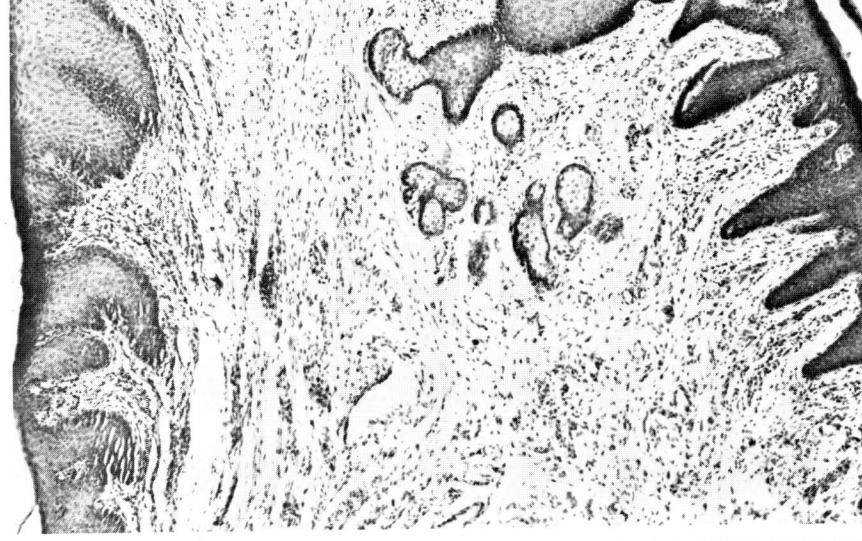

Figure 146. Again two epithelial tissues, but here the core is fibromuscular tissue with a few sebaceous glands and no hairs. *Labium minus* (×50)

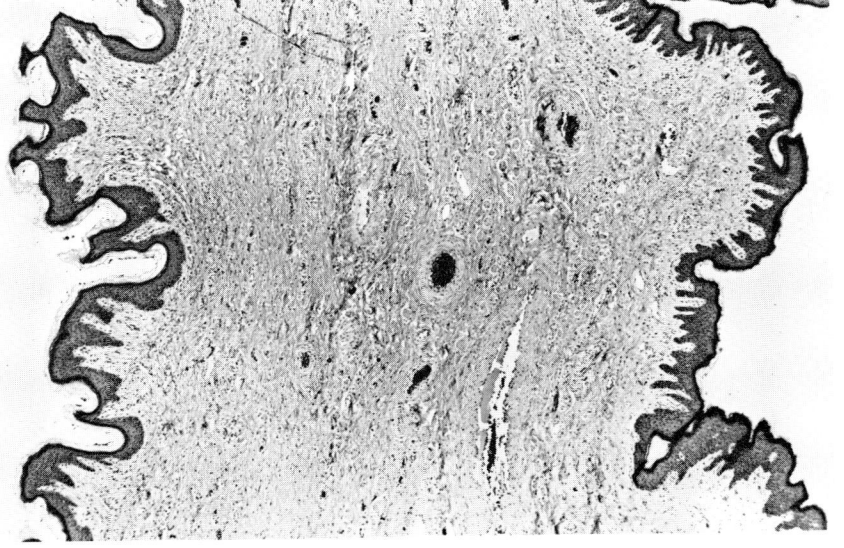

Figure 147. The distinguishing features here are the undulating nature of the epithelium, the lack of skin appendages, and the presence of small nonstriated muscle bundles. A nonkeratinizing type of epithelium may line the inner surface, but this is usually not seen in surgical specimens. *Prepuce or foreskin* (×27)

LINEATES WITH SMOOTH SURFACES

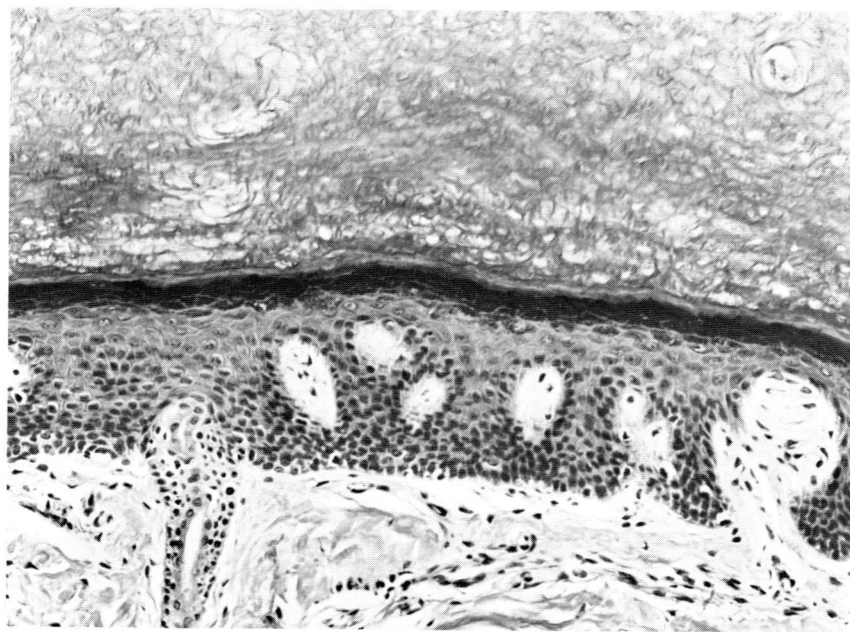

Figure 148. An extremely thick layer of keratin indicates that the epidermis came from a pressure-bearing part of the skin. Between the amorphous cell ghosts in the upper half of the plate and the dark central band, which is the granular cell layer, is a narrow pale band, which by microscopy appears hyalinized and constitutes the stratum lucidum. In the left lower quadrant running vertically is a sweat duct with myoepithelial outer layer. Its passage through the stratum malpighii is not seen, but in the keratin above (stratum corneum) the coiled part of the pore is visible. On the right in a dermal papilla is a laminated Meissner's corpuscle. (This by itself suggests origin from a limited number of sites in the skin — the palmar aspect of the fingers, the soles of the feet, the external genitalia, nipples, lips, or eyelids.) *Finger, pulp* (× 170)

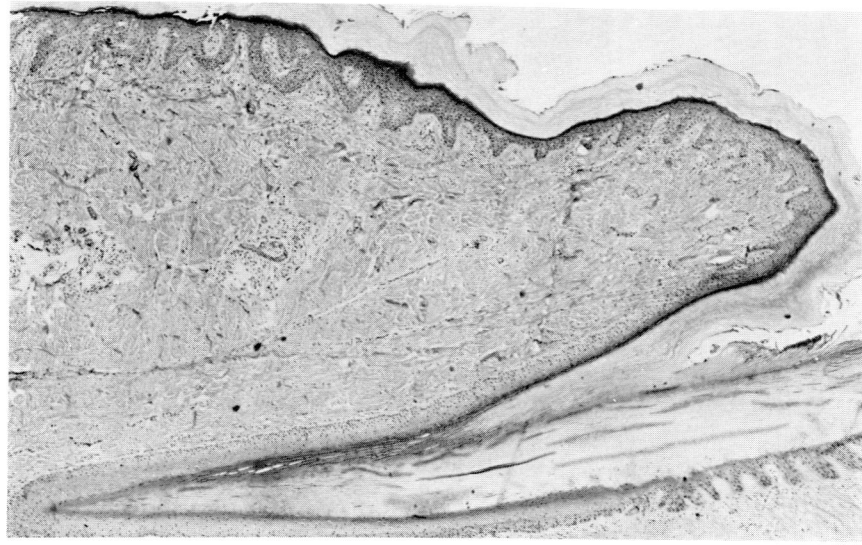

Figure 149. Here a normal keratinizing epidermis runs across the upper part of the plate, turning downwards in an oblique cleft running to the left and then passing horizontally to the right. The epithelium in the upper part and left end of the cleft has no rete ridges, and the keratin material is converted to a thick layer that becomes continous with the nail. In the nail bed the epithelial cells retain their nuclei in parakeratotic fashion, and long regular rete ridges are seen. *Nail and nail bed* (× 50)

LINEATES WITH SMOOTH SURFACES

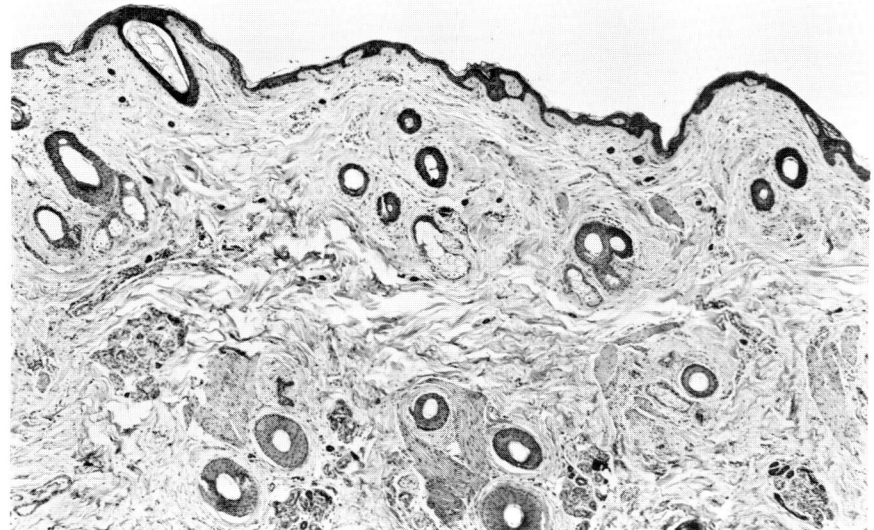

Figure 150. Epidermis can to a limited extent be identified as to the region of origin by considering the type and number of appendages. Numerous hair follicles suggest the scalp. By contrast, completely hairless skin comes from the prepuce, labium minus, palms, or soles. The short broad bundles in the lower field are nonstriated arrector pili muscles. *Epidermis, scalp* (×35)

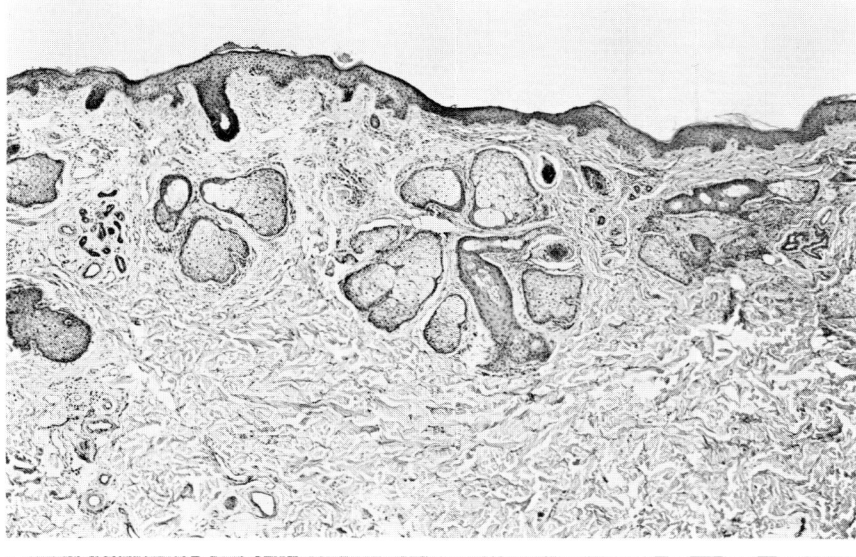

Figure 151. Numerous sebaceous glands but no large terminal hairs indicate origin from a nonhairy part such as face or forehead. A few eccrine sweat glands are included. *Epidermis, forehead* (×31)

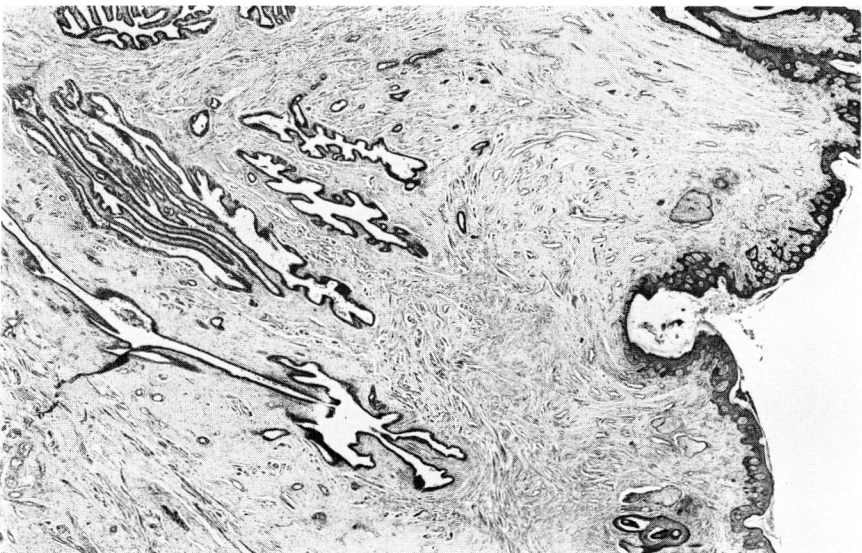

Figure 152. Large ducts running perpendicular to an epidermal surface are found in the nipple. Despite absence of hairs, there is an abundant nonstriated muscle. Numerous muscle fibers are also found in the skin of the scrotum, penis, and perineum. *Epidermis, nipple* (×14)

LINEATES WITH SMOOTH SURFACES

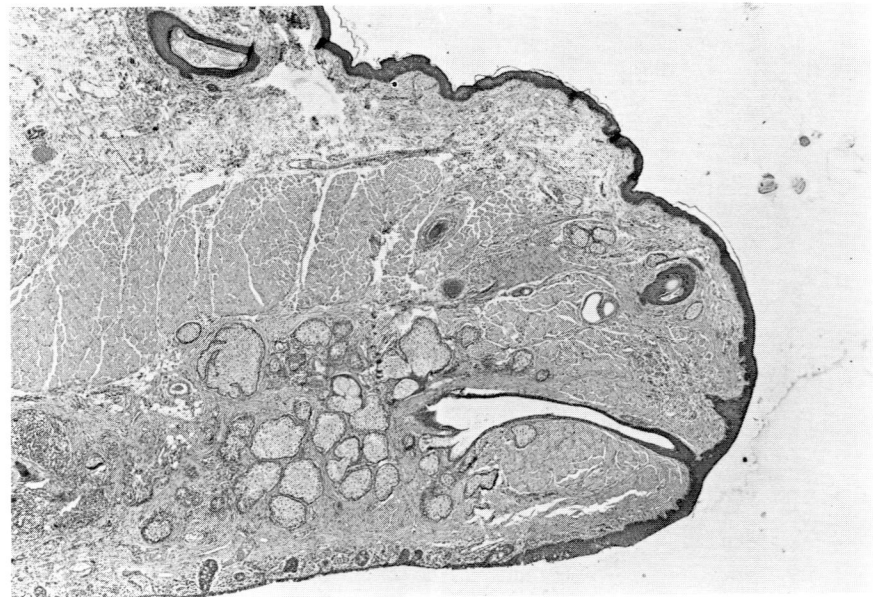

Figure 153. This section has epidermis on the upper and right margins, turning into a stratified columnar epithelium on the lower edge. In the lower third of the figure, there are numerous sebaceous glands (meibomian); these lie in the dense fibrous tissue of the tarsal plate and open into a duct, which is seen running slightly downwards in the lower right quadrant. Above the glands is a dense horizontal band of striated muscle, and in the upper right quadrant, hair follicles and sebaceous glands of the skin are seen. *Eyelid* (× 20)

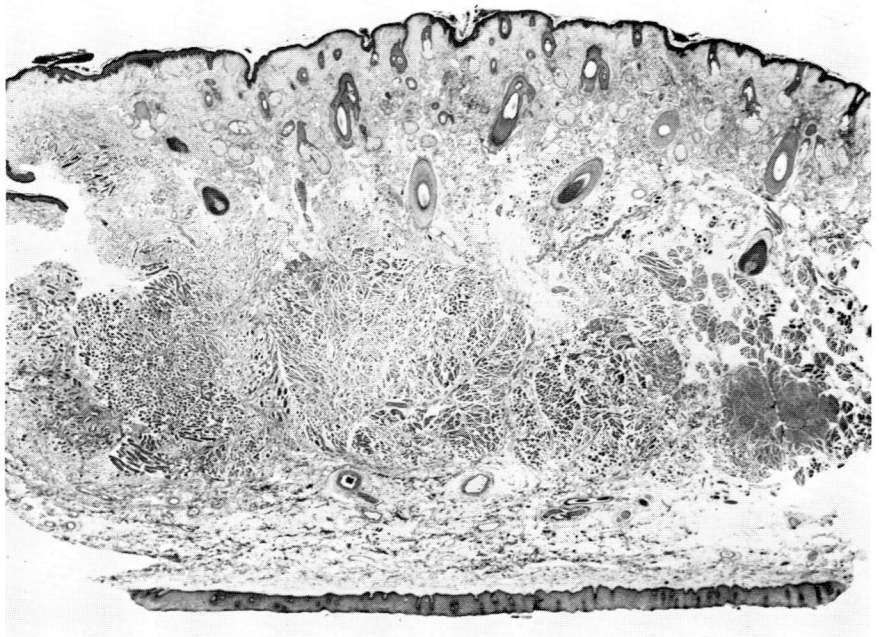

Figure 154. Here the upper surface is epidermis with prominent hair follicles, while the lower margin is a smooth stratified squamous mucosa. The bulk of the supporting tissue in between is striated muscle, the fibers cut transversely. This combination indicates the lip. *Lip* (× 8)

Combinations of epidermis and stratified squamous mucosa come from junctional areas between skin and body openings.

LINEATES WITH SMOOTH SURFACES

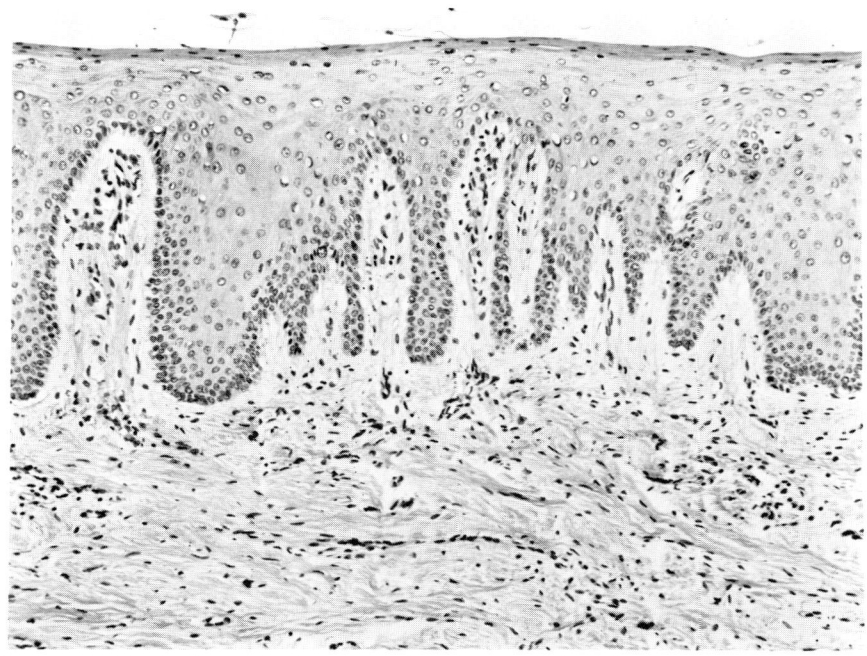

Figure 155. A flat surface with stratified squamous mucosal type of epithelium, showing long downward projections or rete ridges that interdigitate with correspondingly tall connective tissue papillae of the lamina propria is found over the gums. *Gingival mucosa* (×100)

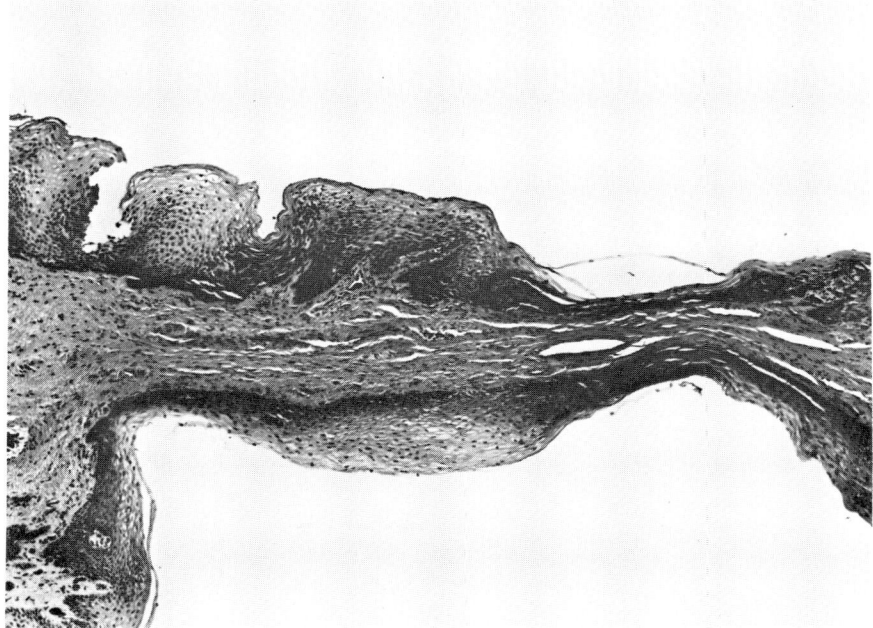

Figure 156. Two surfaces of stratified squamous mucosa with a thin core of fibrous tissue. This lacks glands or muscle fibers and is unique for the hymen. (The compressed area on the right is a forceps mark.) *Hymen* (×60)

Surfaces with stratified squamous mucosa (without a granular cell layer and without keratin) are found in the openings from the skin to the interior of the body (mouth, esophagus, anus, vagina, cornea, and conjunctiva).

LINEATES WITH SMOOTH SURFACES

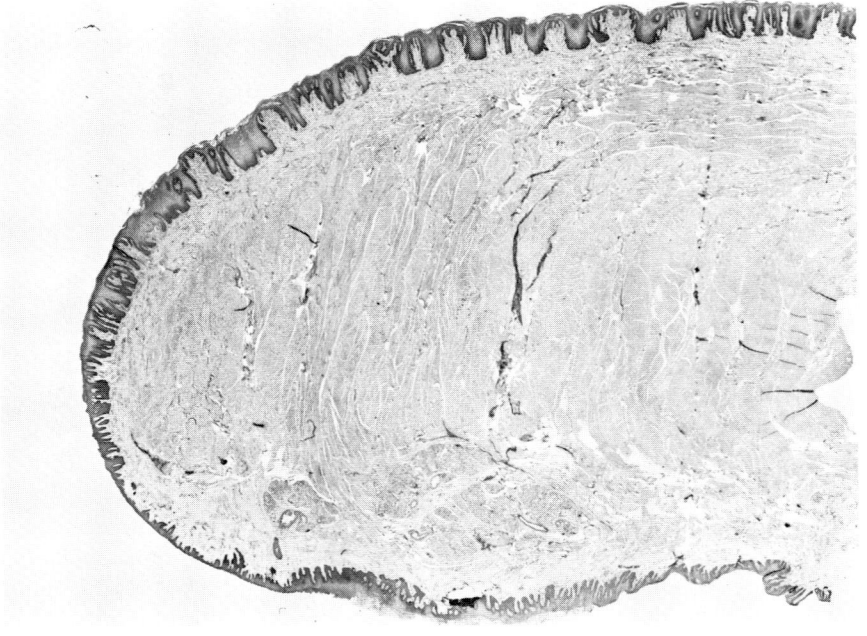

Figure 157. This section is through a free edge with a stratified squamous mucosa continuing from one side to the other. The core tissue is striated mucosa. The looser tissue on the lower margin is the inferior surface *Tongue* (× 8)

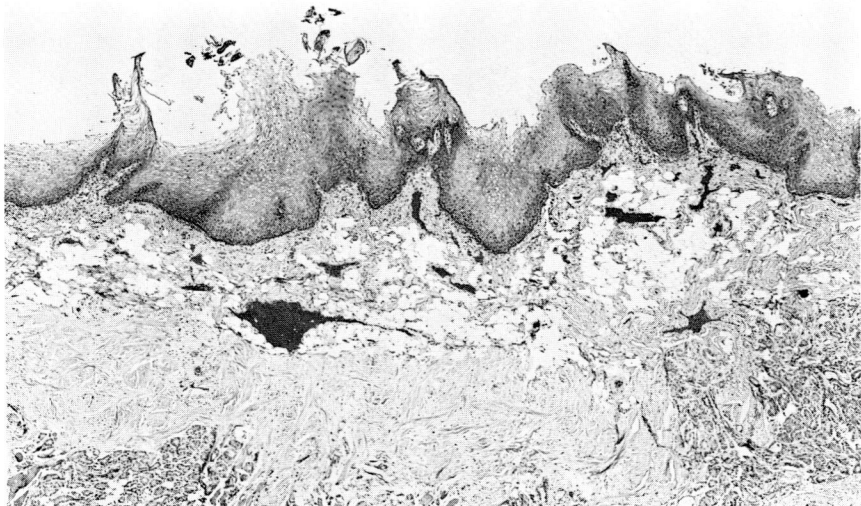

Figure 158. Here the stratified squamous mucosa forms sharp upward projections, composed of degenerating nucleated epithelial cells (parakeratosis). This formation is unique for the papillae of the tongue. *Filiform papillae*, (× 26)

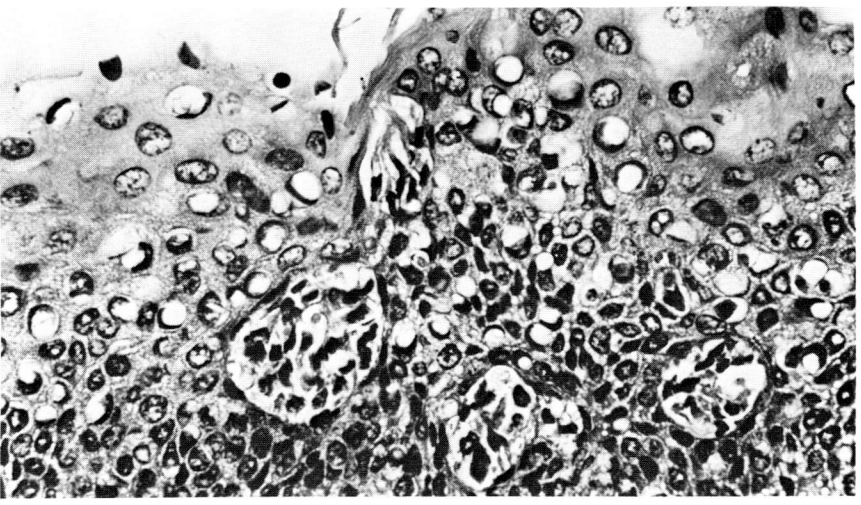

Figure 159. Four islands of epithelioid cells are found here within a stratified squamous mucosa, those in the upper center showing long undulating "hairs". *Taste buds, circumvallate papillae, tongue* (× 400)

LINEATES WITH SMOOTH SURFACES

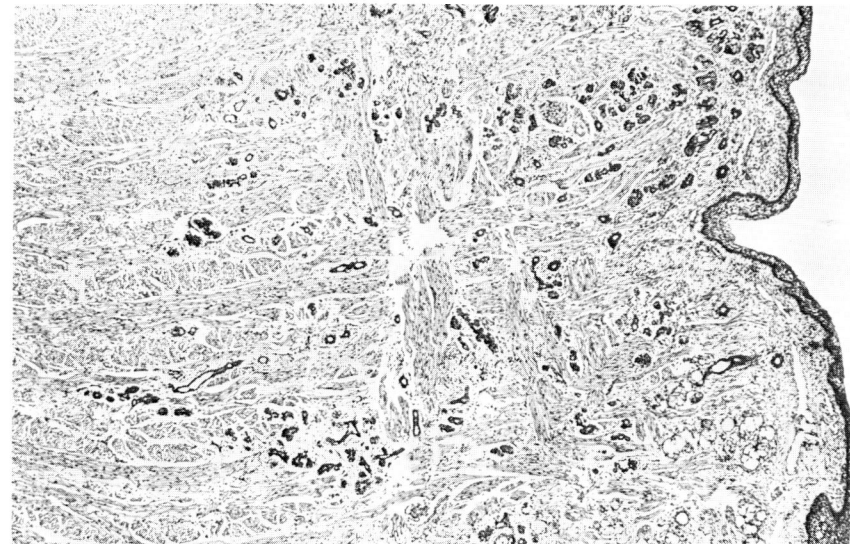

Figure 160. Beneath the stratified squamous mucosa (right margin) are intersecting bundles of striated muscle running in many directions. They are admixed with minor salivary glands. This appearance is unique for the tongue, although sometimes simulated by muscle beneath the buccal mucosa. *Fetal tongue* (× 26)

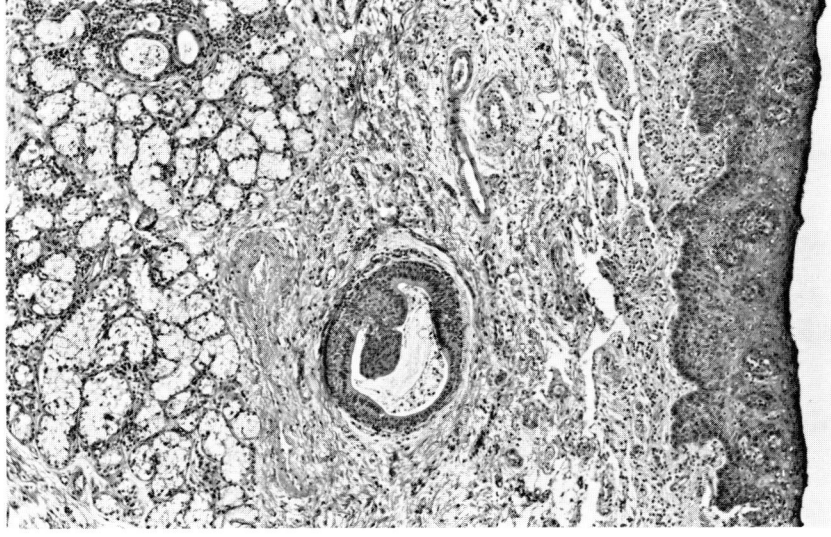

Figure 161. Here the subjacent tissue includes a large duct and a collection of mucus-secreting minor salivary gland acini. No muscle is seen. The appearances suggest the region of the mouth or pharynx. *Pyriform fossa* (× 55)

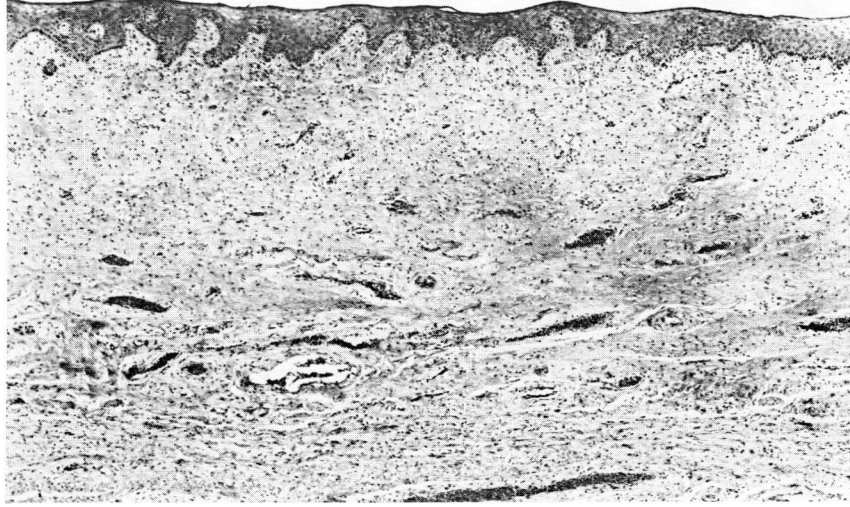

Figure 162. The mucosa in this plate overlies dense fibrous connective tissue in which there are no accessory structures. More deeply nonstriated muscle fibers might be expected. *Vagina* (× 42)

Some stratified squamous mucosal surfaces can be localized by presence or absence of subjacent elements.

LINEATES WITH SMOOTH SURFACES

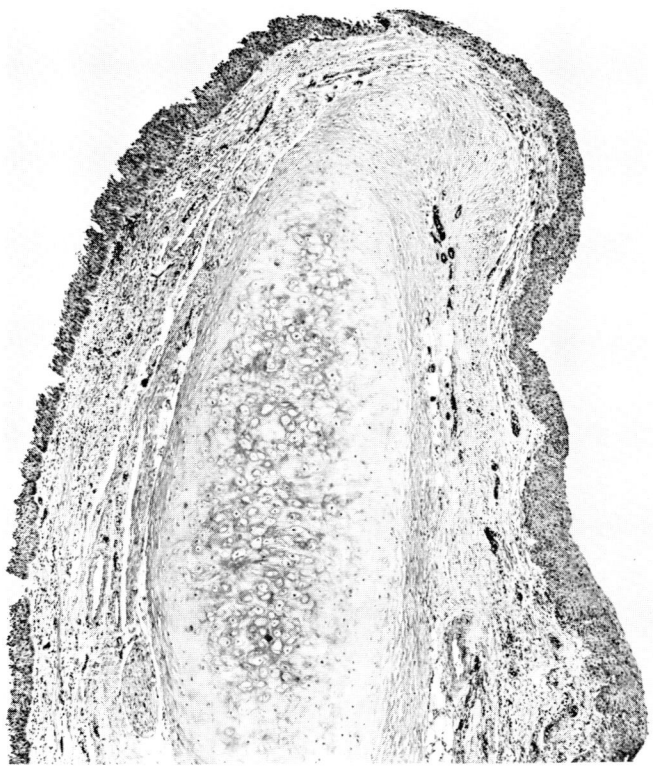

Figure 163. This section has a free edge and must come from the margin of a plate or the edge of an opening. The epithelium on the right is stratified squamous mucosa, merging into a respiratory type of epithelium on the left. The core contains elastic cartilage, and the combination is unique for the epiglottis. In the adult, both surfaces would probably be stratified squamous mucosa. *Epiglottis,* infant (×40)

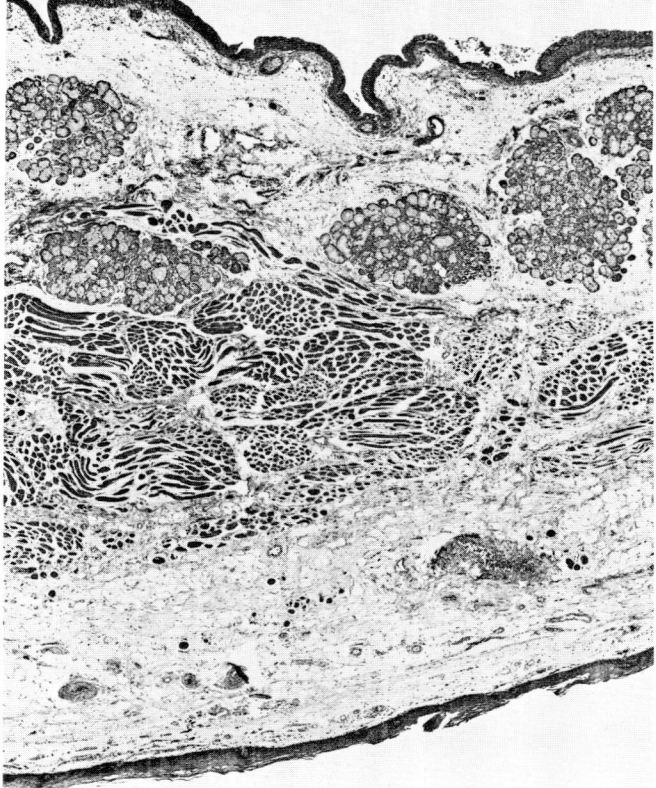

Figure 164. A surface of pseudostratified ciliated columnar cells (above) is here separated from a stratified squamous mucosa (below) by a core of loose connective tissue in which there are striated muscle fibers and, in the upper part, minor salivary glands. *Soft palate* (×20)

Combinations of stratified squamous and respiratory type mucosae enable the identification of certain parts.

LINEATES WITH SMOOTH SURFACES

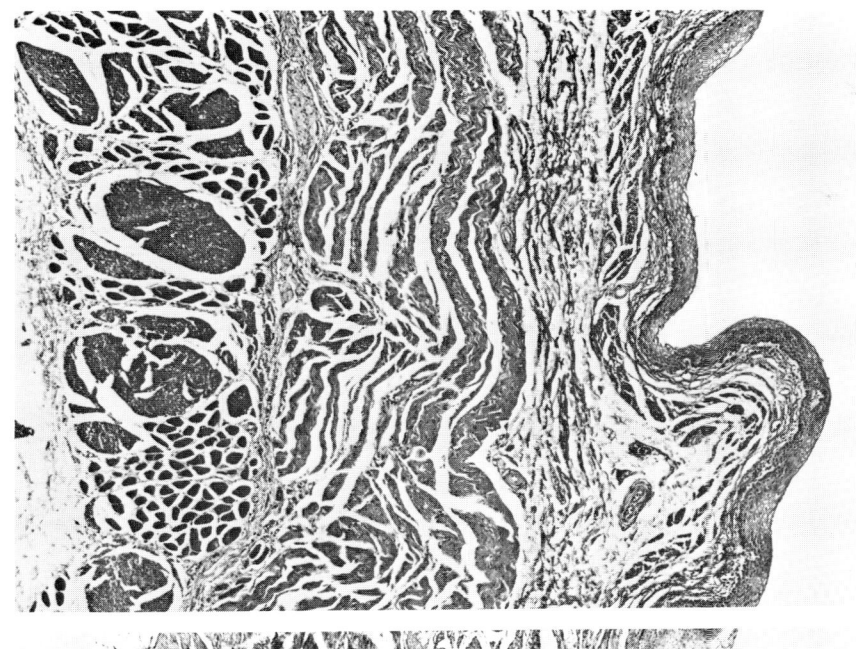

Figure 165. Here there is stratified squamous mucosa on the right margin, overlying a thin layer of nonstriated muscle (the muscularis mucosae) with, more deeply, thick muscle coats, which are partly striated and partly nonstriated. The former are the large triangular fibers seen best in the lower field. In the upper field, striated fibers are admixed with solid masses of visceral muscle, a combination which is unique for the middle third of the esophagus. *Esophagus,* middle third (× 42)

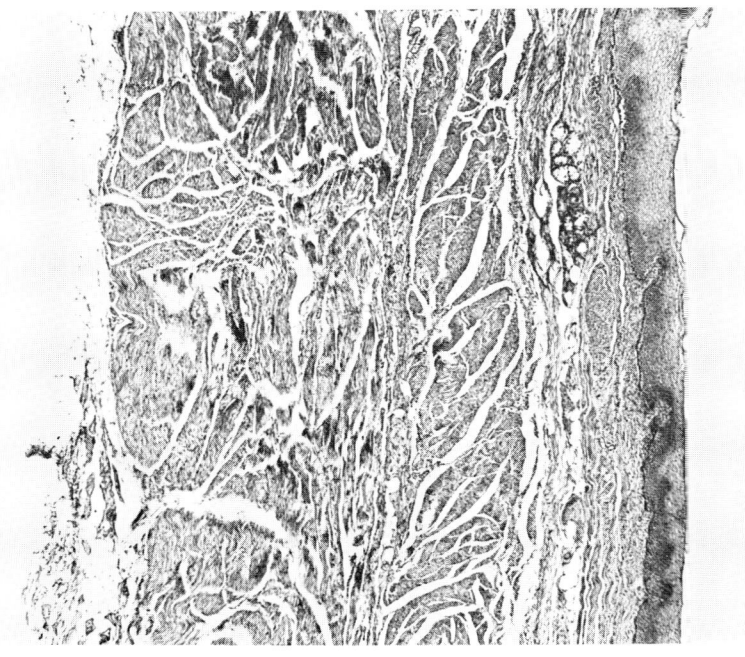

Figure 166. This shows a stratified squamous mucosa on the right, again with a muscularis mucosa, but here there are two muscle coats entirely of nonstriated muscle, typical for the *lower esophagus*. A few glands are seen near the upper margin. (× 27)

A stratified squamous mucosa with muscularis mucosae comes only from the esophagus.

LINEATES WITH SMOOTH SURFACES

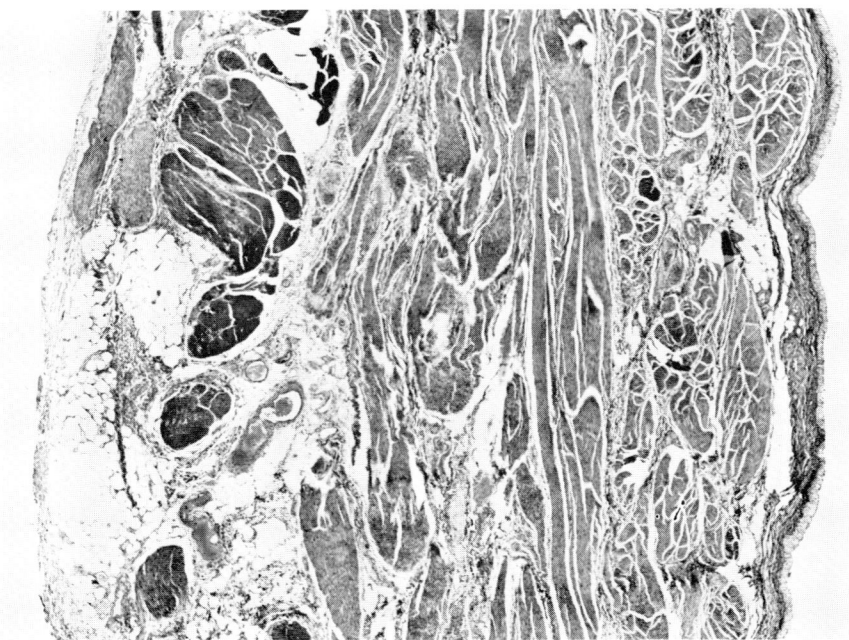

Figure 167. This section has a flat, stratified epithelial surface (right), but the wall is composed of irregular bundles of nonstriated muscle, separated from each other but without showing clear lamination. This arrangement is strongly suggestive of the bladder, and identification will be confirmed if the epithelium proves to be transitional. A full thickness section may include a second epithelial coat, being the serosa from the peritoneum over the dome. *Bladder* (× 11)

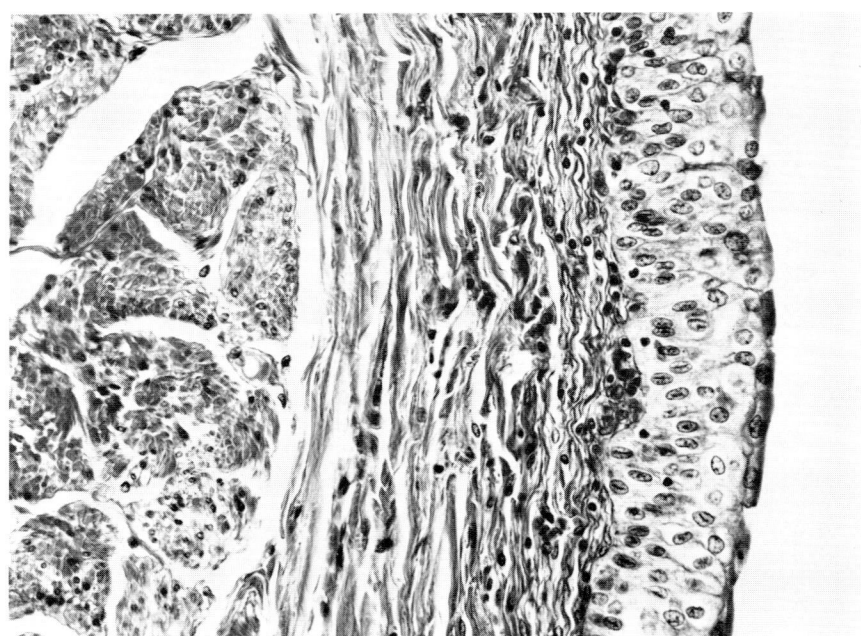

Figure 168. At higher magnification the multilayered epithelium shows no keratin, no prickles, and no mucin. Many of the nuclei have a characteristic bar, and some are indented, an appearance sometimes described as coffee bean. This is typical of transitional epithelium. In the renal pelvis, the same epithelium is seen, but the wall is thinner and more fibrous. *Bladder* (× 250)

LINEATES WITH SMOOTH SURFACES

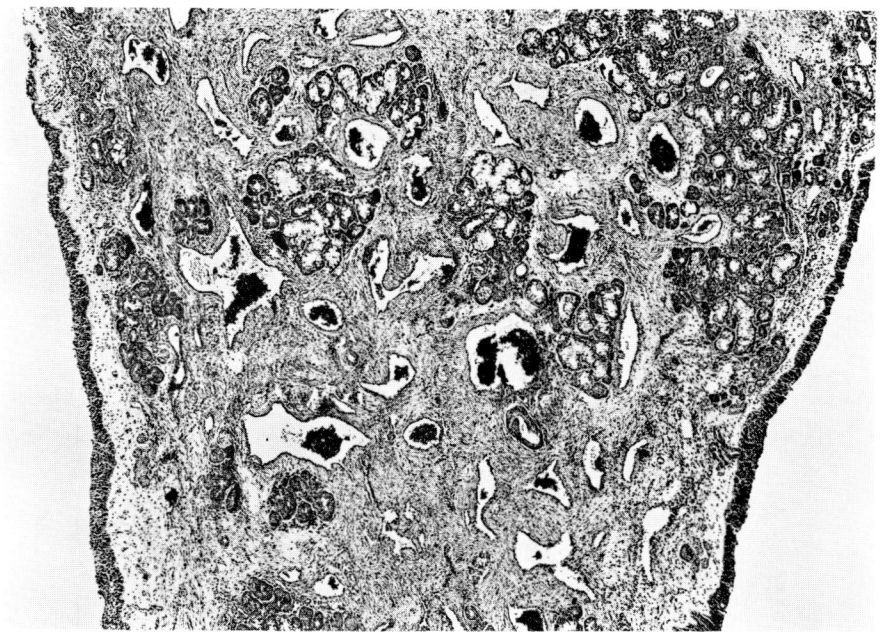

Figure 169. A double-surfaced structure, both epithelia being of respiratory type, can originate only in the nasal passages. The wall is fibrous tissue but is highly vascular with large blood-containing spaces; there are also many minor salivary glands. This section has been deliberately taken from the edge of one of the turbinates, and bone or cartilage would be found in the deeper stroma. *Turbinate* (× 30)

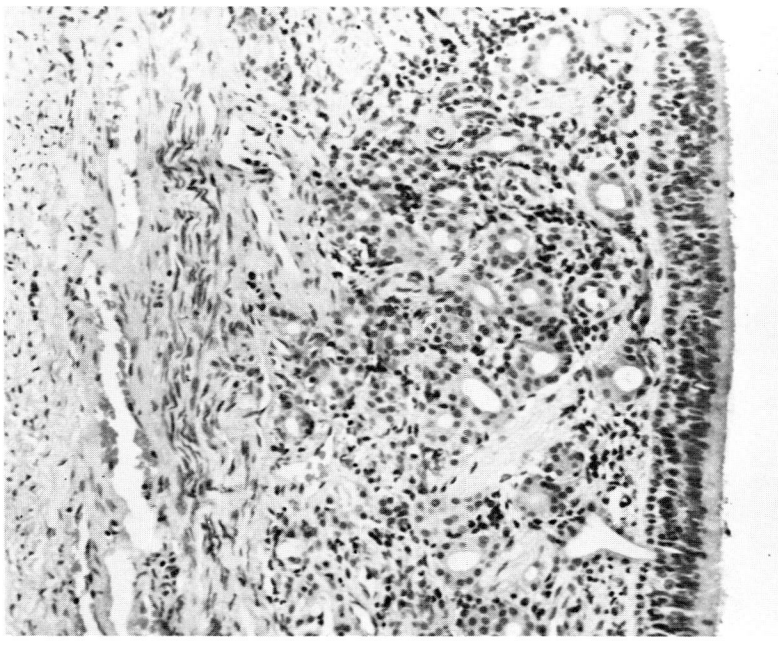

Figure 170. A thick respiratory type of mucosa with nuclei forming rather regular rows, without a definite basement membrane, and with a continuous row of serous glands (Bowman's glands) is unique for the olfactory part of the nose, which includes the roof and sides above the middle turbinates. Vascular spaces and large nerves are also seen. The epithelial cells are of three types — sustentacular cells having their nuclei in the outer layer, ciliated bipolar cells, whose nuclei lie in the midzone, and basal cells more deeply. *Olfactory mucosa* (× 20)

Lineate sections with respiratory epithelium may come from the nasal cavity.

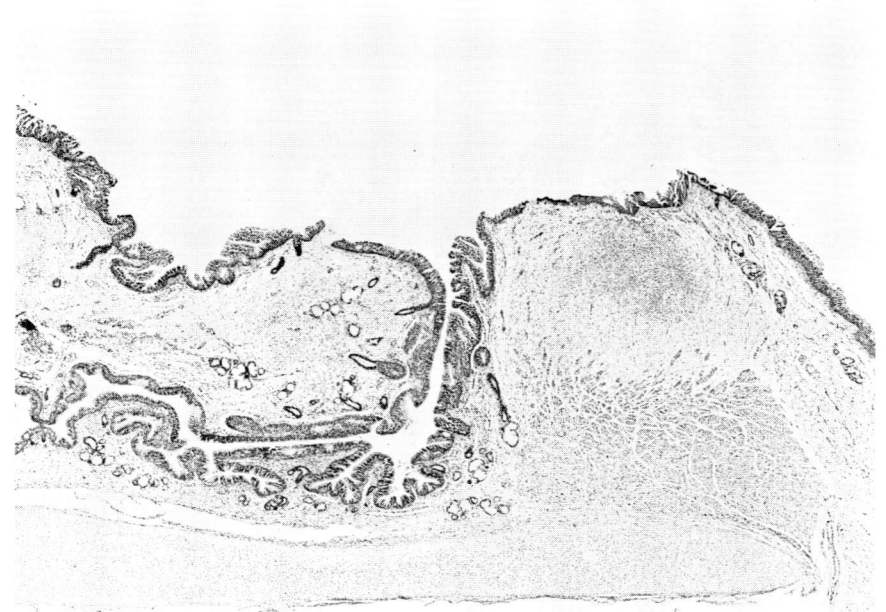

Figure 171. This is a survey picture from the larynx of an infant. The lower margin of the plate shows a solid mass of immature cartilage, and the upper margin is a stratified type of epithelium. In the center of the field, there is a vertical cleft that turns left (cephalad). This is the ventricle of the larynx. To the right of the cleft there is an area of elastic cartilage and fibrous tissue that constitutes the vocal cord. Between the cord and lower cartilage is a broad band of striated muscle. The epithelial lining in the ventricle and on both sides of the cord is respiratory in type; immediately over the cord it is a stratified squamous mucosa. *Larynx* (×16)

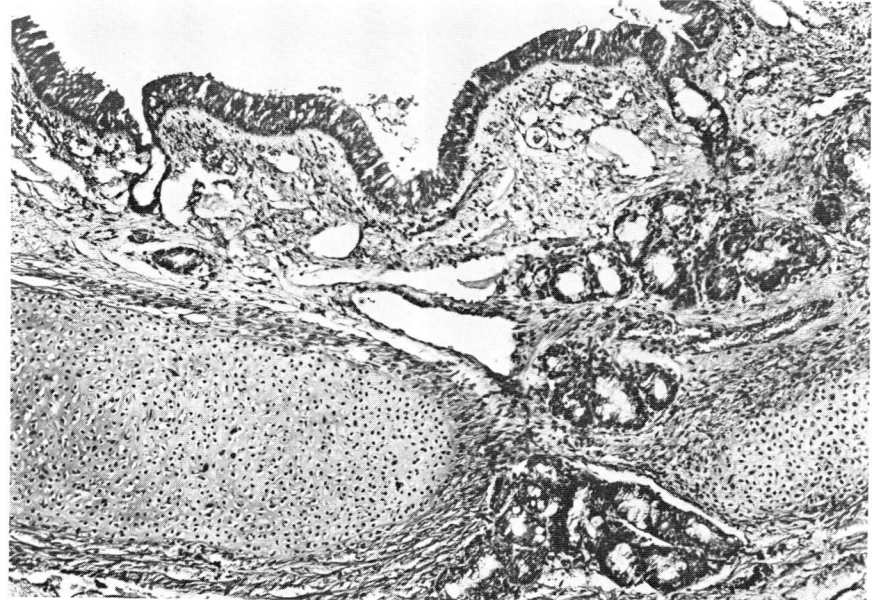

Figure 172. A surface of respiratory type mucosa is seen overlying hyaline cartilage and minor salivary glands, some with ducts that can be seen opening on the surface. Glands pass between the cartilage islands. This combination is seen only in the lower respiratory tract. *Infant trachea* (×80)

Other flat surfaces with respiratory epithelium come from the larynx, from the trachea, or from bronchi cut longitudinally.

LINEATES WITH SMOOTH SURFACES

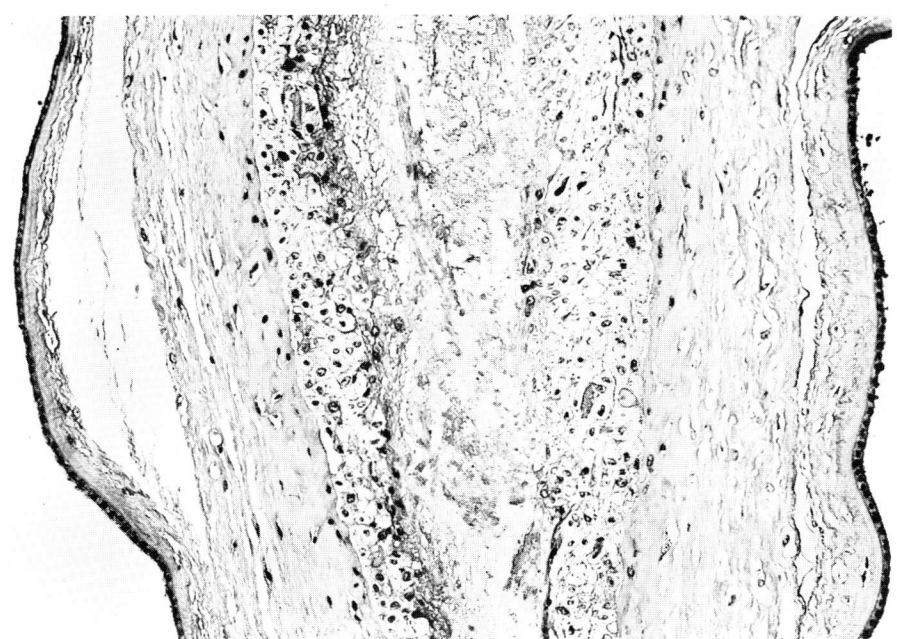

Figure 173. Two surfaces are seen here, each lined by a single layer of cuboidal epithelium. Immediately beneath on each side is a layer of loose connective tissue. More deeply there are two parallel layers of large cells with a central zone of looser myxoid tissue. This combination identifies a diamnionic dichorionic type of fetal membrane, usually associated with dizygotic twins. The outer surface is the amnion; the layers of the large cells are the chorionic trophoblasts. With monozygotic twinning (where the great majority have a diamnionic but monochorionic arrangement) the membranes separating the two fetuses contain no chorionic tissue but a central myxoid zone only. *Diamnionic dichorionic membrane* (×110)

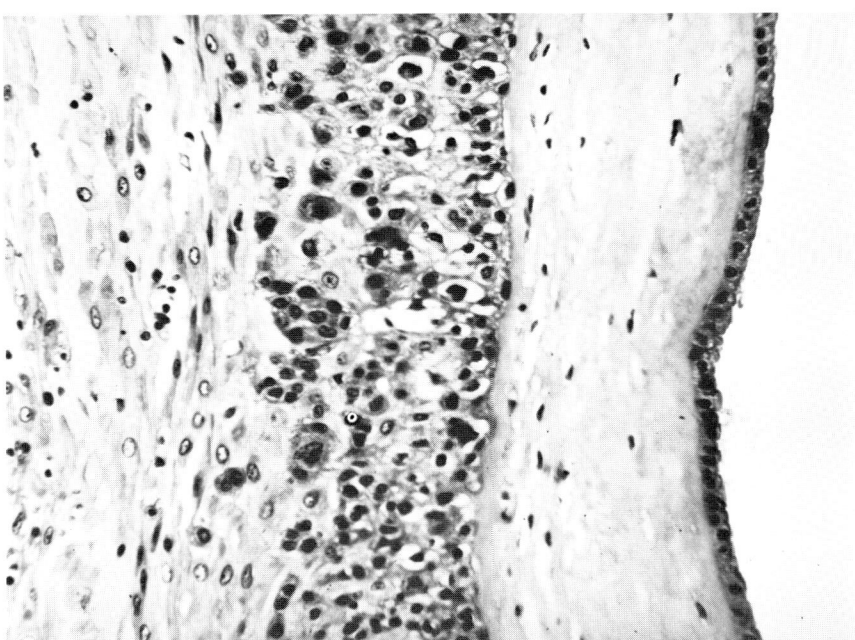

Figure 174. Cuboidal epithelium (right) overlies a single amnion and chorion with large decidual cells from the endometrial mucosa on the left margin. This is the usual appearance of fetal membrane from the uterine wall. *Fetal membrane* (×200)

LINEATES WITH SMOOTH SURFACES

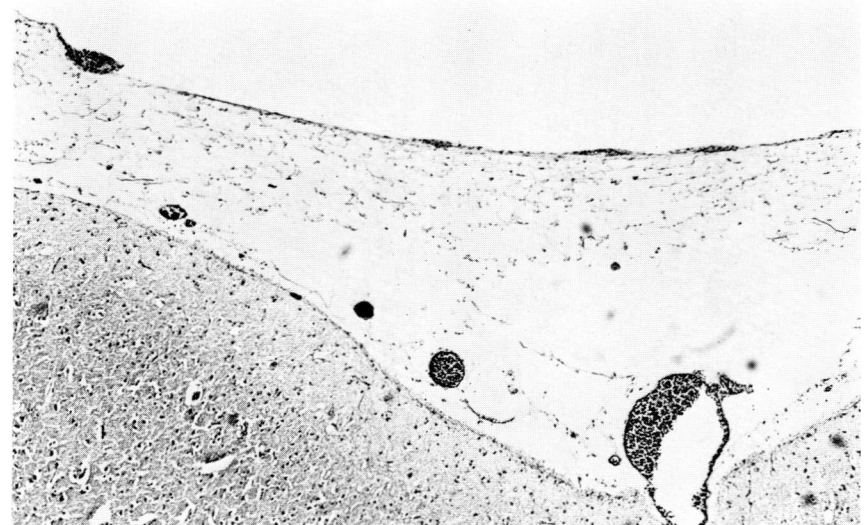

Figure 175. The upper margin here is a thin line of flat squamous cells, which show small characteristic aggregations, or humps, of which four are seen. These are meningocytes of the arachnoid membrane. The tissue immediately beneath is a loose meshwork of fibers joining the arachnoid to the piamater, and within its spaces lies the cerebrospinal fluid. The tissue below is brain cortex. *Meninges* ($\times 10$)

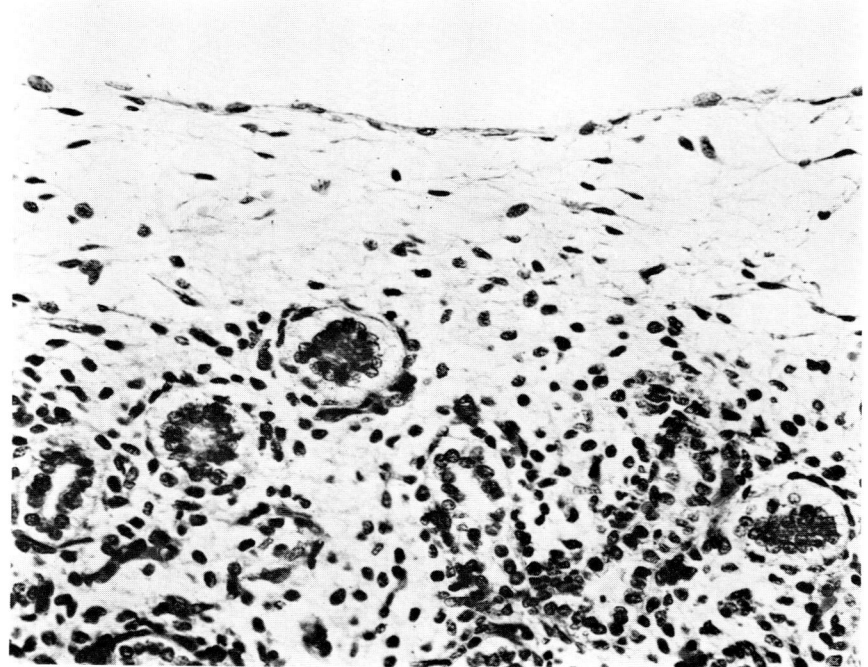

Figure 176. The upper margin here is again formed by flat squamous cells (seen at high magnification) with loose myxoid connective tissue immediately beneath. The more cellular epithelial elements seen as small tubules and annulates in the lower half of the field, in myxoid connective tissue, represent the developing lung of a fetus. In the adult, the mesothelial lining remains, but the pleura is much more dense and fibrous. *Fetal lung, pleura* ($\times 400$)

LINEATES WITH SMOOTH SURFACES

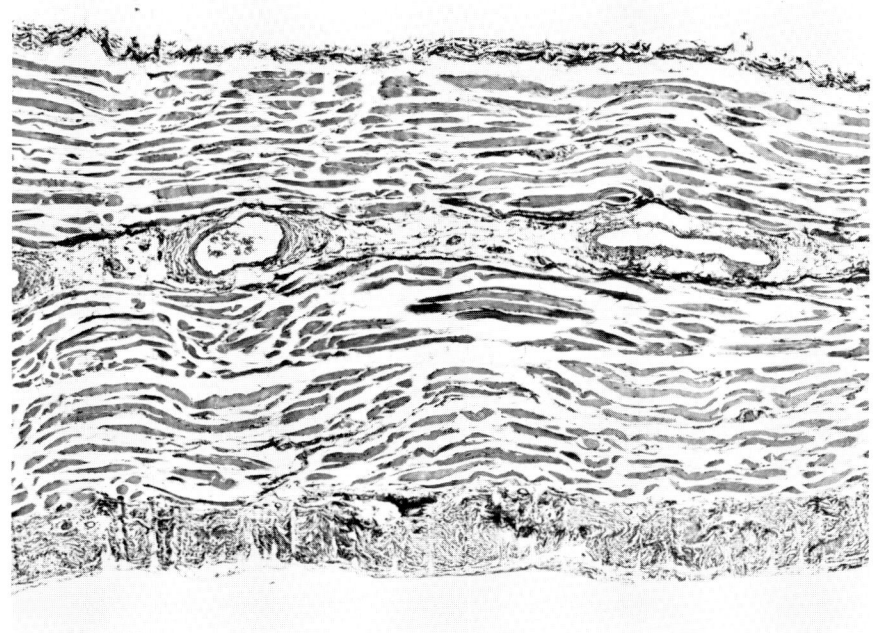

Figure 177. This is a double-surfaced construction, the central part being striated muscle with a narrow rim of fibrous tissue beneath each face. Both surfaces have a flat squamous epithelial lining, and this combination is unique for the diaphragm in its muscular contractile part. (The tendinous central area has a core of dense fibrous tissue.) The upper surface is pleura, the lower is peritoneum. *Diaphragm* (× 36)

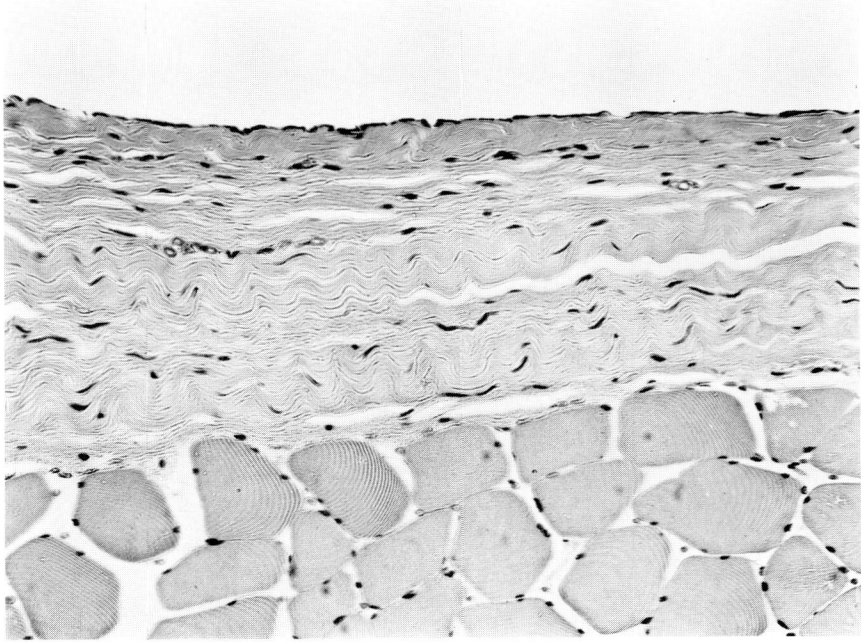

Figure 178. Another flat surface with mesothelial cells overlying dense fibrous tissue and striated muscle fibers comes from the parietal peritoneum, this time from the area immediately deep to the abdominal muscles. In other parts, the serosa may include large amounts of fat and loose myxoid tissue. (In the parietal pleura, striated muscle can be obtained if intercostal muscles are included, but dense fibrous tissue like this would be unexpected.) *Peritoneum* (× 200)

LINEATES WITH SMOOTH SURFACES

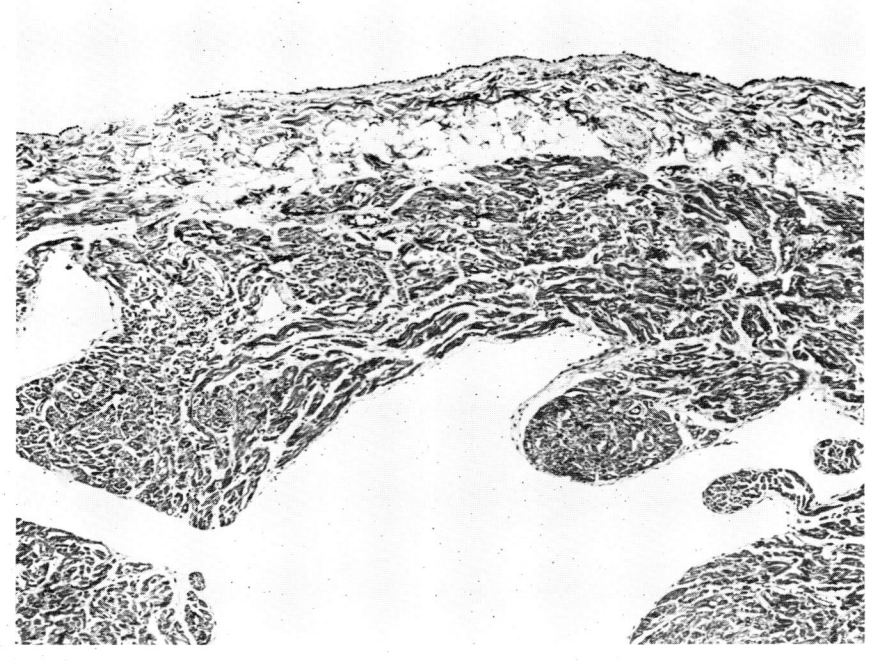

Figure 179. This is a wall whose upper surface is flat and lined by mesothelium (visceral pericardium); the lower surface is quite irregular due to projections of cardiac muscle. The thin wall of very variable thickness is typical of an atrium. *Atrium* (× 50)

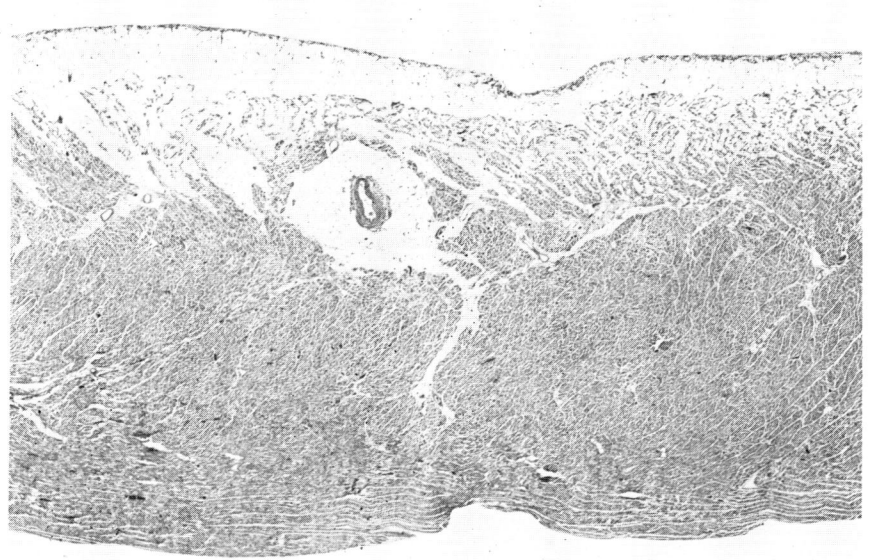

Figure 180. This again is a double-surfaced structure, with simple squamous epithelium (mesothelium), which lies over adipose tissue along the upper margin and is closely adjacent to muscle on the lower edge. The bulk of the tissue is again cardiac muscle, but fat is infiltrating deeply within the fibers. The wall is much thicker than the atrium but not as thick as expected for the interventricular septum or left ventricular wall. *Right ventricle* (× 9.5)

Flat surfaces with simple squamous epithelium (mesothelium or endothelium) come from serous cavities, large vessels, or heart.

LINEATES WITH SMOOTH SURFACES

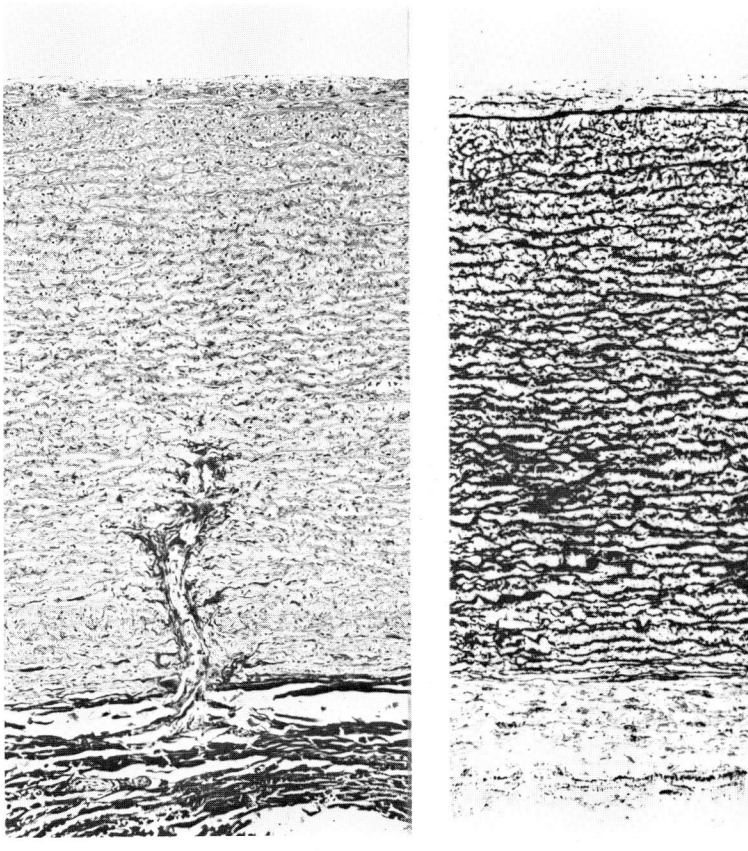

Figure 181. (Left) This figure and Figure 182 show closely interleaved elastic and muscle fibers. Below, a vasa vasorum penetrates the wall to almost midpoint. The adventitial collagen stains darkly. Above, parallel fibers begin with the internal elastica, with other elastic fibers as plates among the muscle elements. *Aorta*, longitudinal section, thoracic area, Masson trichrome, from a nine-year-old subject. (×80)

Figure 182. (Right) Adjacent section to Figure 181, Movat stain. (×80)

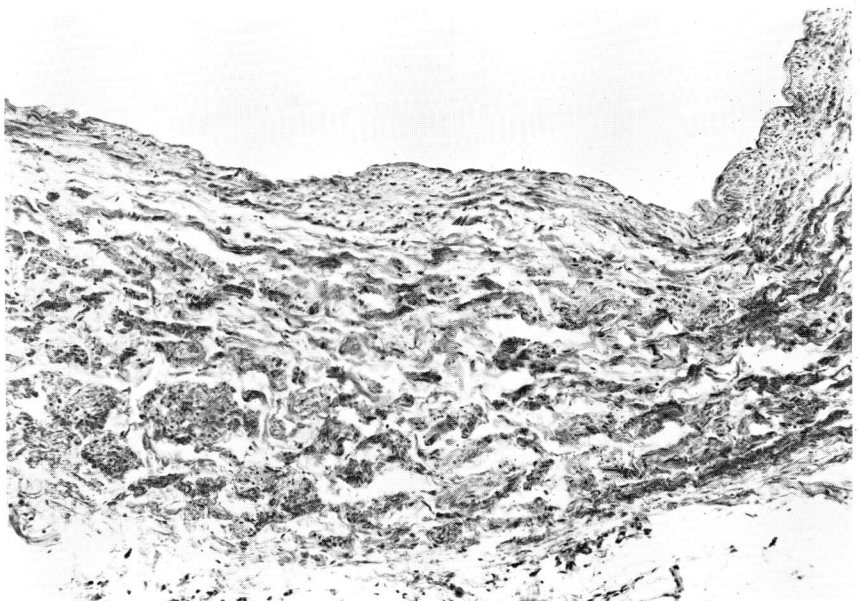

Figure 183. This has a similar flat natural surface with simple squamous epithelium, but the wall is formed of irregular loose bundles of nonstriated muscle and collagen. *Inferior vena cava* (×80)

Flat sections with endothelial surface are vessels, which may be identified according to the muscular or musculoelastic construction of the wall.

LINEATES WITH SMOOTH SURFACES

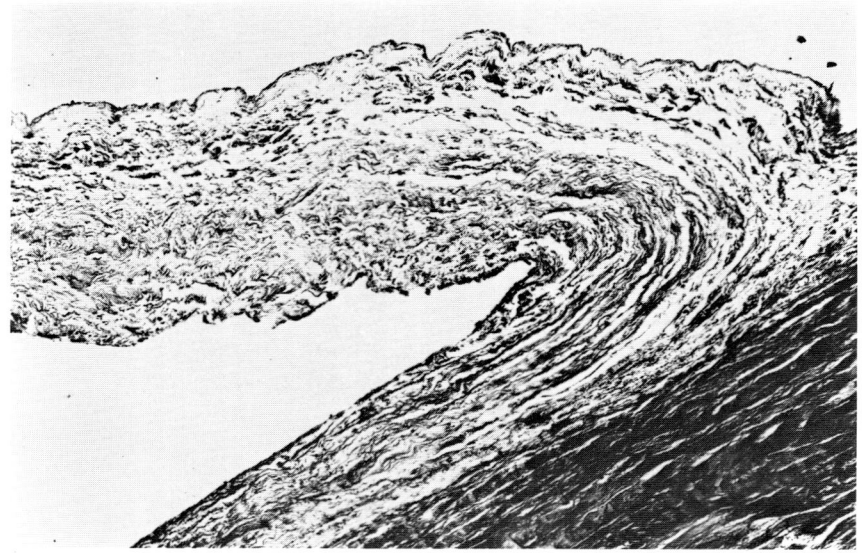

Figure 184. A thin band of myxoid and fibrous tissue with endothelium on both surfaces is a heart valve. In the A-V valves, the subendothelial layer is thicker on lower pressure surfaces (facing the atrial cavities), and in the aortic and pulmonary valves, it is thickest on the arterial faces. *Tricuspid valve* Movat (×80)

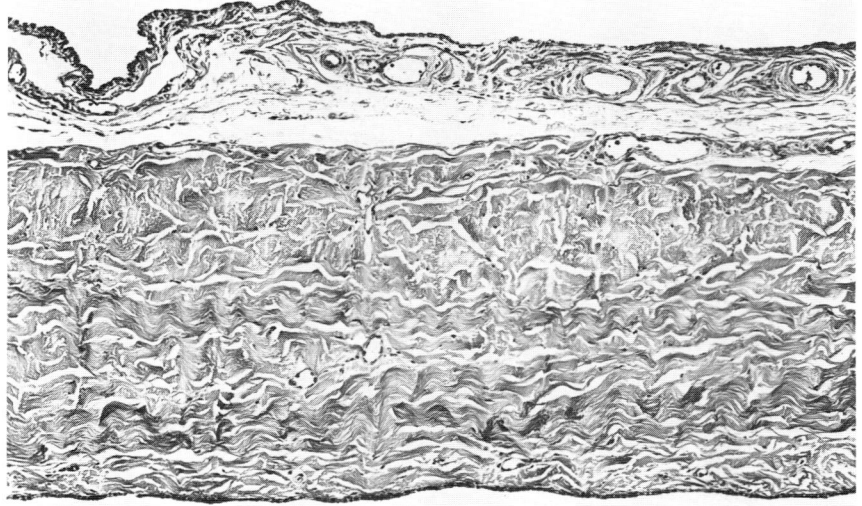

Figure 185. Here the core tissue is dense tendinous fibrous tissue with undulating fibers and some looser tissue along the upper margin. There are two surfaces, both lined by mesothelium. A thin fibrous membrane with these characteristics is *pericardium*. (×200)

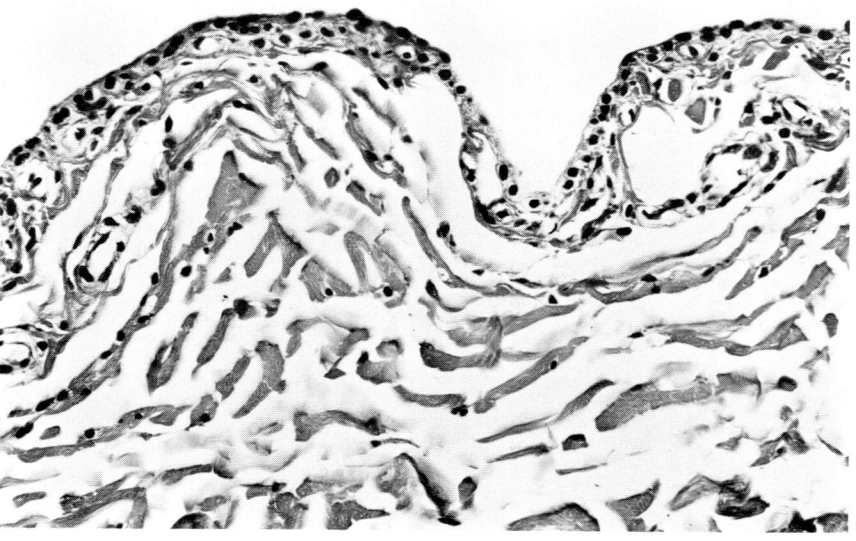

Figure 186. This surface is pseudoepithelial, being formed by an increased number (condensation) of stromal cells. No basement membrane separates them from the underlying fibrous tissue. Joints, bursae, and synovial sheaths are the only open natural surfaces without a true epithelial covering. *Synovium* (×250)

LINEATES WITH IRREGULAR SURFACES

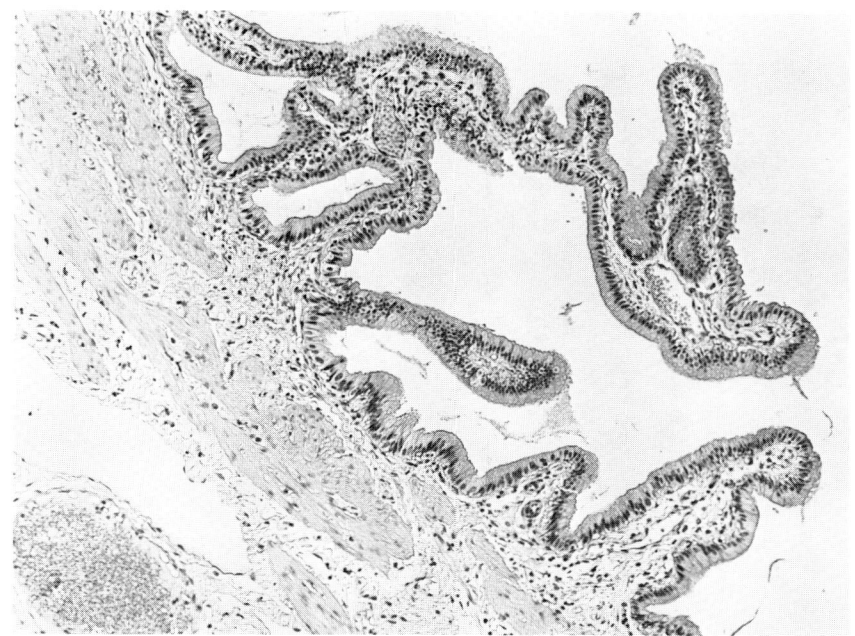

Figure 187. Although virtually flat to naked eye, by microscopy this structure has a highly irregular surface. The epithelium is a single row of columnar cells with clear cytoplasm (sometimes including brown pigment granules) arranged on long, apparently anastomosing processes. These actually represent irregular cuts through partitions which resemble those of an opened honeycomb (as seen by naked eye). There is no muscularis mucosae, and the wall consists of rather irregular and widely separated small bundles of nonstriated muscle. *Gallbladder* (× 100)

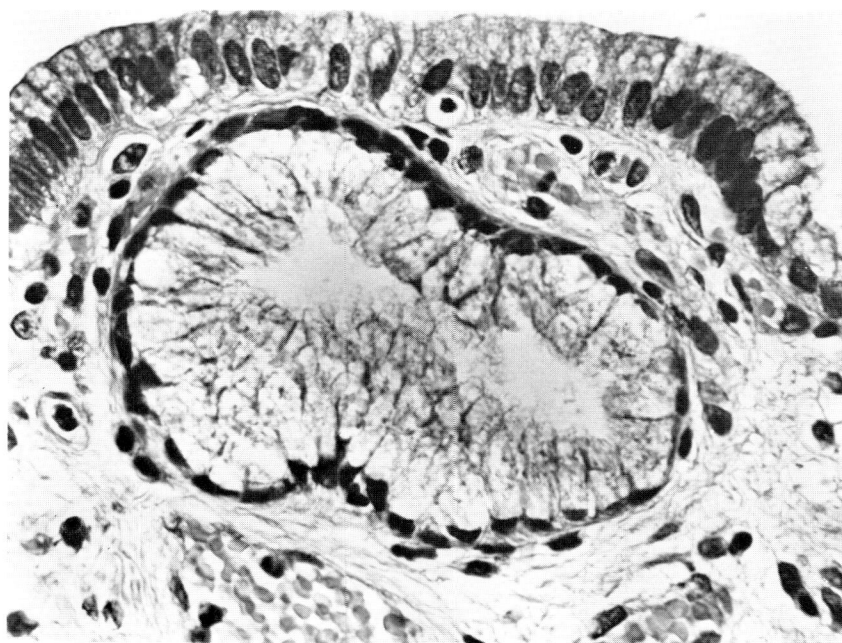

Figure 188. At higher magnification the simple columnar epithelium is well shown. *Gallbladder* (× 480)

LINEATES WITH IRREGULAR SURFACES

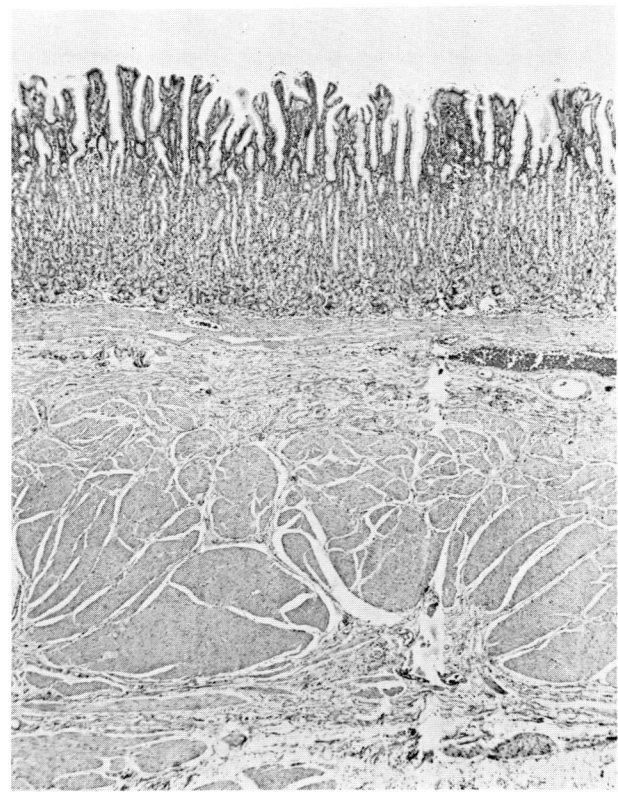

Figure 189. The surface mucosa (above) forms a thick fringe lying on a narrow muscularis mucosae. Between this and the thick muscularis propria (which begins about the center of the plate), there is a zone of loose connective tissue containing blood vessels and nerves. The slightly funnel-shaped dents in the surface of the mucosa are the fovea; these are relatively shallow at the cardiac end and deeper at the pyloric end. *Body of Stomach* ($\times 27$)

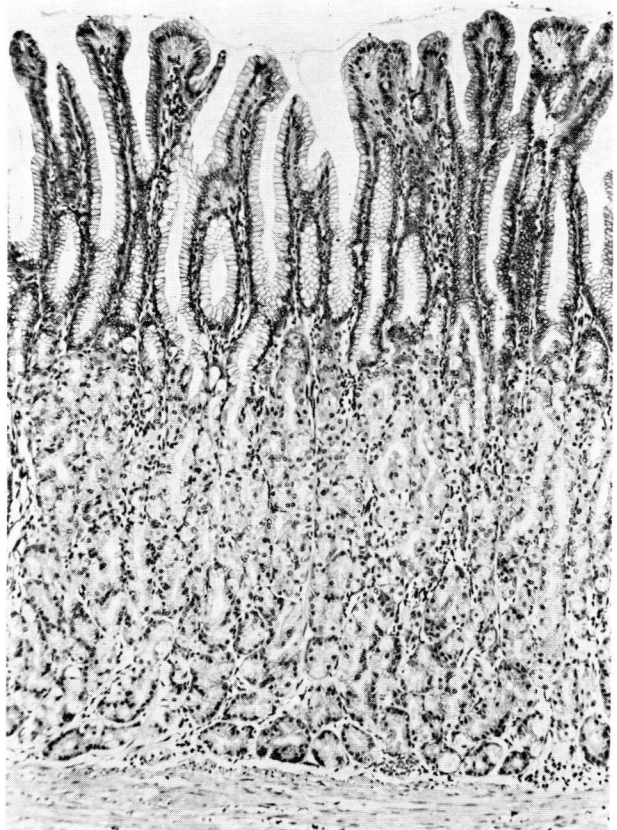

Figure 190. This shows the fovea and the clear cells that line them at higher magnification. Deeper are tubular glands with parallel and circular profiles (depending on how they are cut). The muscularis mucosae is seen at the lower margin of the plate. *Body of stomach* ($\times 80$)

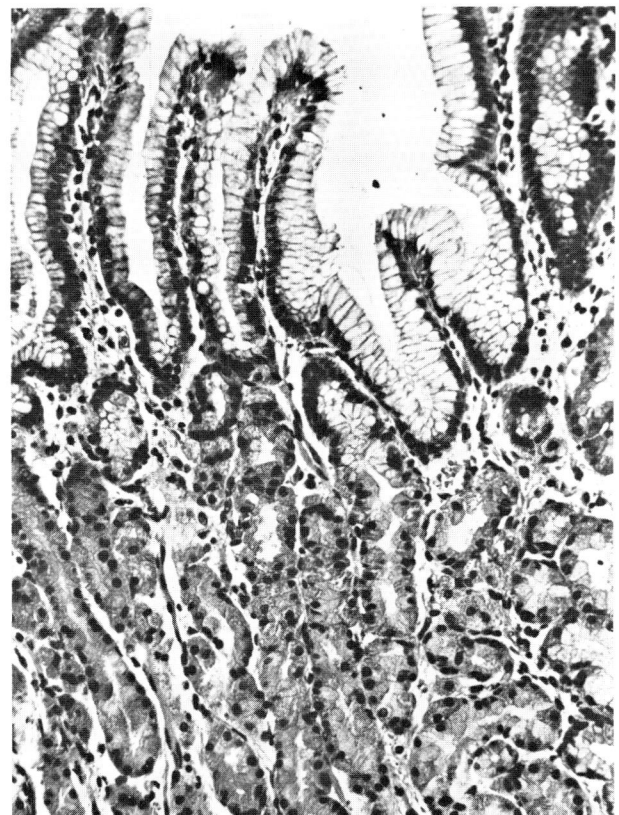

Figure 191. At higher magnification, more cytoplasmic details can be appreciated. The acid-secreting (oxyphilic) parietal cells have a triangular shape, with their bases lying against the basement membrane. In this black and white reproduction of an H & E stain, it is difficult to see them among the relatively gray chief, or zymogenic, cells, which dominate the picture. There is a difference in the quality of the mucus produced by epithelium of the fovea and that of the deeper neck zone, although this requires special stains to be appreciated. Scattered paracrine cells are found in the stomach, again requiring special stains. *Body of stomach* (× 200)

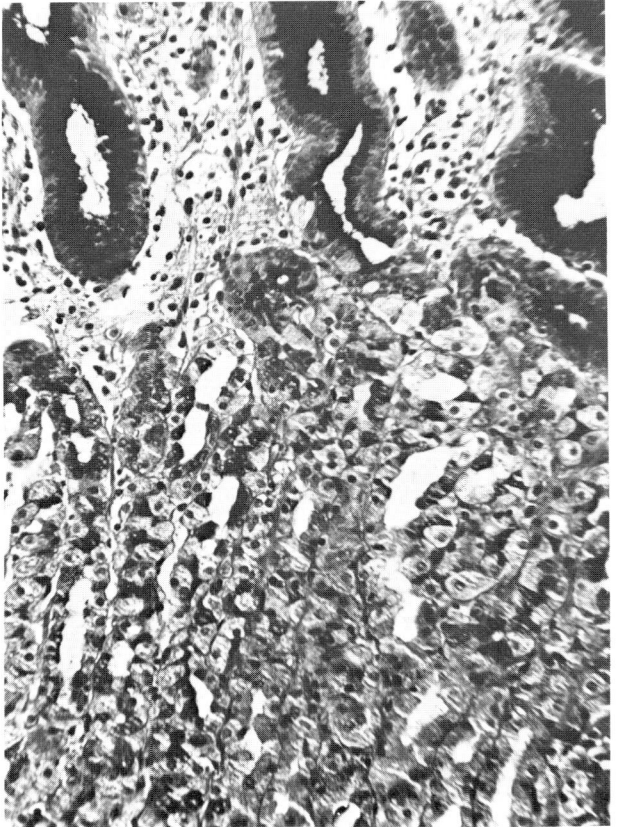

Figure 192. This PAS preparation attempts to accentuate the differences between chief cells and parietal cells. The latter are now darkly staining and triangular, in contrast with the pale acid-secreting units. The three fovea along the upper margin have very dark cytoplasm because of the glycoprotein nature of their mucus and its reaction in the PAS stain. In the lower half of the figure the very dark cells are mucous cells, the round or triangular cells with clear cytoplasm and central nuclei are the acid-secreting cells, and the gray rather more columnar cells are the chief (zymogenic) cells. *Body of stomach* PAS-Orange G stain (× 200)

LINEATES WITH IRREGULAR SURFACES

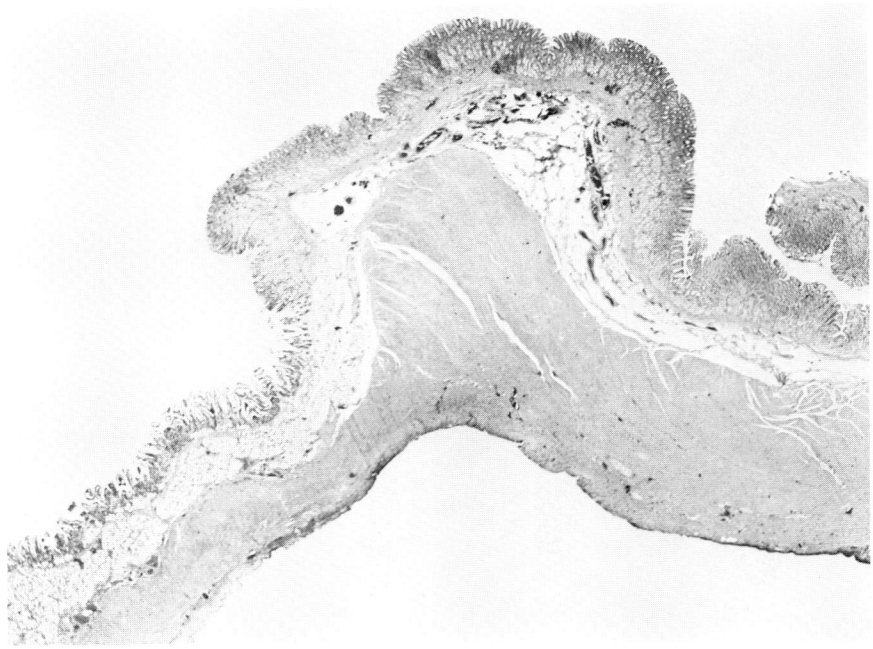

Figure 193. Gastroduodenal junction with thick areas of pyloric sphincter muscle in the center; stomach to the right, and duodenum to the left. (×6.5)

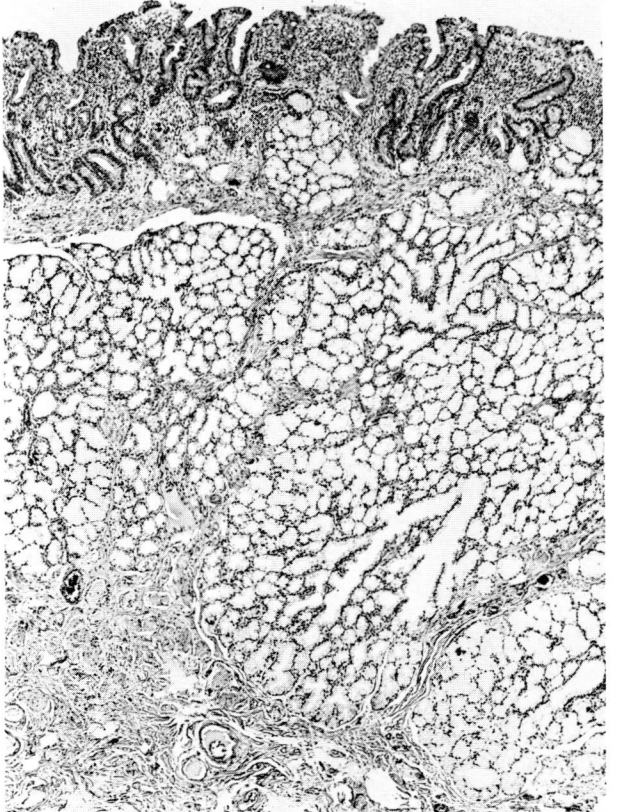

Figure 194. The fringed mucosa contains goblet cells indicating intestinal origin. Beneath is a large mass of glands with small acini and clear cells, both above and below the muscularis mucosa, which is disrupted; this arrangement identifies the duodenum. The glands are Brunner's glands. *Duodenal mucosa* (×31)

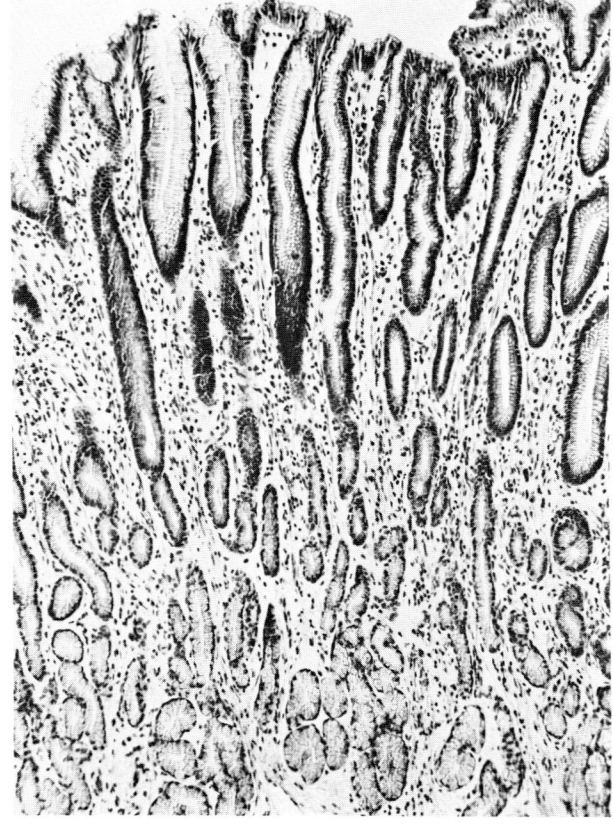

Figure 195. The pyloric fovea are long; there are no goblet cells. Although there are tubuloalveolar glands with clear cytoplasm, these lie above the muscularis mucosa. The antrum contains G (gastrin) cells, demonstrable by immunocytochemistry. *Pyloric mucosa* (×80)

LINEATES WITH IRREGULAR SURFACES

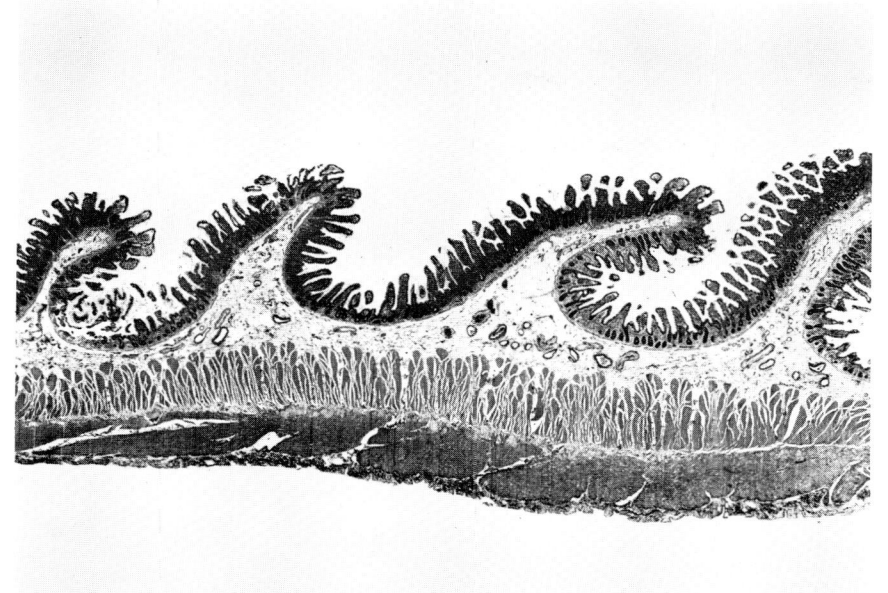

Figure 196. This is a survey of the small intestine showing four folds, or rugae, each surmounted by numerous hairlike villous processes. The sharp line following the contour of the surface mucosa is the muscularis mucosa, and projecting into the rugae is loose connective tissue with numerous vessels. Across the bottom of the figure lie two thick bands of nonstriated muscle, the upper (circular) coat being cut transversely and the lower (longitudinal) being cut in its long axis. Parasympathetic nerve plexuses run in the submucosa (Meissner) and between the inner and outer muscle coats (Auerbach's plexus). *Small intestine* (× 10)

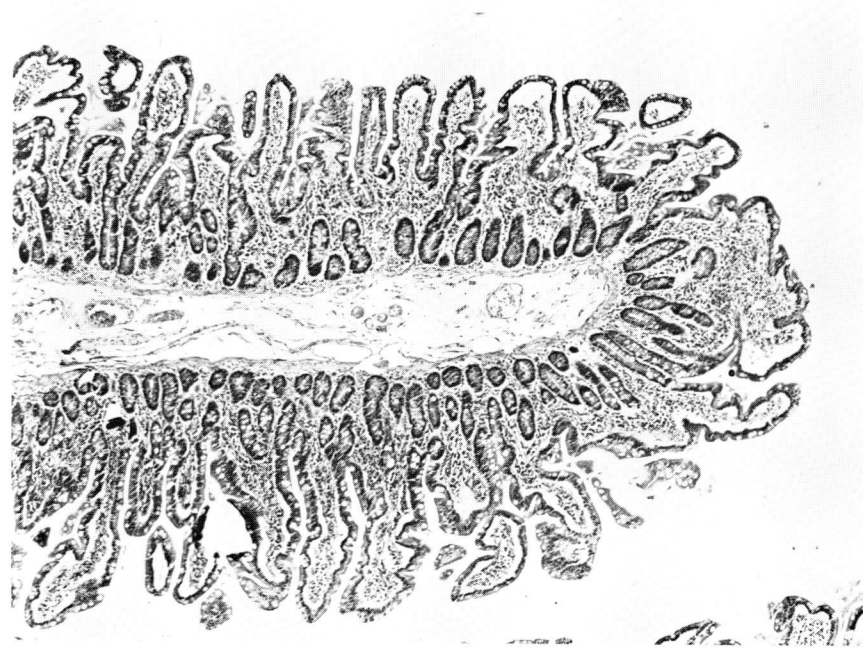

Figure 197. This is a higher magnification of one of the folds with its villi. The intervillous clefts lead to one or often two crypts, and the clear goblet cells, which are interspersed throughout the mucosa, are clearly seen. The thin line of muscle fibers at the base of the glands is the muscularis mucosae, while the center of the field is loose connective tissue with blood vessels. It will also be noted that the loose connective tissue of the mucosa itself contains many small nuclei; these are chiefly lymphocytes, which are normally present in the lamina propria of the intestine. *Small intestine* (× 36)

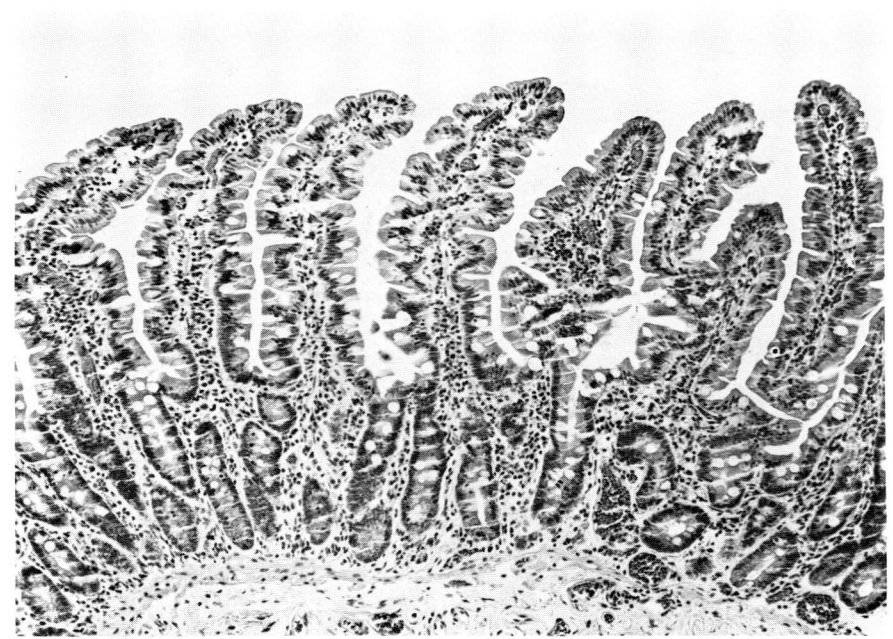

Figure 198. At higher magnification the villi, crypts, goblet cells, lymphoreticular infiltrate, and thin muscularis mucosae can be better appreciated. *Small intestine* (×100)

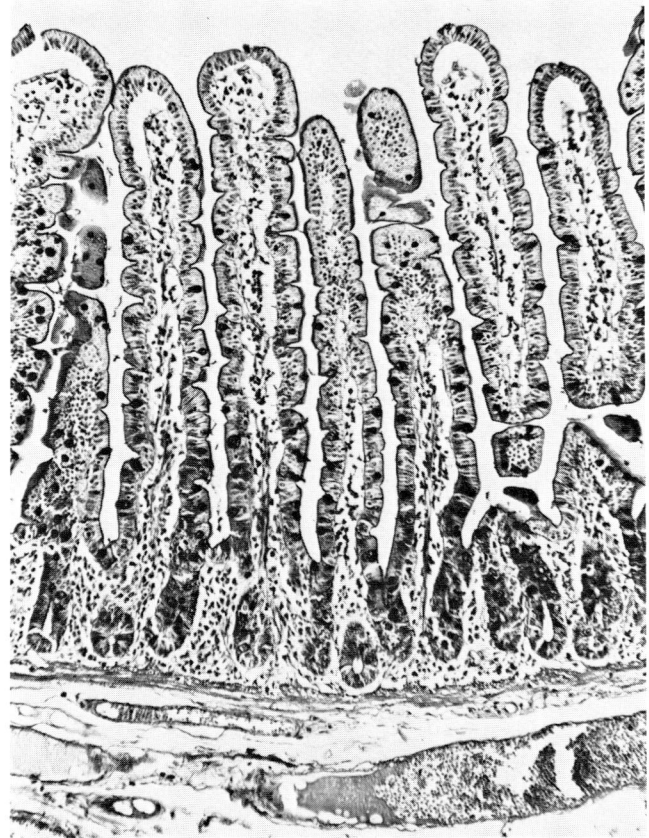

Figure 199. This is a PAS (undigested) preparation to show the glycocalyx (the thin dark line that covers the epithelial surface of the villi), a superficial layer of glycoprotein nature. The goblet cells stain a magenta color and are represented by black circles and rectangles interspersed among the lining epithelial cells. PAS (×100)

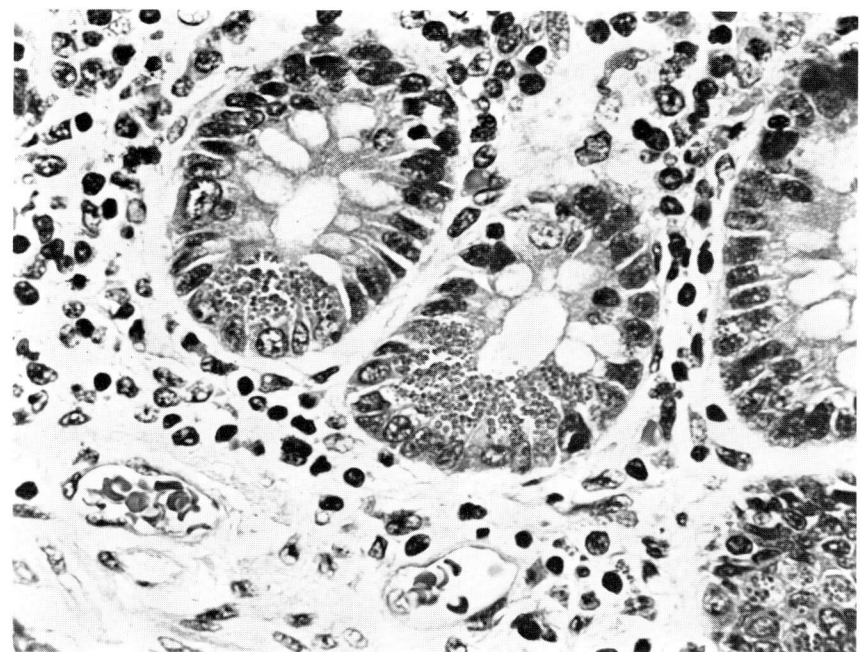

Figure 200. This figure shows the bottom ends of three crypts of Lieberkühn. In the left and center crypts, the cytoplasm of the lowermost cells is occupied by numerous coarse granules; in an H & E preparation these are brightly eosinophilic and identify Paneth's cells (associated with lysozyme). In normal adults these are restricted to the small intestine, but in infants they may be seen in the large intestine. *Paneth's cells* (×300)

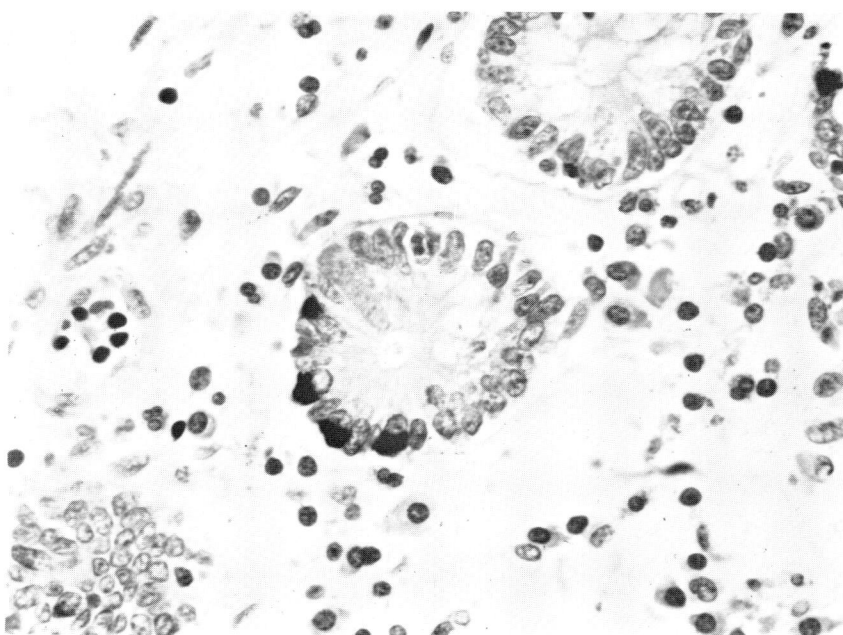

Figure 201. The crypts of Lieberkühn contain other cells, some of which have the ability to reduce silver preparations directly. These are argentaffin cells, which are associated with serotonin and substance P. They are part of the "diffuse endocrine system" (paracrine) described by Feyrter (1958). In this figure the argentaffin granules are seen as dense black masses peripheral to the nuclei in four cells at the bottom and left side of the lower crypt. The old name for these cells is Kulchitsky's cell; a newer name is EC_1 (enterochromaffin). *Argentaffin cells,* Masson-Fontana (×490)

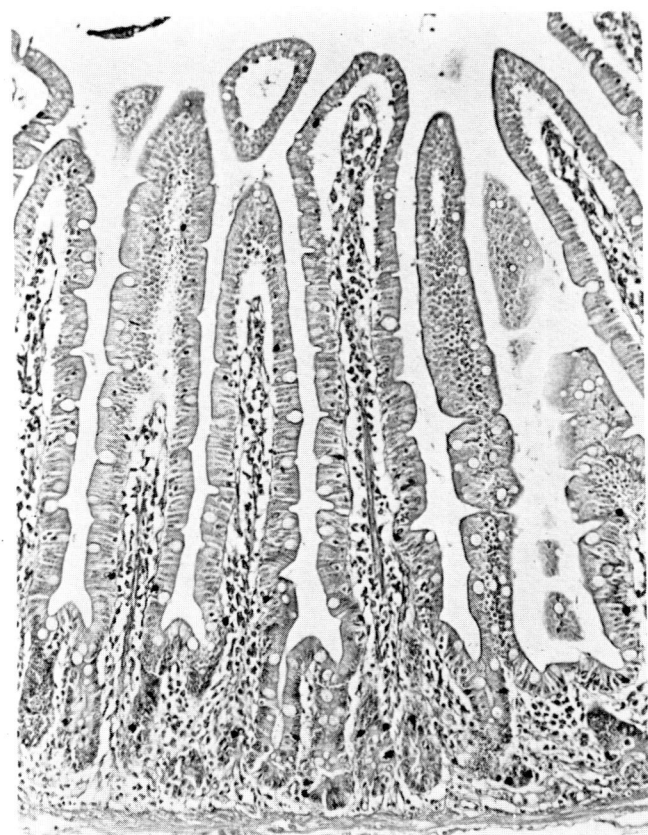

Figure 202. If small intestine is examined by argyrophil methods (where silver deposits are induced by including reducing agents in the reaction mixture), paracrine cells other than those of the base of the crypts can be seen. The additional cells correspond to those which have been found by immunocytochemical methods to be associated with polypeptide and biogenic amine production (Pearse, 1977). They are termed EC_2 cells and have been related to motilin. *Small intestine, paracrine cells,* Grimelius silver reaction (×120)

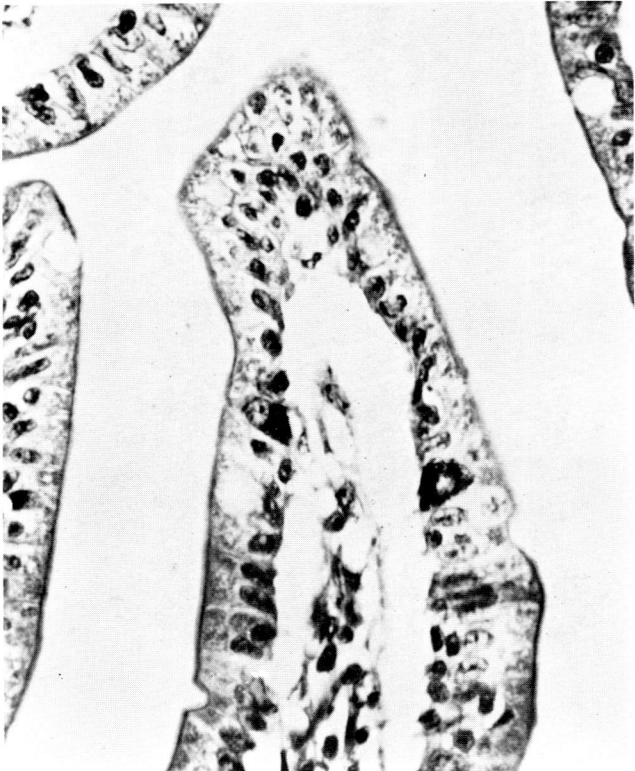

Figure 203. This is a lead hematoxylin preparation of small intestine, which also outlines certain paracrine cells by a black precipitate as seen in two cells, one on the right and one slightly higher on the left side of the central villus towards its apex. Both silver and lead methods are relatively nonspecific. *Paracrine cells,* lead hematoxylin (×480)

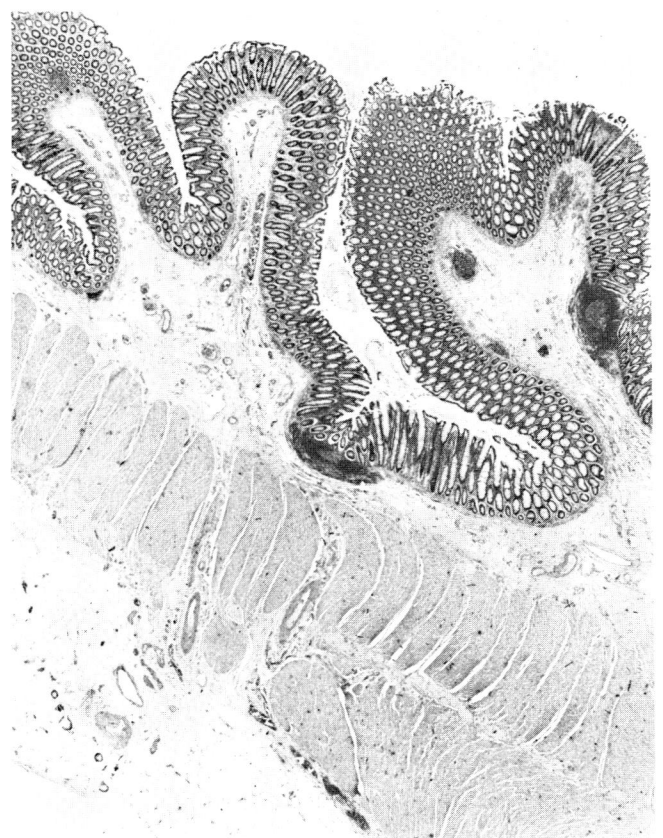

Figure 204. This fringed mucosa is thrown into coarse folds, again demarcated by a thin muscularis mucosae, with loose connective tissue containing vessels and with a thick band of circular muscle (cut transversely) running obliquely across the lower field. Part of a second longitudinal muscle coat is seen in the lower margin with serosal connective tissue in the lower left corner. This is one of the taeniae or thick longitudinal bands dominating the muscularis externa, which is otherwise very thin relative to the inner circular coat. The mucosa contains innumerable tubules (crypts) many seen as slits, but others (where glands have been cut obliquely) seen as oval or rounded profiles. *Colon* (× 10)

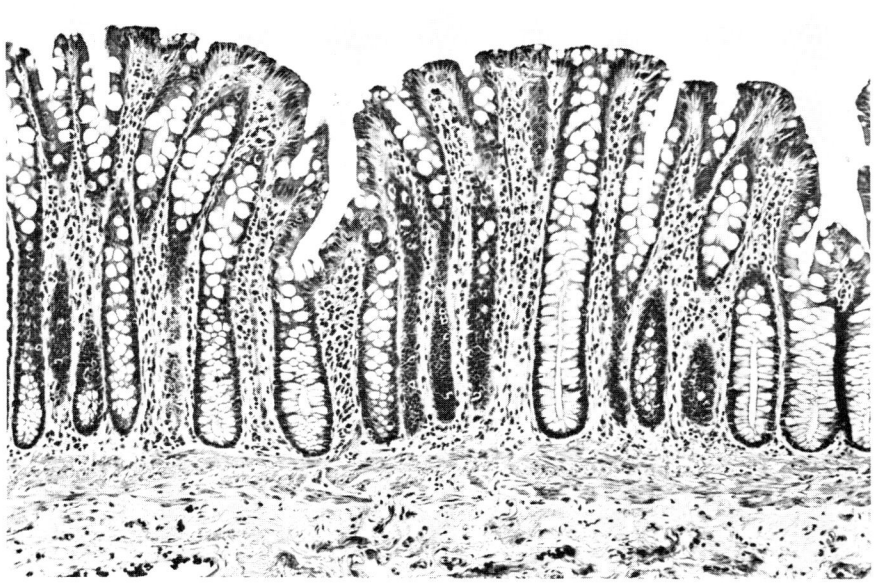

Figure 205. At higher magnification the regular tubular glands contain many goblet cells, here seen as clear, round holes. (These increase in number from the ascending colon to the rectum where they predominate.) To show the EC_1 cells argentaffin reactions would be needed. The upper margin of the crypts is taken to be the surface level, and in contradistinction to the small intestine, there are no projections above this line. The muscularis mucosa is clearly seen running along the base of the crypts. Again myeloid and lymphoid cells are present in the lamina propria. *Colon* (× 200)

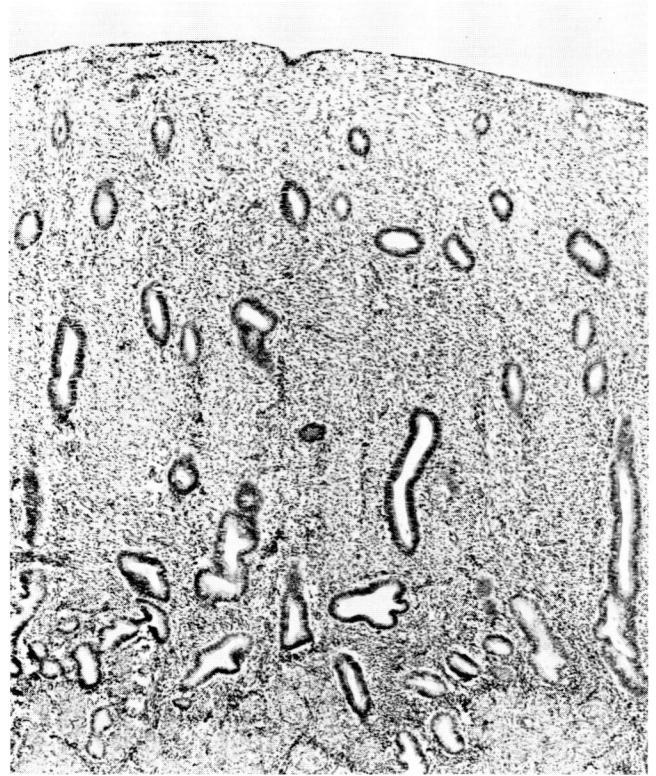

Figure 206. An epithelial surface is seen running across the upper part of this plate, and in the loose somewhat myxoid stroma beneath, there are circular and parallel gland profiles (regenerating glands in proliferative phase). Just above the lower margin, there are less regularly arranged glands, part of the basal layer from which regeneration occurs. This section is from the wall of the uterine cavity three days after a curetting. *Endometrium* (× 42)

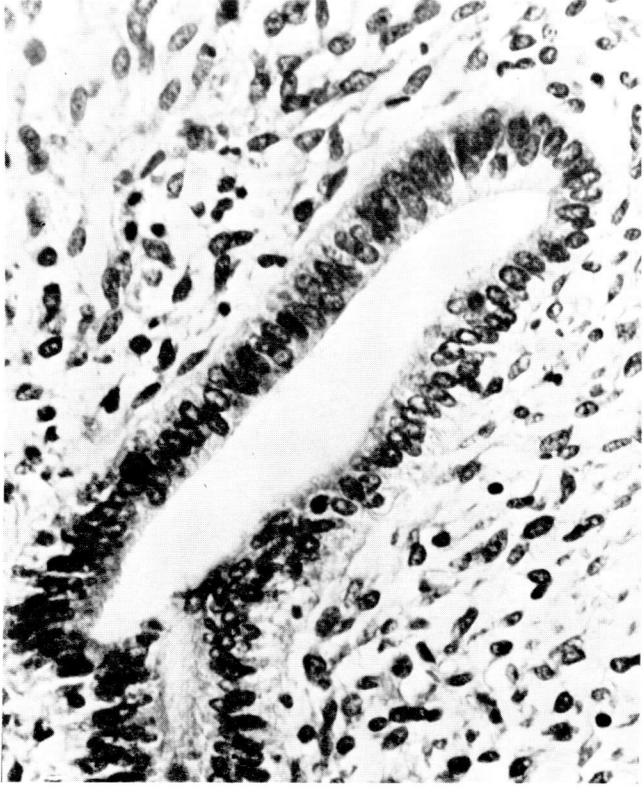

Figure 207. At higher magnification these glands have a single layer of columnar cells, and occasional mitotic figures can usually be seen. The stroma is loose and fibrillary, and it is difficult to distinguish intercellular matrix from mesenchymal cell cytoplasm because both are watery in appearance. *Proliferative endometrium* (× 350)

LINEATES WITH IRREGULAR SURFACES

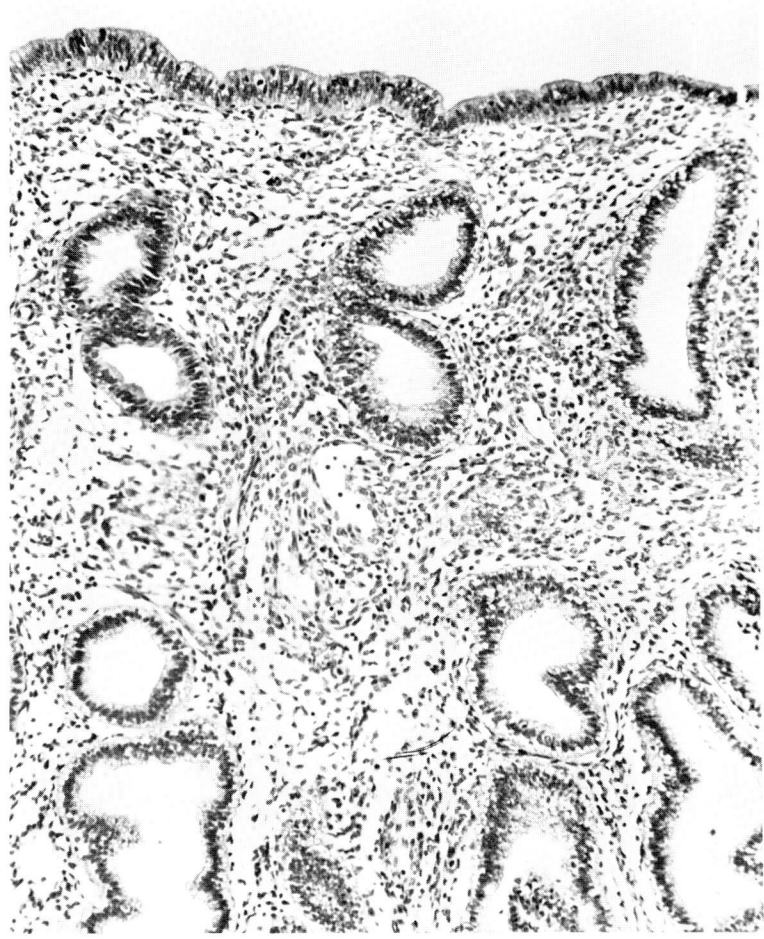

Figure 208. In this figure endometrial surface glands and stroma are seen as before, but there is a striking increase in the diameter of the gland lumens, more glands appear to be present per unit area, they are slightly convoluted so that they are cut across more often, and there is some evidence of clear vacuoles in the cytoplasm beneath the nuclei. *Midphase endometrium* (× 110)

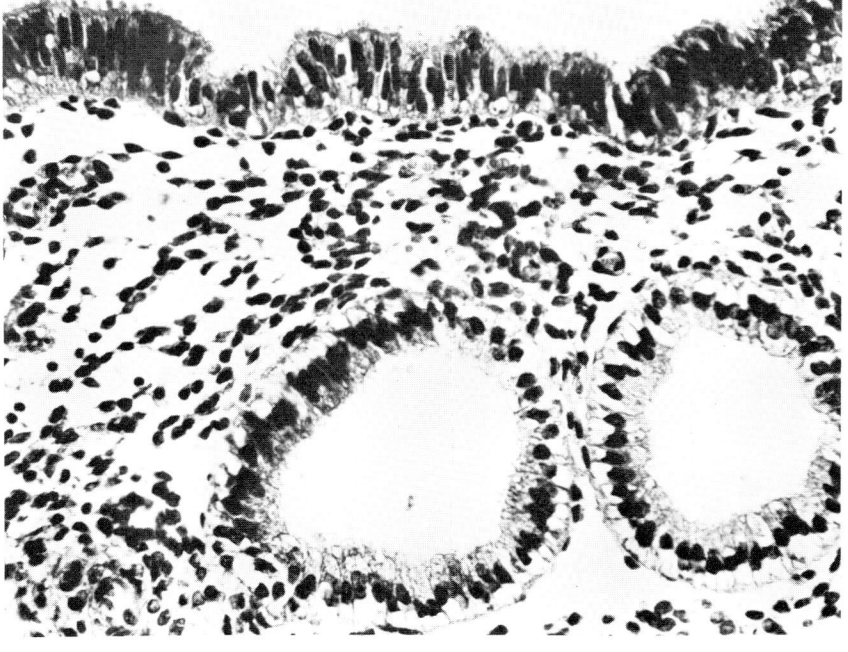

Figure 209. At higher power, clear vacuoles are present peripheral to the nucleus in virtually every cell; this represents the secretion of glycogen. When subnuclear vacuoles of this sort are found in a majority of the glands, it is an indication that ovulation has occurred, and it marks the earliest secretory phase of the cycle. *Early secretory endometrium* (× 300)

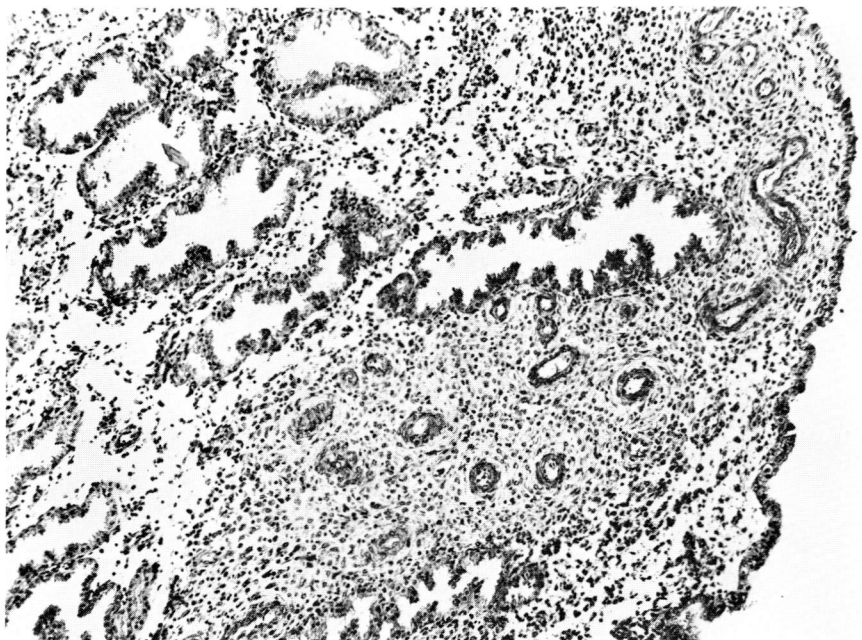

Figure 210. At a later stage of the cycle, glands are even further dilated and more tortuous, and the secretory vacuoles are found on the luminal aspect of the epithelial cells. The stroma has become edematous. In the lower half of this figure the stroma has an epithelioid appearance indicating pseudodecidual change. The numerous small arteries are the spiral arteries cut transversely. It is these vessels which are believed to constrict and produce ischemic necrosis with desquamation at menstruation. *Late secretory phase endometrium* (× 80)

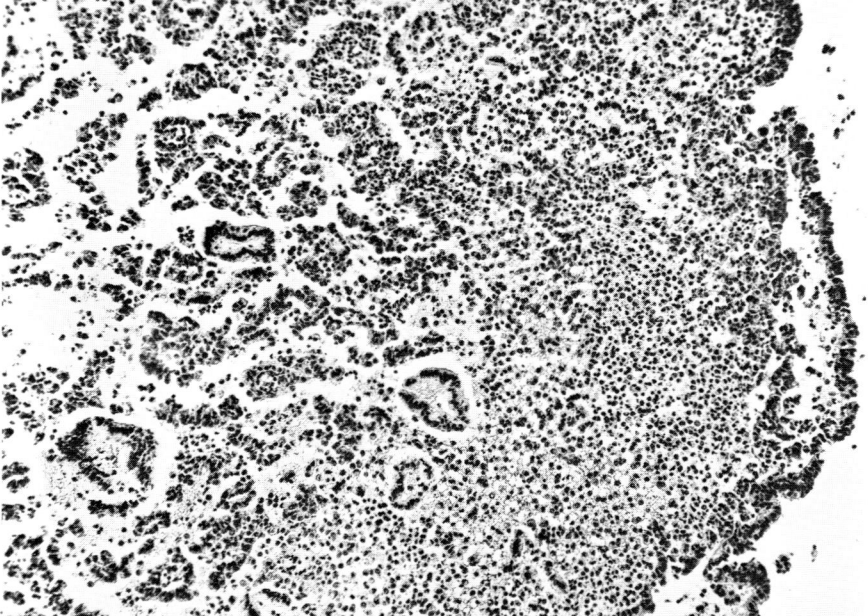

Figure 211. The stroma next appears to disintegrate and is infiltrated by numerous polymorphs as well as by extravasated red cells. The glands are fragmenting, and the surface mucosa is being shed. *Menstrual endometrium* (× 90)

Table 4

CYCLIC CHANGES IN ENDOMETRIUM

Short narrow glands Mitoses Loose spindle stroma	Early proliferative
Longer glands Stratification of epithelial nuclei	Late proliferative
Mitotic activity maximal Stratification of nuclei Subnuclear vacuoles in most glands	2 to 3 days post ovulation
Disappearance of mitoses Supranuclear vacuolation	4 to 5 days post ovulation
Tortuous glands Luminal secretion Disappearance of vacuoles Stromal edema	6 to 8 days post ovulation
Spiral arteries Predecidual changes in stroma	9 to 11 days post ovulation
Polymorphonuclear infiltration Stromal disintegration Hemorrhage	12 to 14 days post ovulation

LINEATES WITH IRREGULAR SURFACES

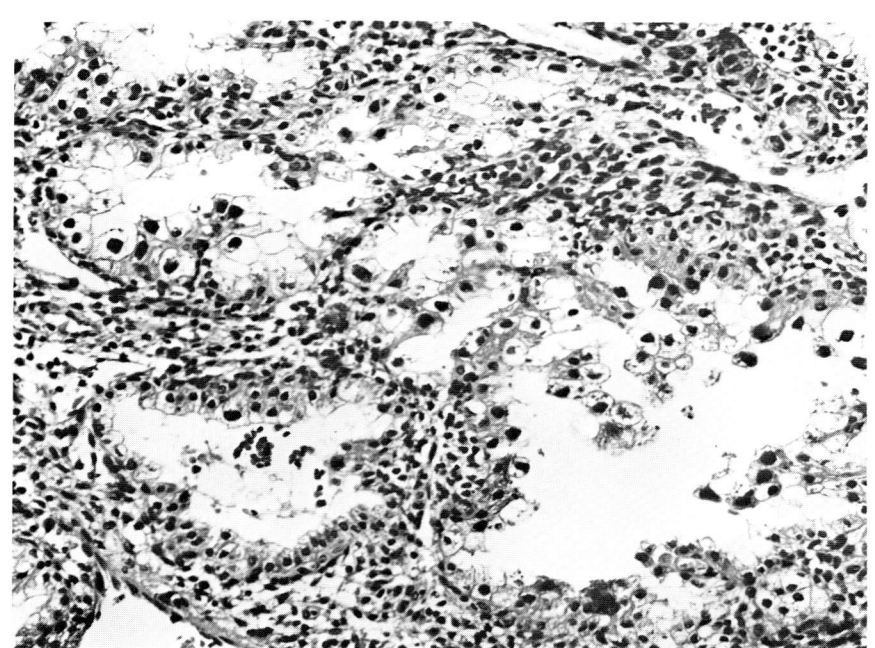

Figure 212. These glands are widely dilated and somewhat tortuous. The cells are characterized by empty cytoplasm on their luminal aspects and by large hyperchromatic nuclei of irregular size. This is the type of change seen in early pregnancy. *Pregnancy endometrium* (× 160)

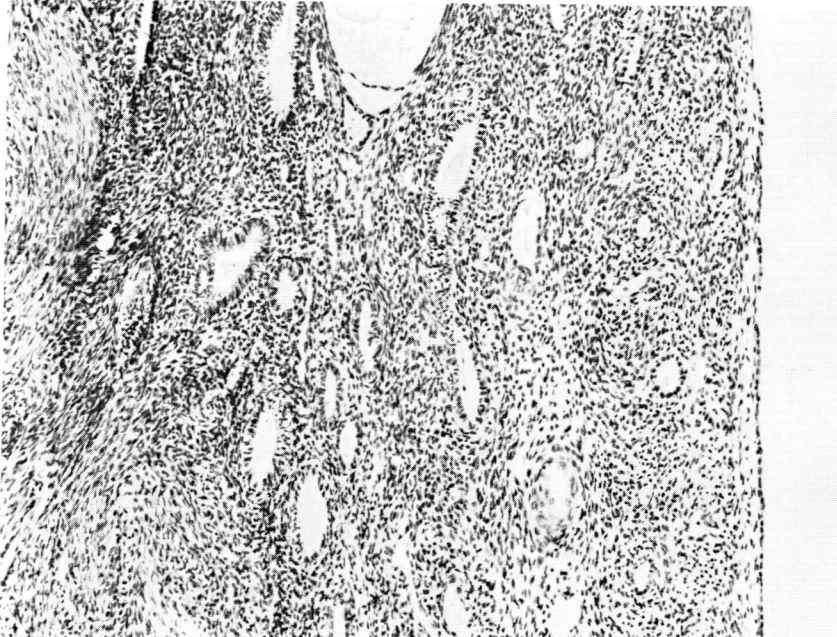

Figure 213. Changes opposite from those in Figure 212 are here apparent. The endometrium as a whole is thin, and the stroma is rather fibrous and spindle cell in type. The glands are dilated but show no sign of projections and are lined by a single layer of low columnar epithelium. *Atrophic endometrium* of the postmenopausal state (× 100)

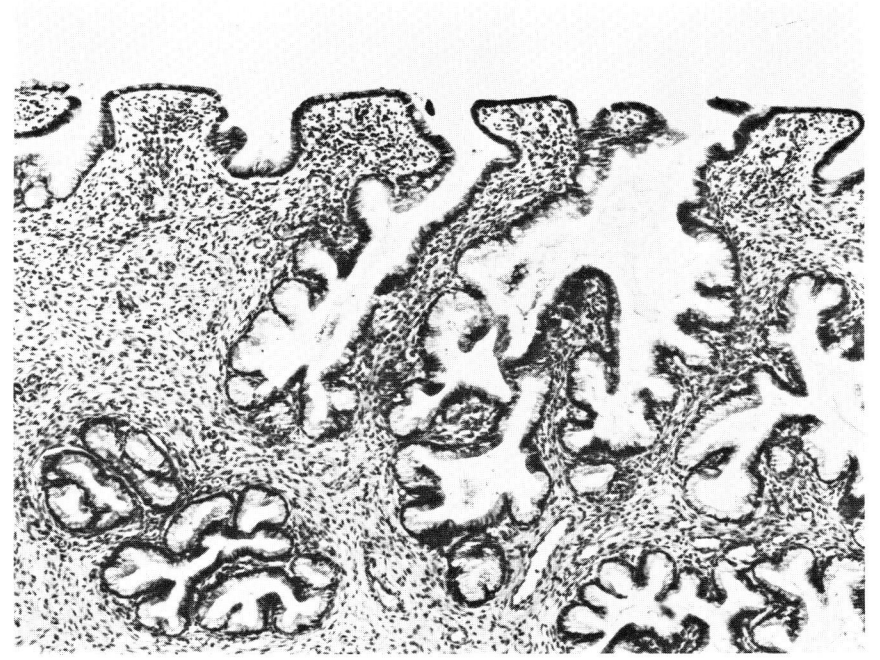

Figure 214. This wall is interrupted by numerous glands growing down from the surface and branching in an irregular racemose fashion (like a bunch of grapes). The lining cells are tall and columnar with clear mucus-containing cytoplasm. The stroma is more compact and cells more spindle shaped than in the endometrium. The combination of epithelial and stromal characteristics is typical of the endocervix. *Endocervix uteri* (×70)

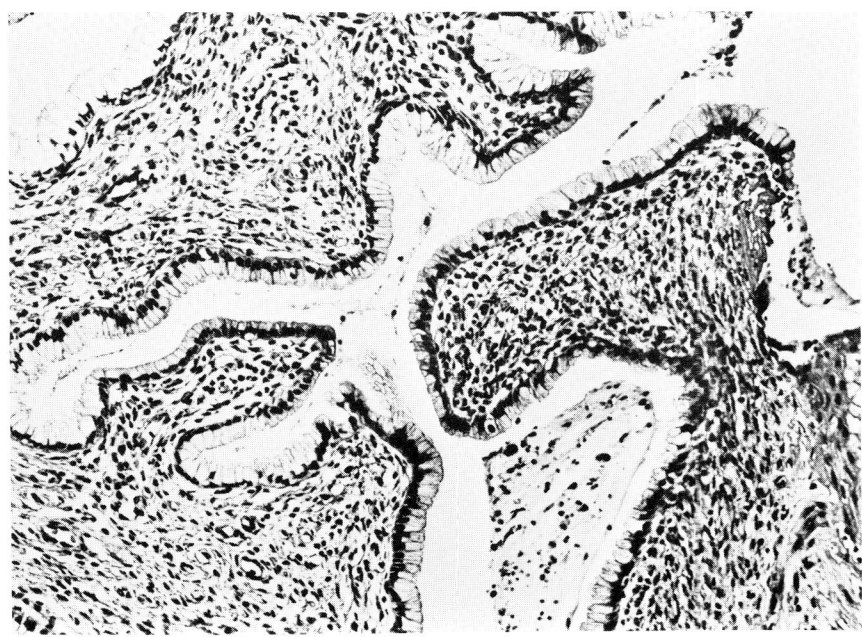

Figure 215. At higher power the clear cytoplasm and the branching glands are more apparent. In the lower center, the gland contains mucus and debris of inflammatory cells. On the extreme right is a fragment of stratified squamous mucosa, a very frequent finding in otherwise unremarkable cervices, which is due to metaplasia. *Endocervix uteri* (×140)

Annulate Sections (From Tubular Laminated Parts)

Hollow cylinders of the size of the appendix, oviducts, ureters, vasa deferentia, bile ducts, bronchi, and most blood vessels are usually cut across to give an annulate type of section. The eyeball, which is a hollow spheroid, also appears ringlike. Very small blood vessels, bronchioles, ducts, and ductules appear as enclaves within some other structure. There are also a number of small vestigial tubules, inconstantly present and identified chiefly by their location. These include bile ducts (Luschka's ducts) in the bed of the gallbladder, remnants termed the epoophoron in the mesosalpinx, and similar tubules in the broad ligaments, representing remnants of the mesonephric or wolffian tubules or ducts. That part which runs down the side of the uterus and cervix is termed Gartner's duct. In the male, comparable remnants of the müllerian duct may be found in the groove between the testis and epididymis and are known as the appendix testis. Connected to the head of the epididymis may be an appendix epididymis of wolffian derivation. (These are often less tubular than solid structures.)

In identification, chief importance attaches to the contour of the inner surface and the type of epithelium. Some tubes have a smooth lining, as with blood vessels, others have an irregular surface, as in the appendix or fallopian tubes. The type of epithelium ranges from a stratified squamous keratinizing epithelium (seen in the external ear) through all other types down to endothelium of blood vessels. Again, supporting tissues are important. Cartilage, minor glands, a muscularis mucosae, and the number and arrangements of definite muscle coats are all looked for. Elastica has a prominent role in the construction of blood vessels.

The eye is included here because of its configuration. Actually, it is a highly specialized part with unique characteristics both in its entirety and in all areas of its substructure.

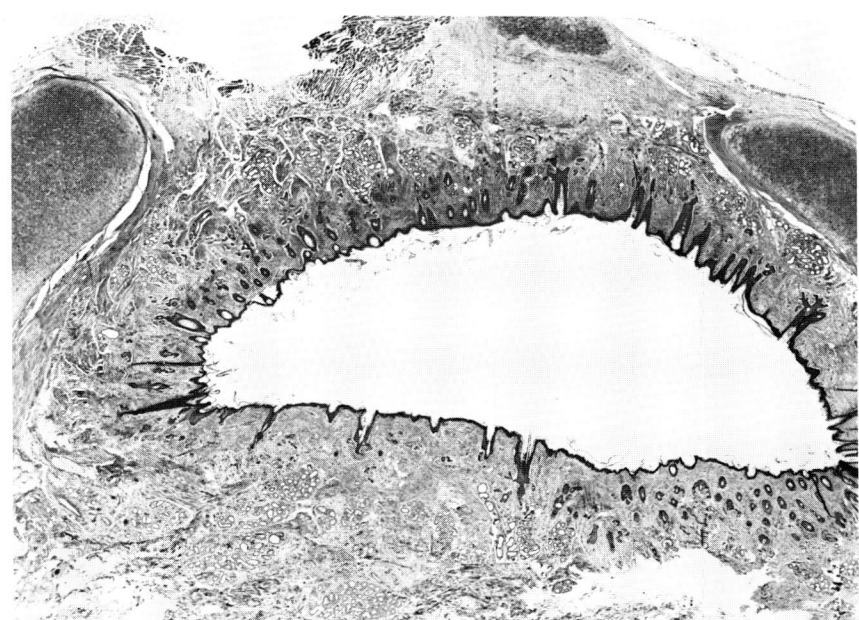

Figure 216. A tube lined by epidermis is found in one place only – the external auditory canal. Cartilage is seen in the wall, although close to the tympanic membrane, bone may be present. *External auditory canal* (× 8)

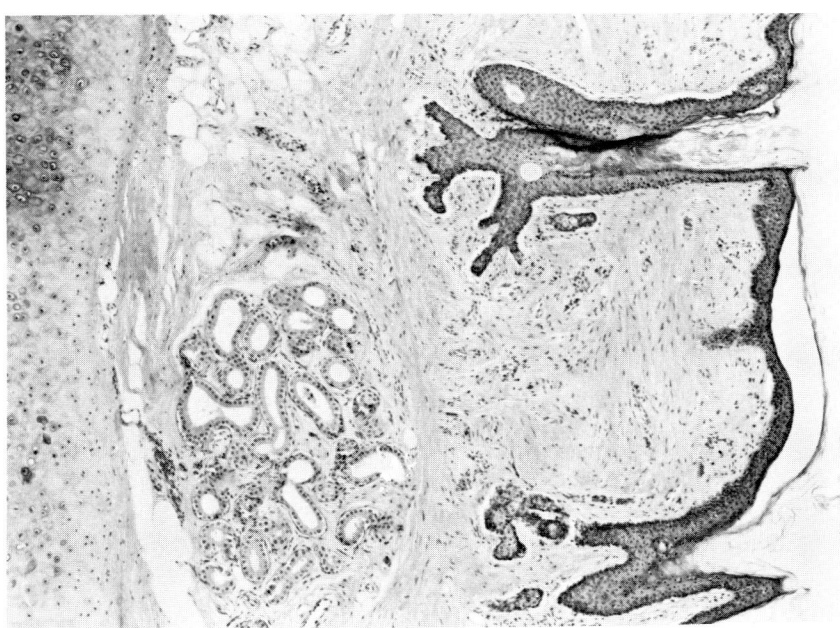

Figure 217. At higher magnification the epidermis gives rise to hair follicles projecting downwards. In the left field is elastic cartilage and immediately next is a collection of apocrine glands, which contribute to the formation of wax and are therefore termed ceruminous. *External auditory canal* (× 50)

ANNULATES

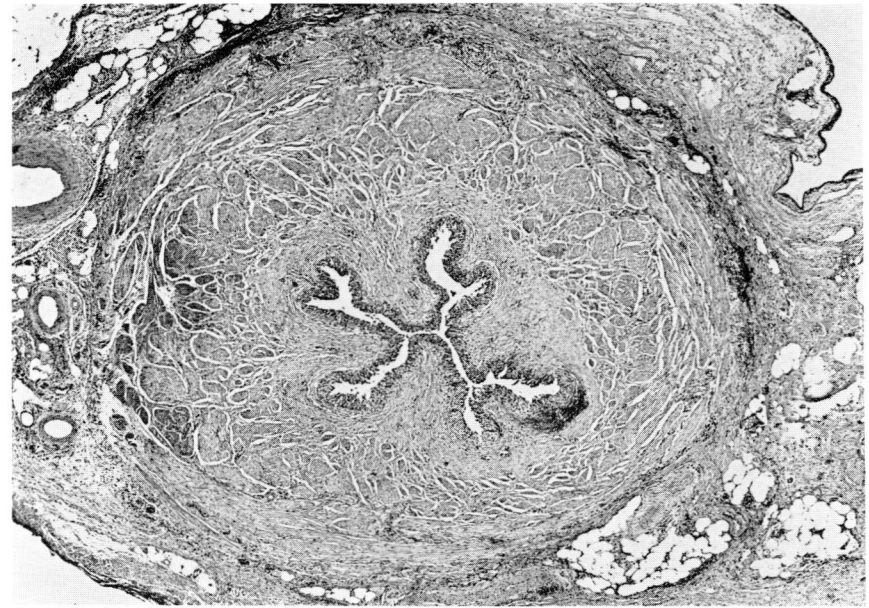

Figure 218. There is only one muscular tube lined by transitional epithelium, arranged (in the contracted state) on broad processes to form a stellate lumen. This is the *ureter* (×22)

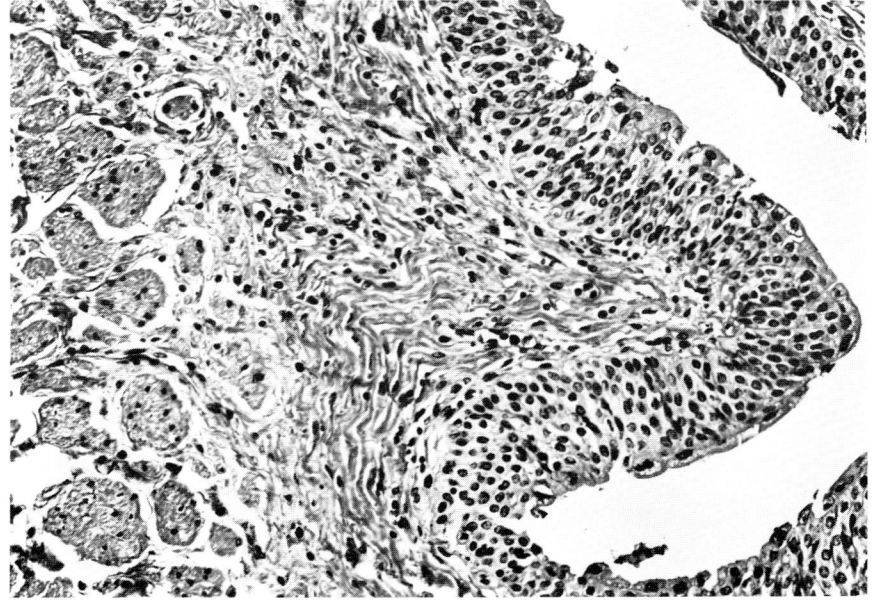

Figure 219. At higher power the stratified polygonal (transitional) epithelium is seen (without keratin, prickle cell, or mucin formation). Within the left field are parts of the inner layer of muscle. In the lower third of the ureter there may be three coats, an inner and outer longitudinal and a middle circular layer. *Infant ureter* (×190)

ANNULATES

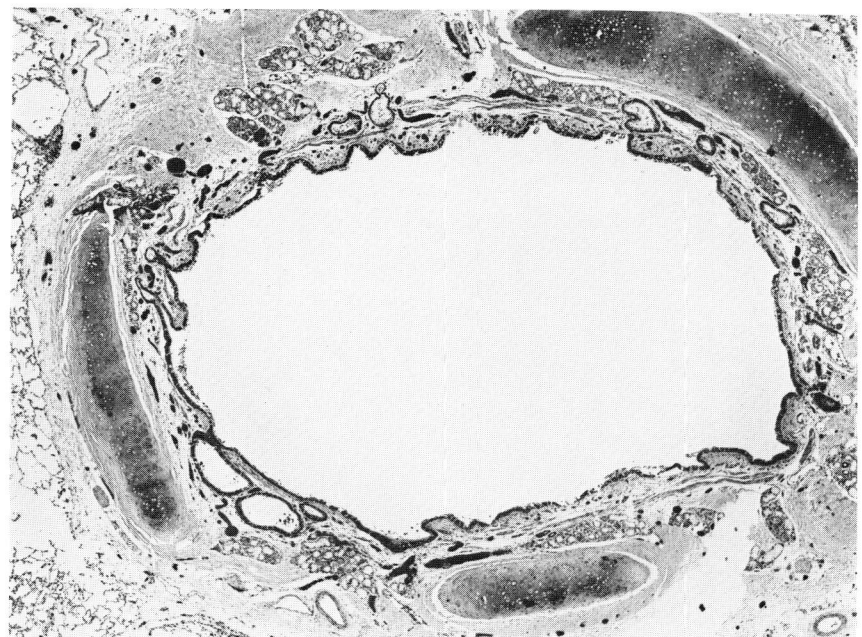

Figure 220. A tube lined by pseudostratified ciliated epithelium and having minor salivary glands and cartilage in the wall is a bronchus. Strands of muscle (not a complete coat and thus not a true muscularis mucosae) may be seen running circumferentially beneath the mucosa. *Bronchus* (×16)

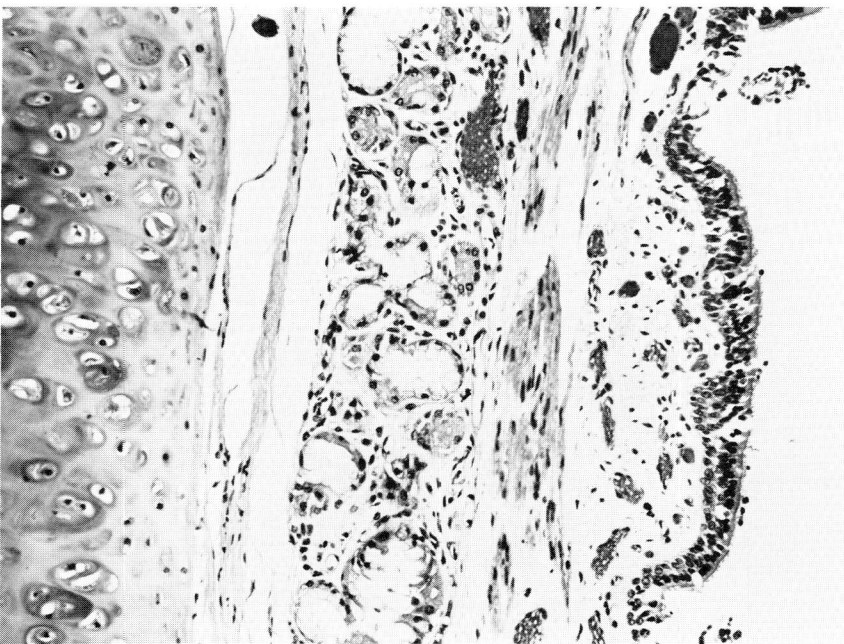

Figure 221. The different layers are more clearly seen here. The fine hairlike processes on the right surface are cilia; muscle bundles run vertically across the field just to the right of the minor salivary glands, which show both serous (dark cytoplasm) and mucous (clear cytoplasm) cells. Hyaline cartilage is seen at the left margin. *Bronchus* (×120)

ANNULATES

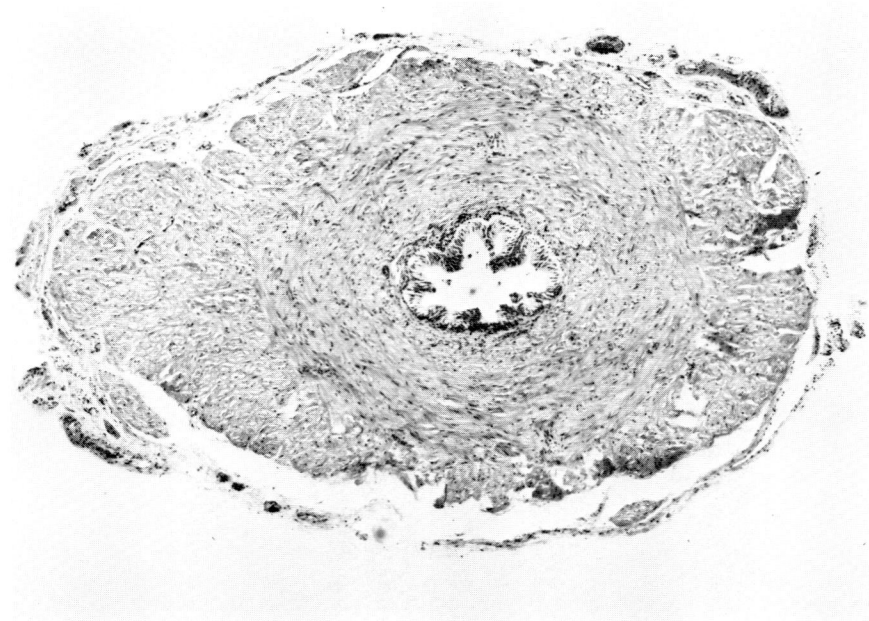

Figure 222. A thick muscular tube with three coats (outer and inner longitudinal and a middle circular layer) is either the lower ureter or vas deferens. There is a relatively narrow lumen, and the lining is a stratified columnar epithelium on broad folds, identifying the *ductus deferens*. (×12)

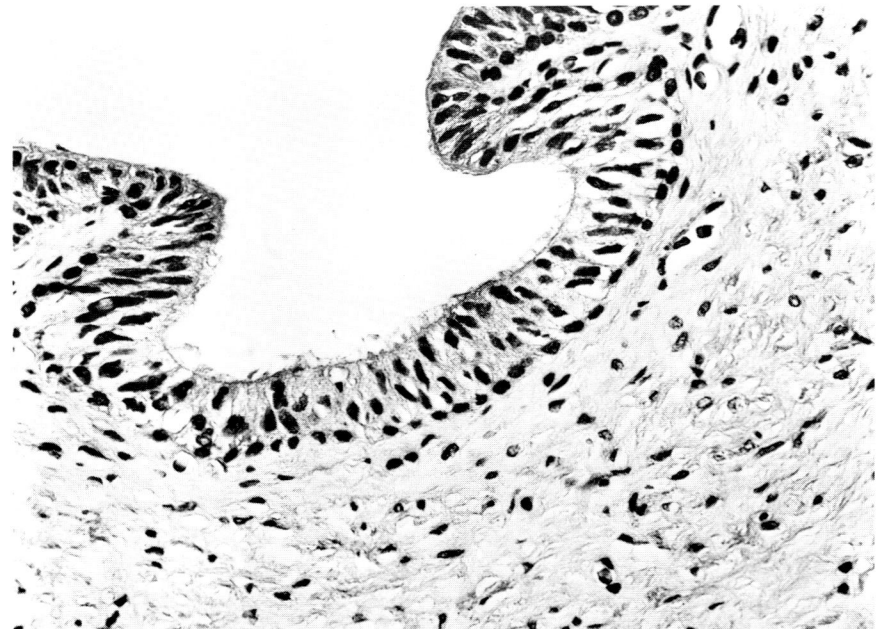

Figure 223. At higher power the stratified columnar epithelium shows long surface processes (stereocilia). Within several nuclei (e.g. at nine o'clock) are oval inclusions seen normally and of uncertain significance. *Ductus deferens* (×320)

ANNULATES

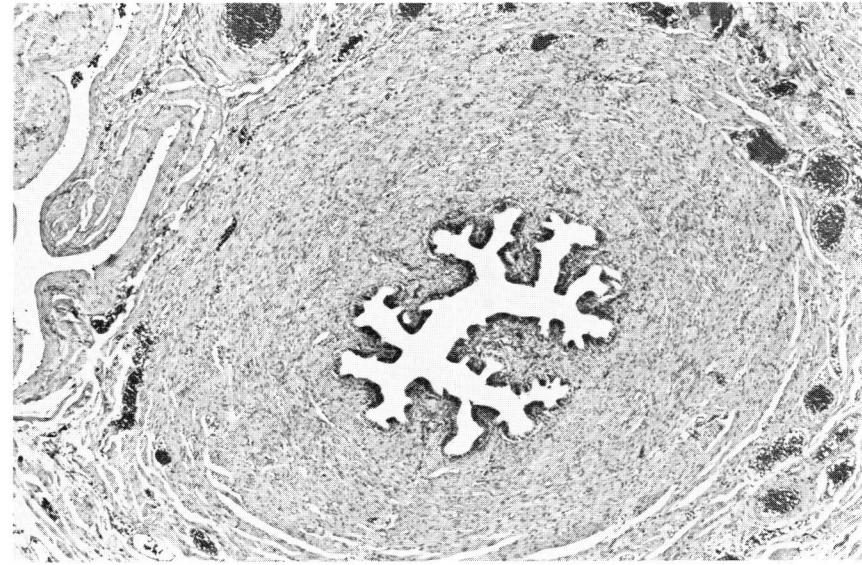

Figure 224. A muscular tube with intraluminal projections covered by a single columnar epithelium is the fallopian tube. The lumen is narrow in this particular section, and the muscle extending into the mucosal folds shows little evidence of lamination. An external serosal surface may sometimes be included. *Oviduct, isthmus* (× 30)

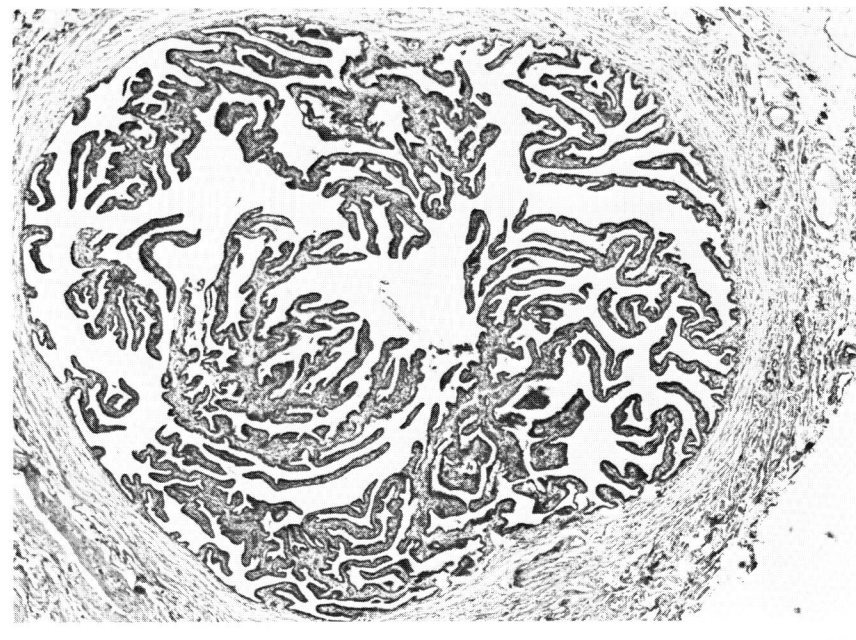

Figure 225. The arrangement and height of folds in the fallopian tube varies along its length. Here the lumen is wide, and the mucosal folds are long and thin, identifying the ampullary end. *Oviduct* (× 30)

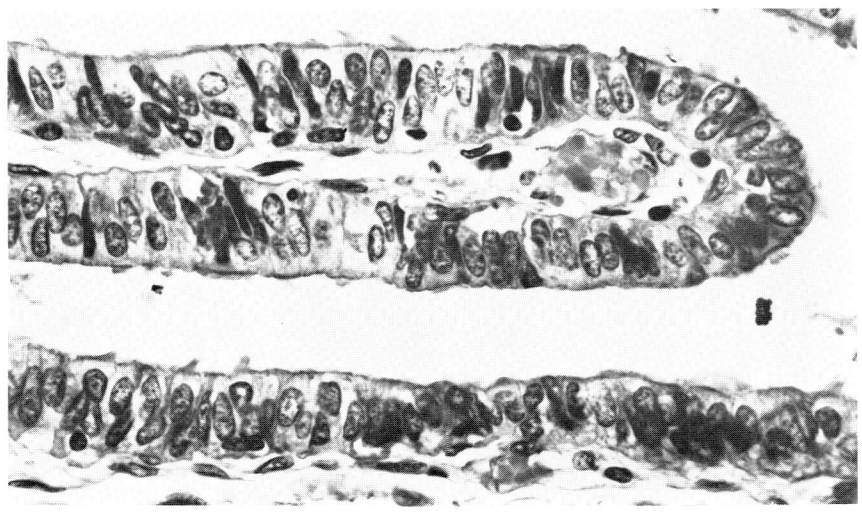

Figure 226. The epithelium is a single row of cells, some of which are ciliated. Those with dark narrow nuclei have been described as peg cells. They are variants of the nonciliated mucous cells. *Oviduct* (× 480)

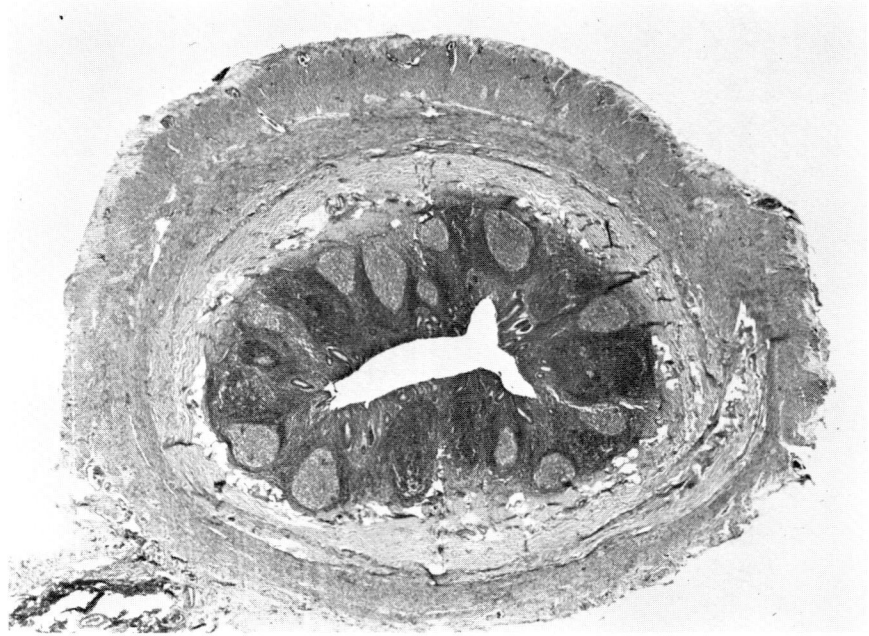

Figure 227. A laminated muscular tube with a simple columnar epithelium, having outward evaginations rather than inward projections, is the appendix. Lymphoid masses are prominent around the lumen. In this figure part of the inner circular muscle coat is seen above. Serosa may cover part of the surface. *Appendix* (× 14)

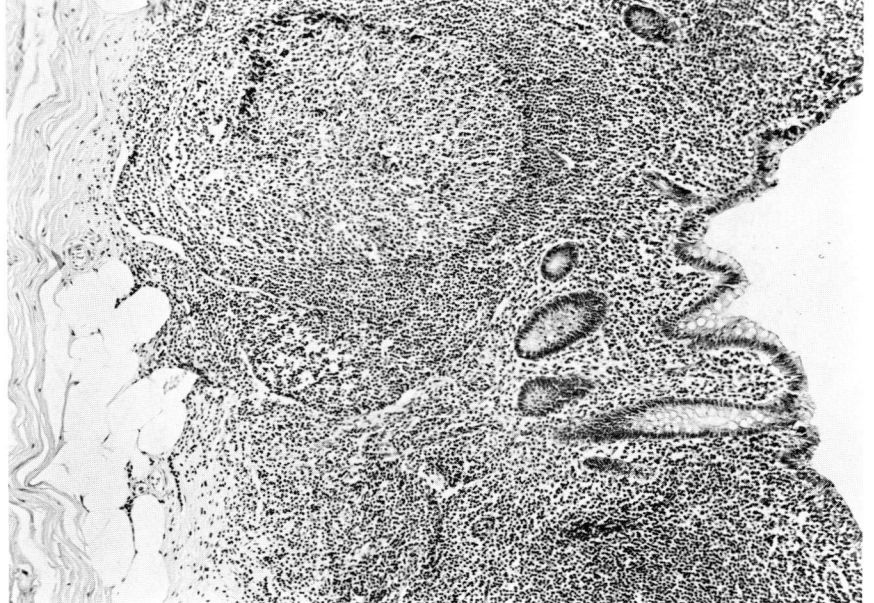

Figure 228. At higher power the epithelium is a simple columnar type with goblet cells (most easily recognized by the clear cytoplasm). The epithelium forms intramural crypts, which are surrounded by lymphocytes, in both diffuse and nodular aggregates. A germinal center is seen in the upper left. The muscularis mucosae is interrupted by the lymphoid tissue to the extent that it is not visible. Fat is seen in the lower left. *Appendix* (× 80)

ANNULATES

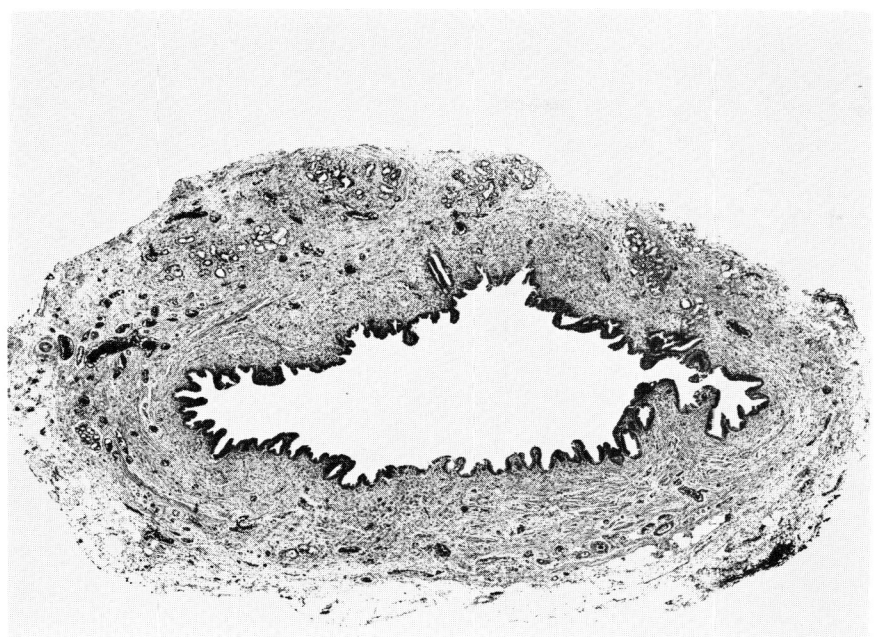

Figure 229. In this tube, the wall is relatively thin, and the lumen relatively large. The lining shows irregular, short intraluminal projections; the wall has very little muscle but is chiefly fibrous tissue with scattered glandular aggregates, seen as small spaces chiefly in the upper part of the circumference. *Common bile duct* (×22)

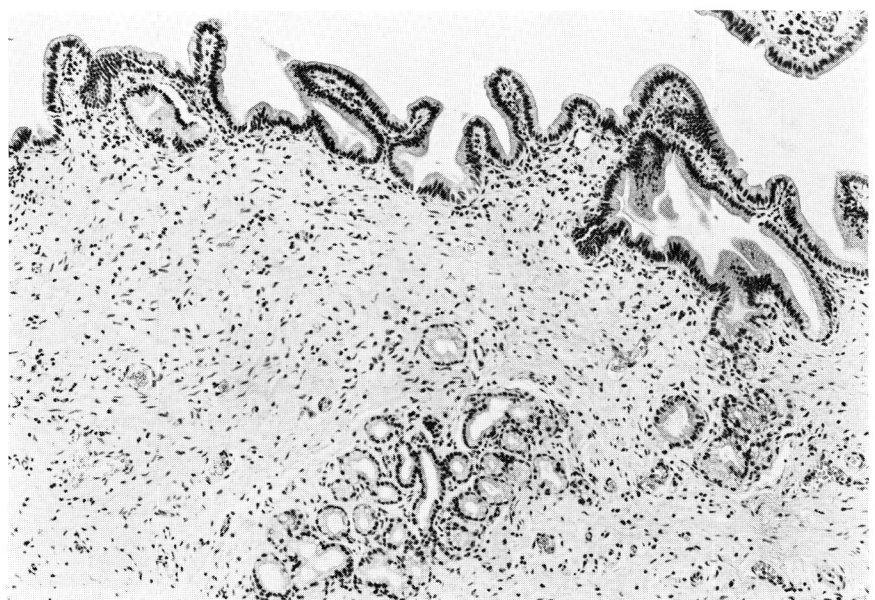

Figure 230. The lining cells are a single layer of tall columnar cells with clear cytoplasm. There is no muscularis mucosae; the wall is fibrous and contains small glandular collections, again with clear cells. *Common bile duct* (×100)

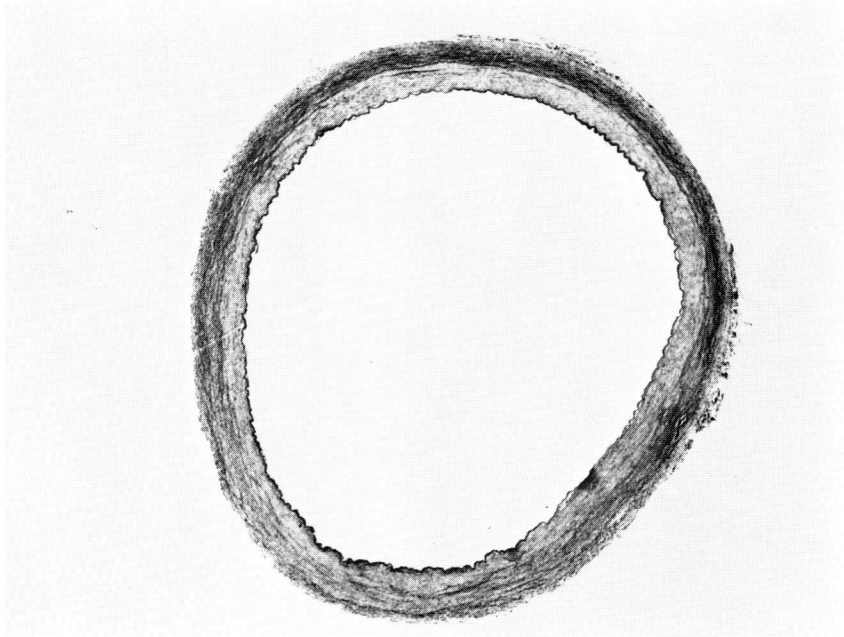

Figure 231. This tube has a relatively thin wall and very large lumen. The inner surface is finely crenated by a dark band, which is the internal elastic lamina. The inner pale-staining part of the wall is predominantly muscular, while the outer dark zone has a large component of elastic fibers. This specimen comes from the common carotid artery close to the aorta, from a twenty-one-year-old male. *Carotid*, hybrid artery — partly muscular, partly elastic ($\times 9.5$)

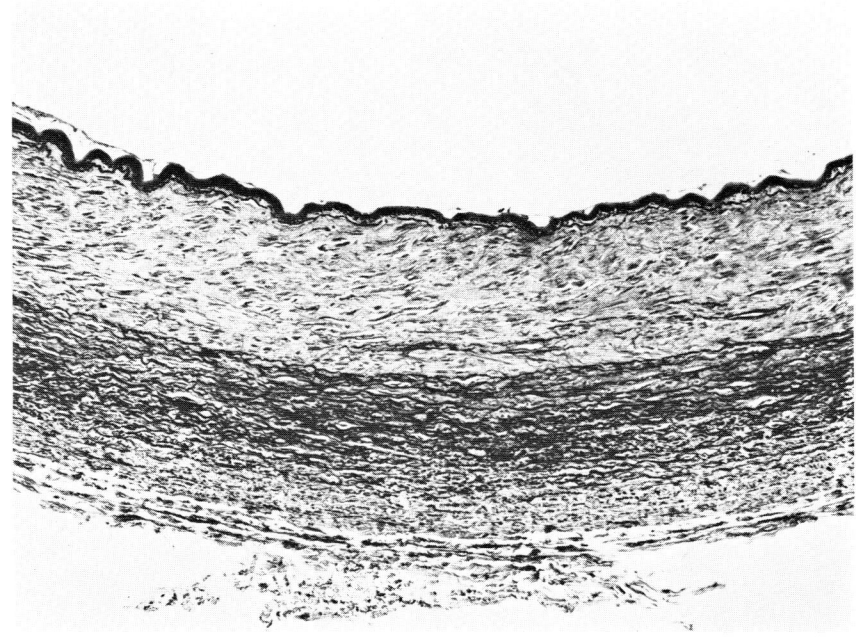

Figure 232. At higher power the internal elastica is thick, but the endothelium is not visible. Parts of the loose adventitia are seen below. These two preparations were stained with Movat. (The only artery without an internal elastica is the umbilical artery, where its occurrence is quite variable.) *Carotid* ($\times 65$)

ANNULATES

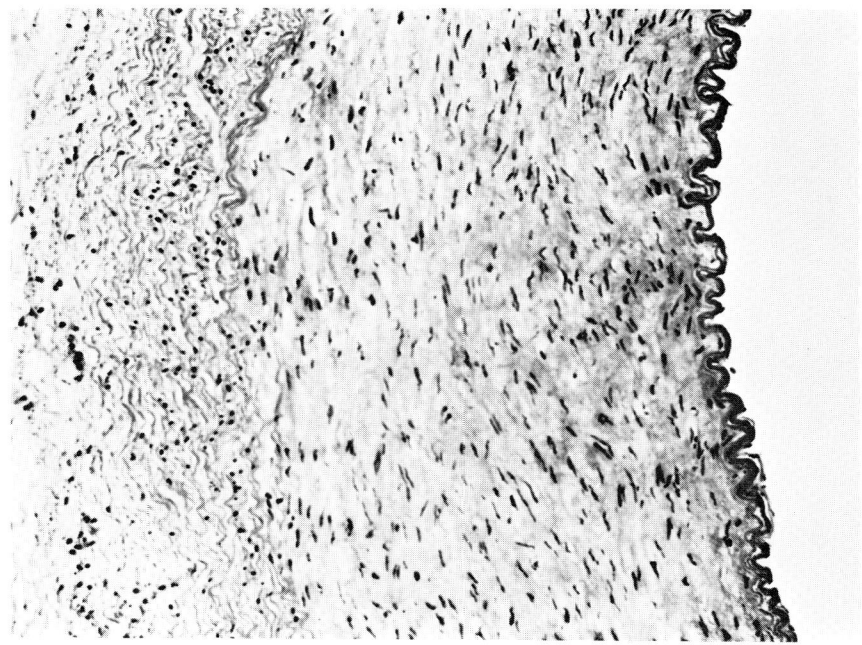

Figure 233. This is again an artery, as indicated by the thick internal elastic lamina running down the right margin. The left of the field shows undulating fibers of collagen and elastica from the connective tissue of the adventitia. The tissue between adventitia and the internal elastica lamina is dominated by nonstriated muscle. *Muscular artery* (× 80)

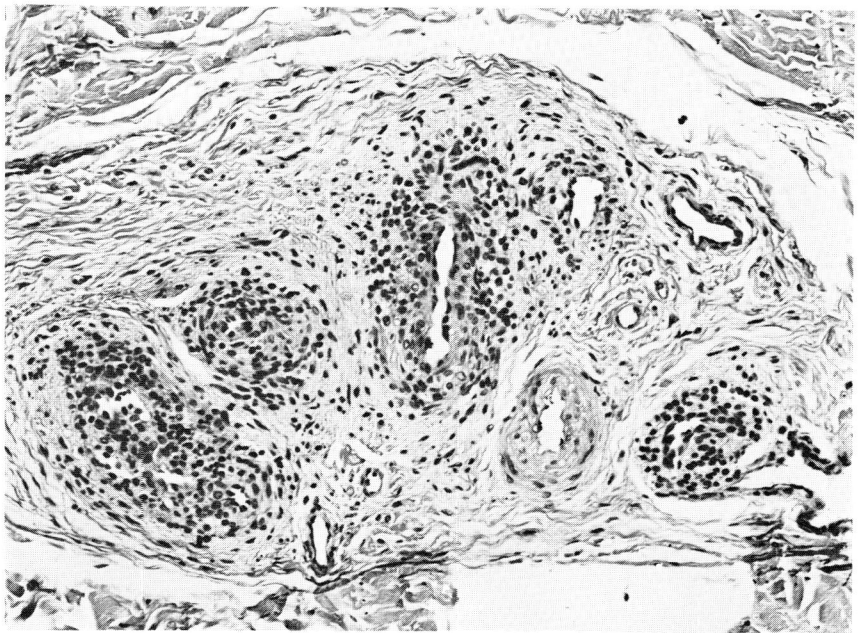

Figure 234. This figure shows a small artery (below and to the right of center) with four more cellular structures, which represent vessels cut several times because of tortuosity. These are modified arteries with no internal elastica and with numerous myo-epithelial cells in the wall. They are seen fraying off into the surrounding connective tissue. This is a glomus, a shunt mechanism between artery and vein, allowing for control of circulation. Glomera are found under the nails, in the pulp of the fingers and toes, in the external ear, and in other places. One is named: — the glomus coccygeum, which lies in front of the tip of the coccyx. *Glomus, fingertip* (× 150)

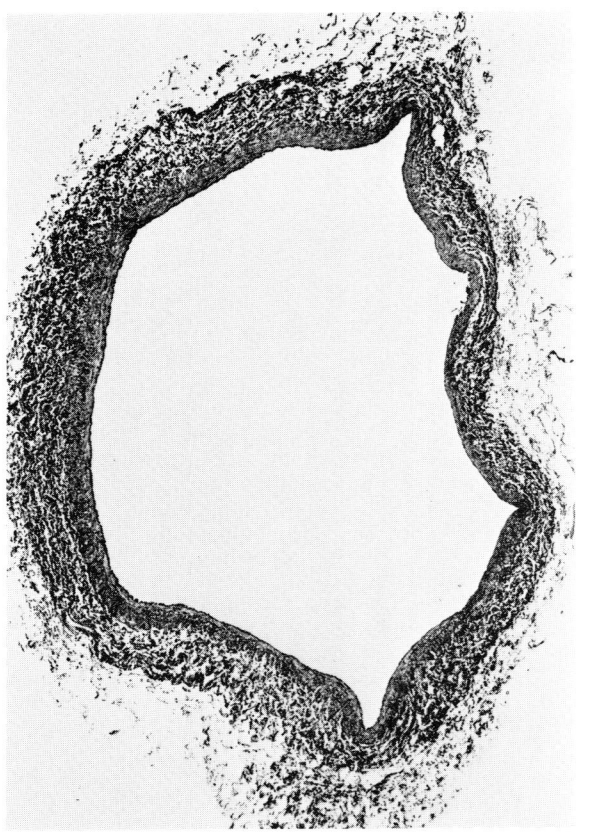
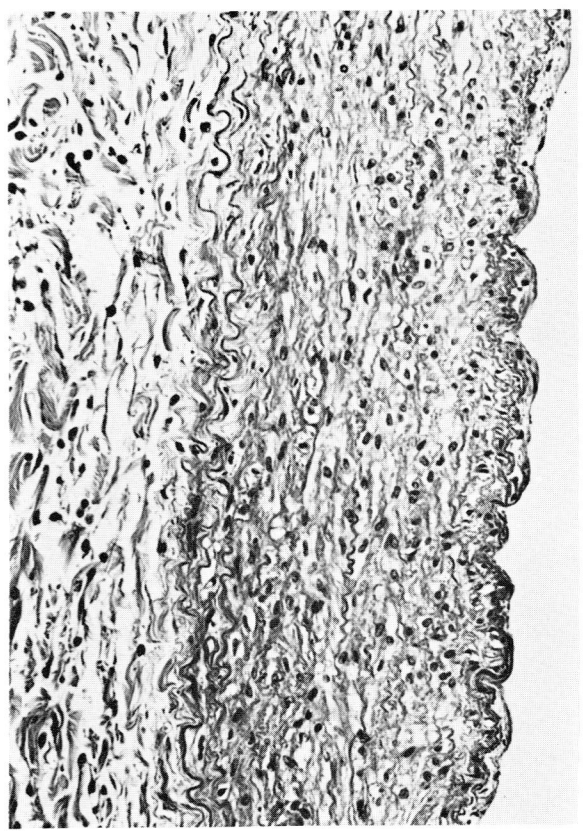

Figure 235. Vessels whose muscle coats are thin relative to their total diameter and that lack a distinctive internal elastica are veins. The muscular elements have a looser arrangement than those of an artery, with occasional irregular elastic fibers, which become more prominent towards the adventitia. Veins from the legs may closely resemble arteries; the superior vena cava may include cardiac muscle, and splenic veins may have irregular nonstriated muscle thickenings in their walls. *Vein*, fifteen-year-old girl, Movat stain (× 12.5)

Figure 236. *Vein* (× 120)

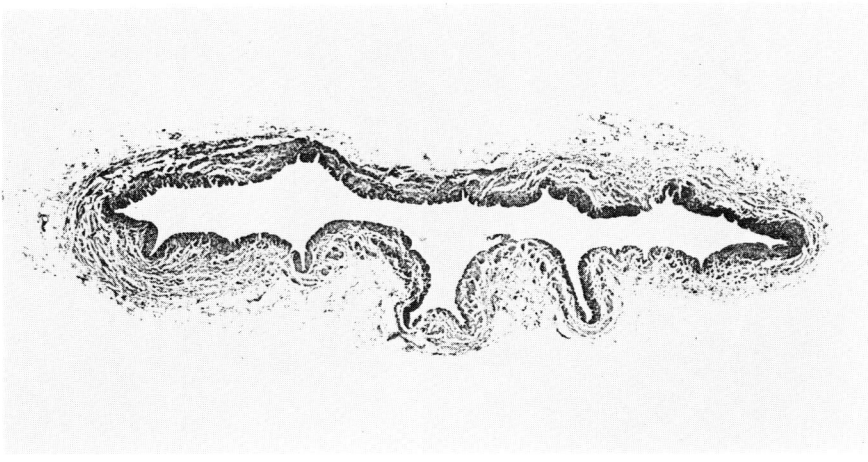

Figure 237. The thoracic duct is not commonly encountered in sections and can be confidently identified only by macroscopic dissection, as at its termination at the junction of the left subclavian and left internal jugular vein. The wall is lined by endothelium, lying on muscle. The general features are those seen in a vein, but amounts of muscle may be quite irregular, and the content of the duct is lymph rather than blood. *Thoracic duct* (× 27)

ANNULATES

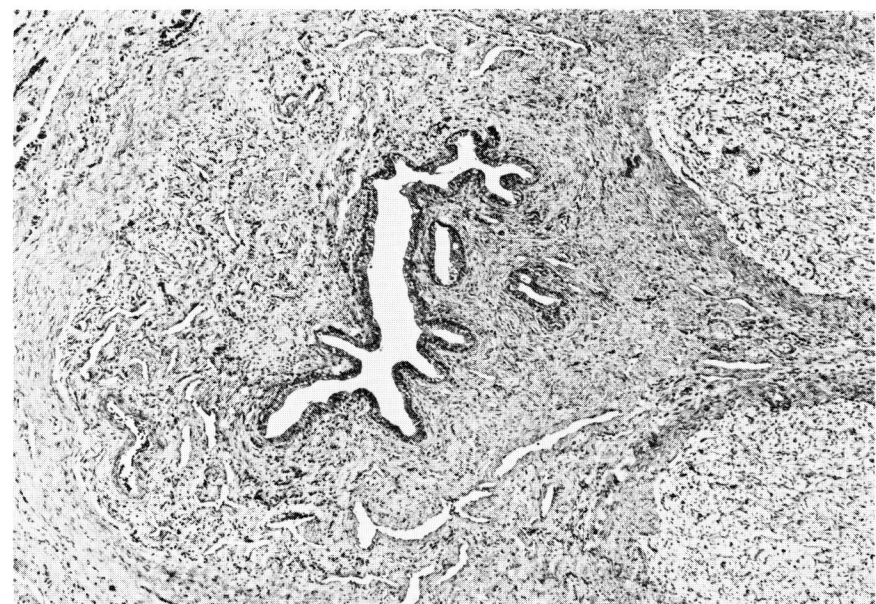

Figure 238. This tube has a lining of stratified columnar epithelium but has no organized muscular wall. Rather, it is surrounded by erectile tissue, recognized as such because of the anastomosing slitlike spaces and the intervening nonstriated muscle. Two other pale masses of similar nature on the right margin are the corpora cavernosa, from the dorsal aspect of the penis. This combination identifies the urethra. The urethral epithelium varies in type from transitional to stratified columnar to stratified squamous in passing from its proximal end to the external meatus. Small glands arising from the urethra are Littre's glands. *Infant penis, corpus spongiosum and urethra.* (× 60)

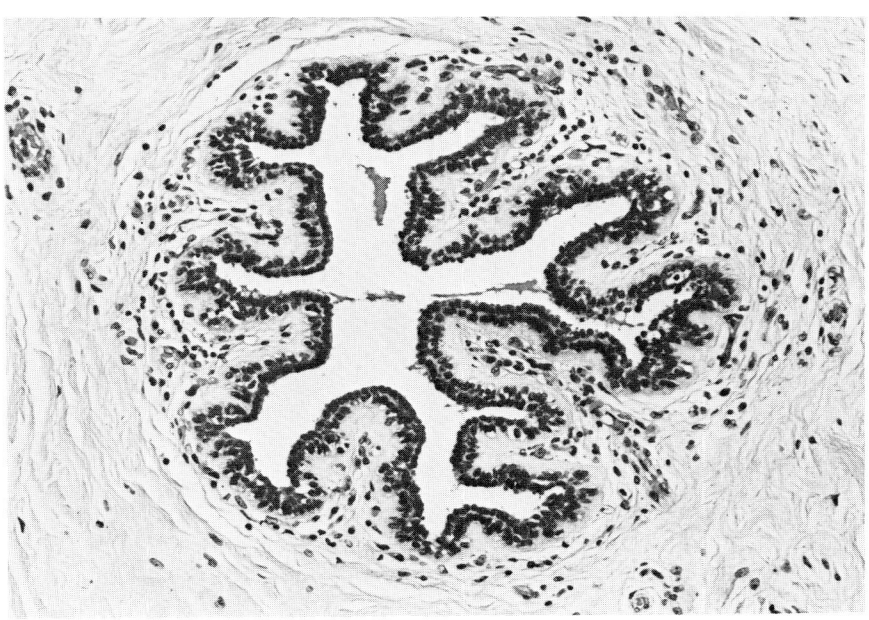

Figure 239. A duct with convoluted outline and a distinct double layer of lining epithelium, including a peripheral myoepithelium, again without organized muscular wall but embedded in rather loose fibrous tissue, is found in the breast. *Duct, mammary gland* (× 150)

Annulates of microscopic dimensions are found within certain parts, by which the nature of the duct itself is identified.

ANNULATES — EYE

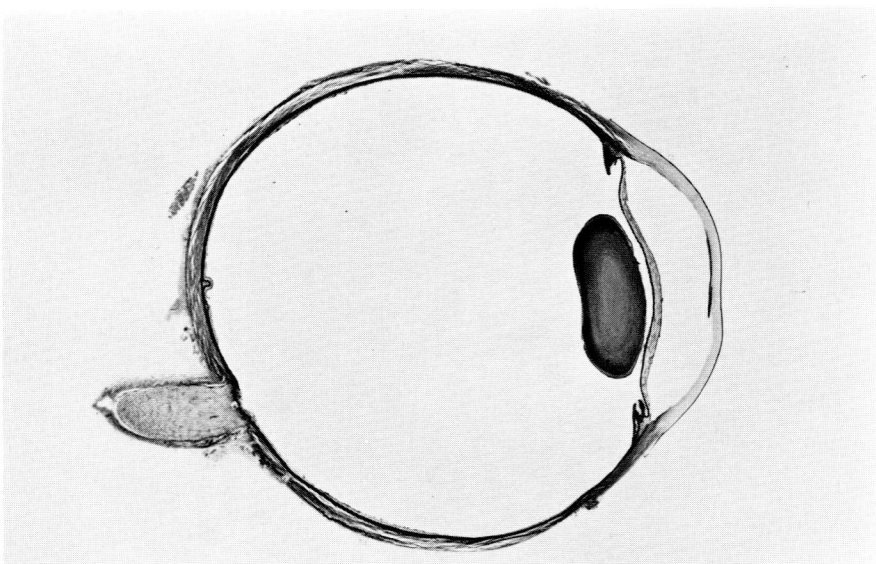

Figure 240. This is a horizontal section, for purposes of orientation. The short side (from optic nerve to cornea) is the nasal side. The cornea and anterior chamber are on the right; the dark disc is the lens. Projecting from the wall above and below the lens are the ciliary bodies, whose long membranous extensions form the iris diaphragm. (Suspensory ligaments are not visible but run from the ciliary processes to the lens.) The space between the ciliary processes and the iris is the posterior chamber; the space in front of the iris and lens is the anterior chamber. Behind the lens is the vitreous cavity with the optic nerve projecting to the left. The wall of the globe shows the fibrous sclera externally. The dark line is the pigment layer of the retina, within which some of the retinal epithelium can be vaguely made out. *Eye from child* (× 4.2)

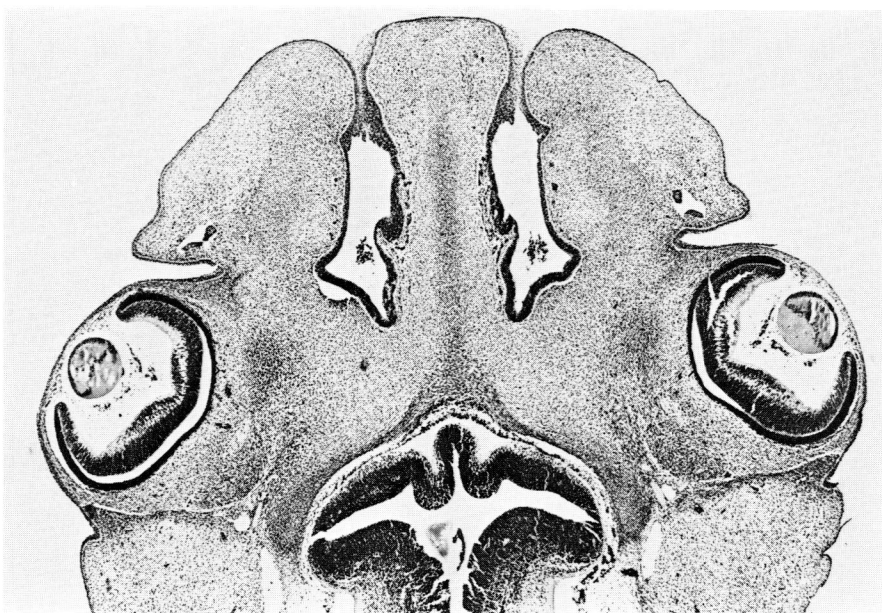

Figure 241. This is a horizontal section through the developing fetal head, with nose above and central nervous system below. The cuplike optic vesicles on each side are most conspicuous because of the heavy pigmentation in the external layer. Within the concavity is myxoid vascularized tissue, which will subsequently be replaced by vitreous. The globular body is the lens, with the epithelium over its anterior half turning inwards to form a nuclear line across the equator. The epithelium that will form the cornea is seen as a continuation from the skin. *Fetal eye development* (× 26.5)

ANNULATES

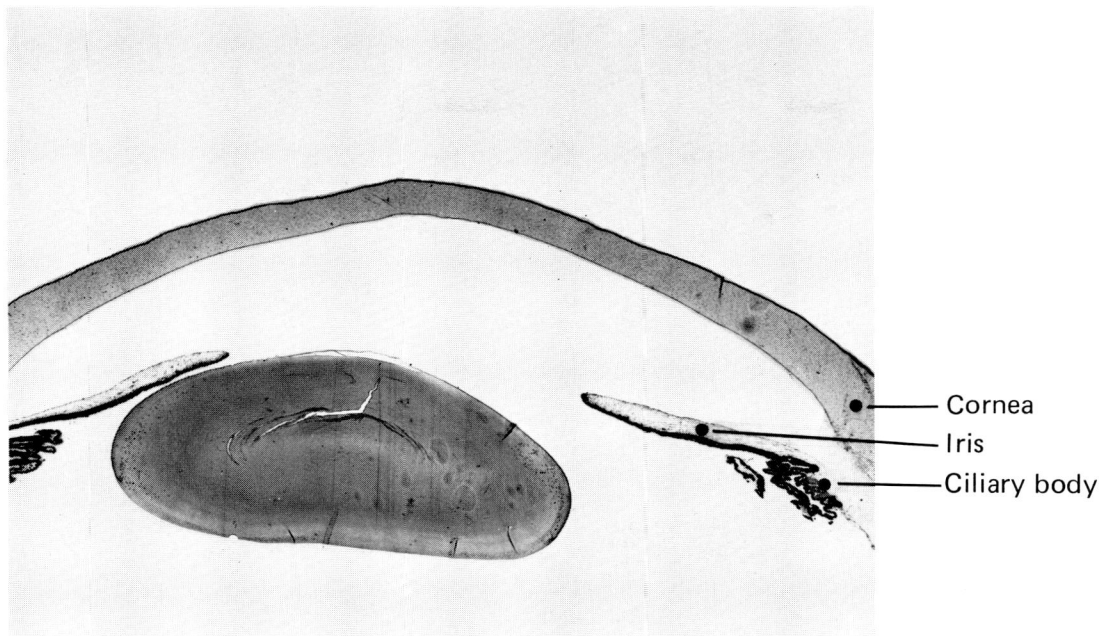

Figure 242. The anterior and posterior chambers are shown again here. The arching band of tissue across the upper part is the cornea with a dark line or corneal epithelium external to the substantia propria and a second thin dark line of endothelium beneath it. Immediately beneath the surface epithelium is an amorphous membrane (Bowman), while the comparable membrane related to the endothelium is Descemet's membrane. The lens epithelium is seen as a thin dark line in front and on both sides the nuclei fray off into the lens substance. On the posterior surface of the iris is a dark line of pigmented epithelium, which continues over the ciliary processes. *Infant eye* (× 12)

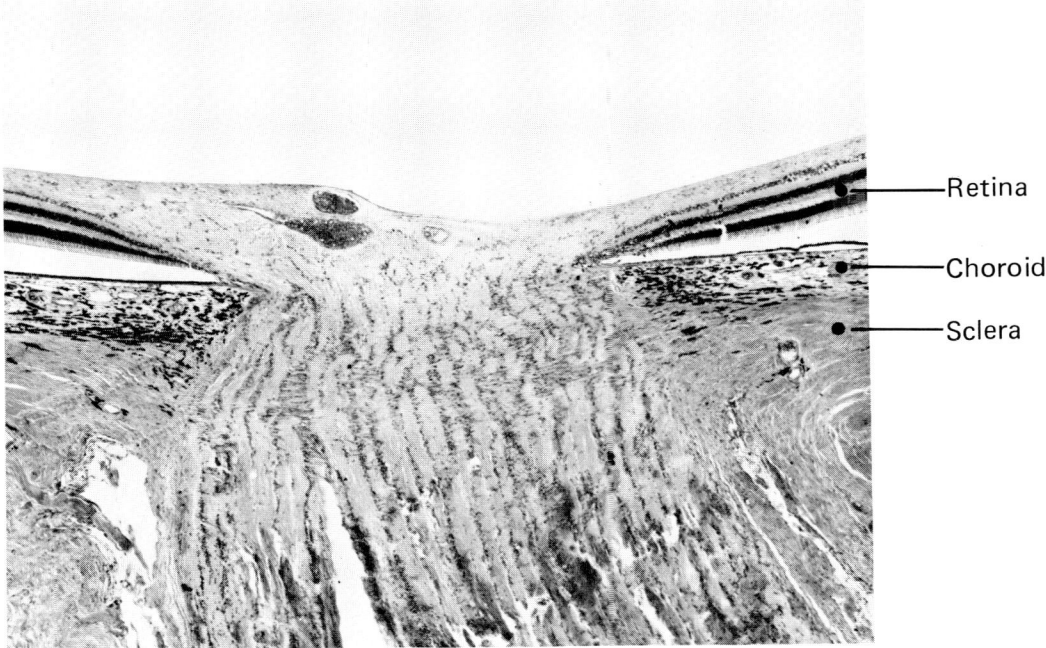

Figure 243. This is the posterior part of the vitreous chamber, where the axonal fibers that arise from the ganglion cells in the retina exit through the choroid and between the collagenous fibers of the lamina cribrosa sclerae, which pass from one side of the sclera to the other. The nerve head corresponds to the optic disc; it contains no ganglion cells. *Adult eye, optic disc* (× 36)

ANNULATES

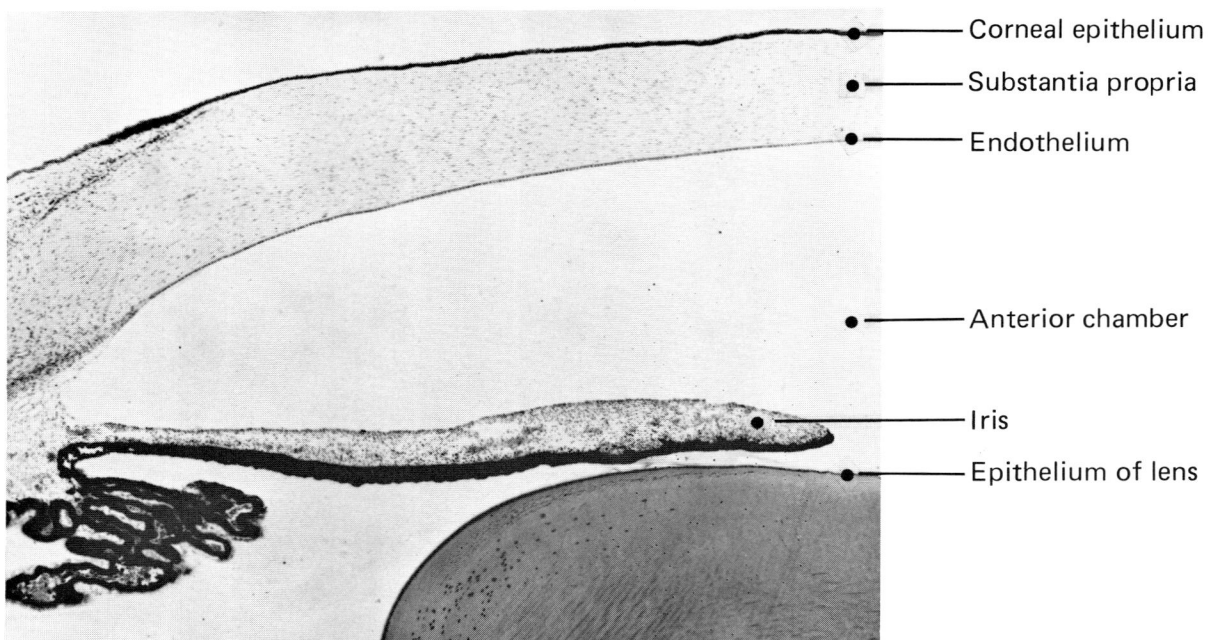

Figure 244. The angle formed between the cornea and the iris as it arises from the ciliary body is the filtration angle. Loose fibrous tissues in the anterior wall of the angle constitute the pectinate ligaments, where aqueous humor filters out to enter Schlemm's canal. *Infant eye* (× 20)

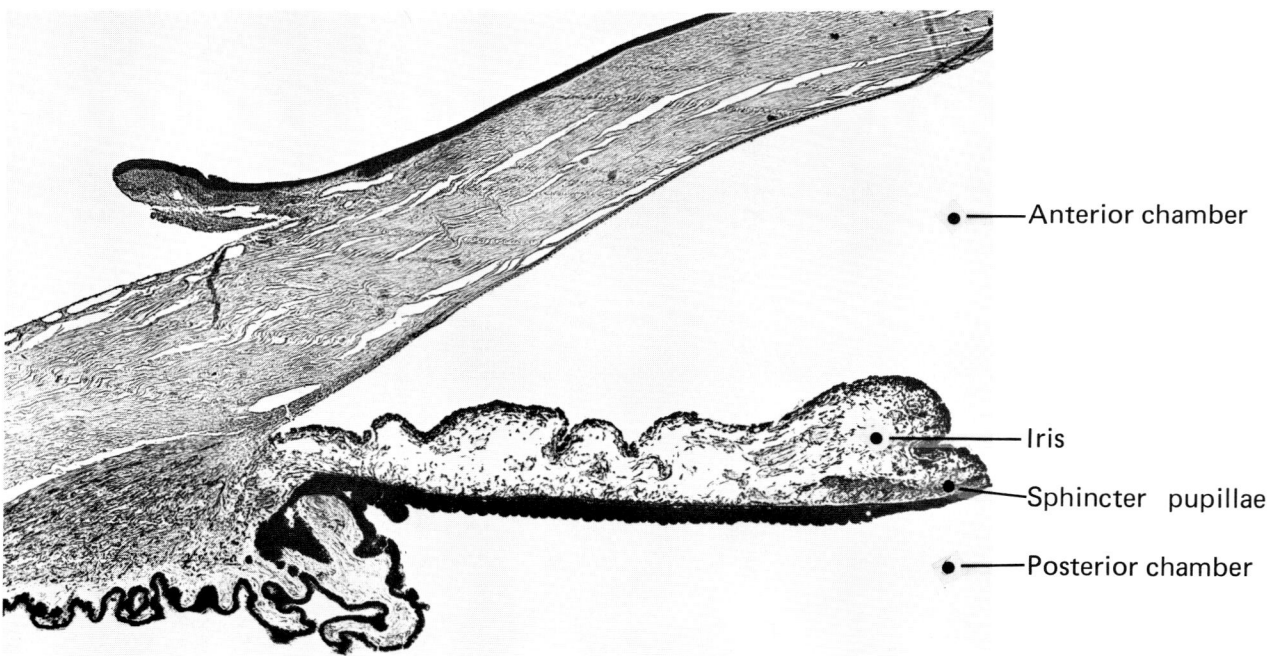

Figure 245. In the left quadrant just above the horizontal undulating line of pigmented cells is a triangular wedge of ciliary muscle. Just above the filtration angle is an oval space, Schlemm's canal. The dark line of fibers at the medial tip of the iris belongs to the sphincter pupillae muscle. *Adult eye* (× 31)

ANNULATES

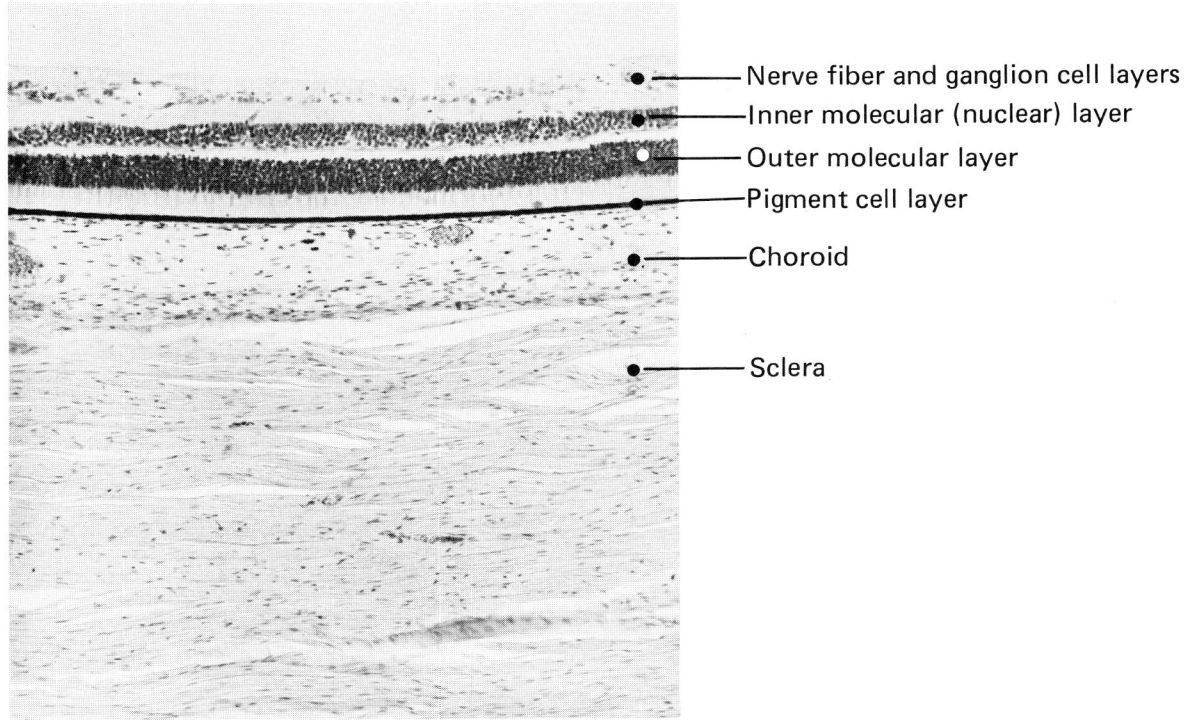

Figure 246. This figure shows the three major coats of the eye, with retina above. Between the ganglion cell layer and the inner molecular layer of the retina is the inner plexiform layer. Between the two molecular (or nuclear) layers of small neurones is the outer plexiform layer, and just above the pigment layer are the rods and cones. The loose connective tissue below this is the choroid, and the dense collagenous bundles belong to the sclera. (The small neurones are bipolar.) *Wall of globe* (× 100)

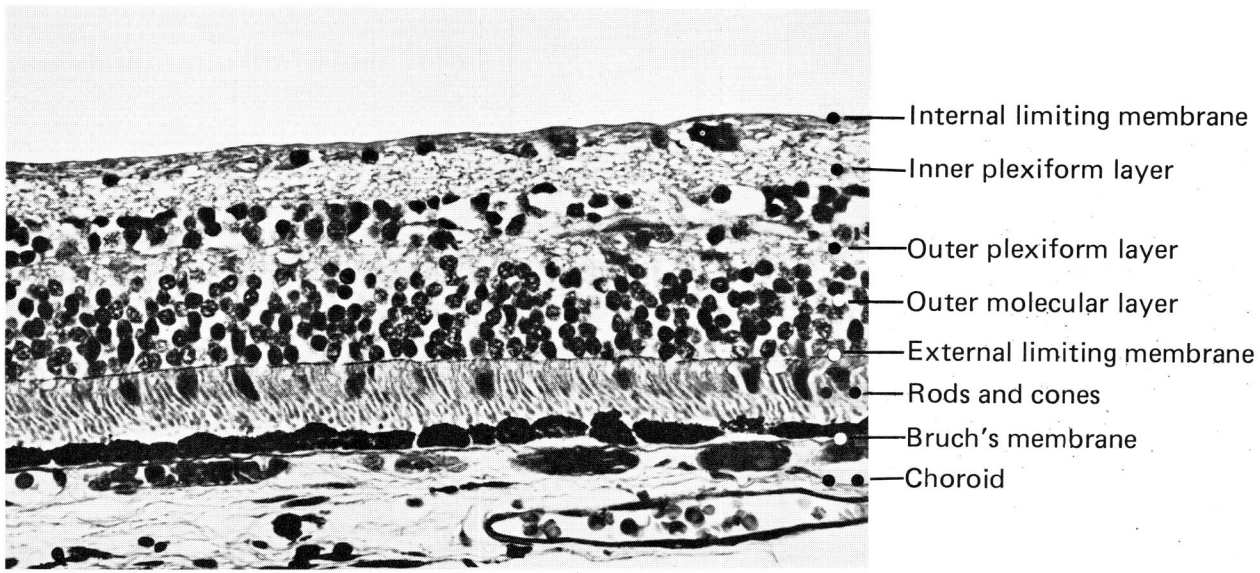

Figure 247. This is specially stained to show the membranes of the retina; at the same time the shape of the cones is much more easily appreciated. The thinner longer lines are the rods. *Retina*, Masson trichrome (× 400)

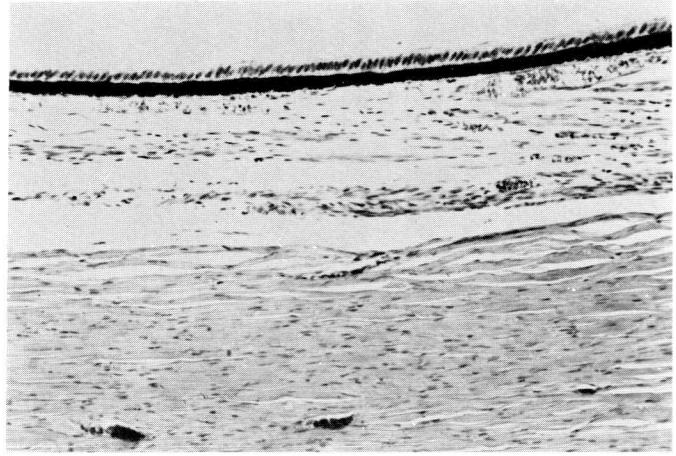

Figure 248. In its extreme anterior part, the retina is reduced to a layer of epithelial cells and of pigment cells. The loose choroid and the dense sclera are seen beneath. *Retina, pars plana* (× 100)

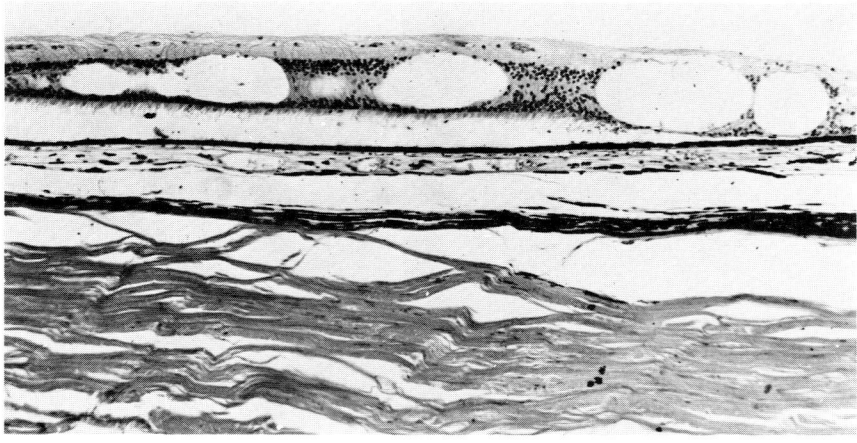

Figure 249. Just posterior to pars plana is an area where ganglion cells are not present, the nuclear layers tend to fuse, and cystoid degeneration is seen, even in relatively young adults. *Retina, ora serrata* (× 80)

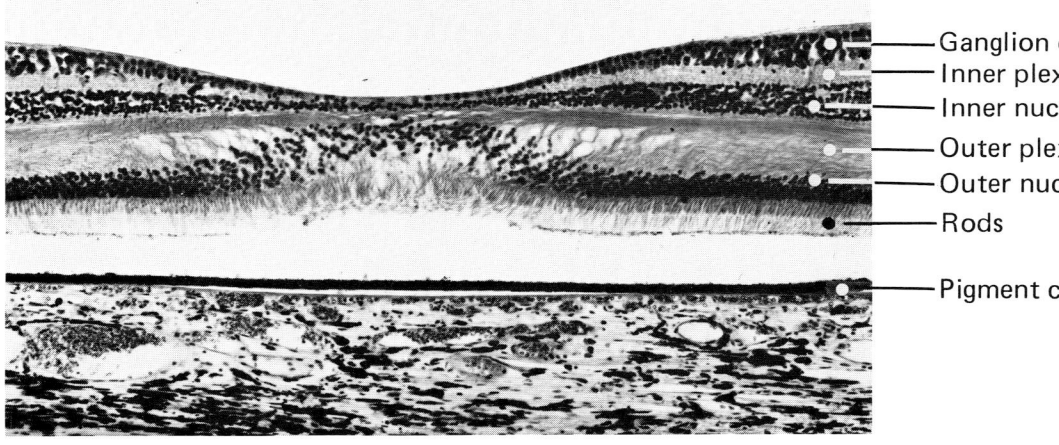

Figure 250. At the fovea or pit, there is a sharp thinning of the retina, with virtual disappearance of the ganglion cells (which, however, form an unusually thick band in the immediate periphery). The inner and outer nuclear layers become thin, and rods disappear (the retina here shows artefactual separation where it usually occurs, between the rods and cones and the pigment cell layer). *Fovea or macula lutea* (× 100)

Multiperforate Sections

In most multicavitary parts, the spaces are reasonably uniform throughout the section, as with thyroid, breast, and so forth. However, sometimes there are unique and different types of subunits. For example, the inner ear is a complex system of tubes and sacs known as the membranous labyrinth lying within the tunnels of the petrous temporal bone. Hearing is mediated by Corti's organ, balance by the otolith organs, and sense of position by the cristae of the semicircular canals, all very different. The ovary, which is multicystic in the reproductive period of life, shows a unique combination of follicles of various sizes, in a matrix of dense fibrous tissue in which there are also hyalinized remnants or corpora albicantia. More than this, distinctive ova may be seen in the subcapsular layer of fibrous tissue. In general, the ovary is a solid structure before puberty and again in the postmenopausal state, but even at birth there may sometimes be numerous small cortical cysts believed to reflect the effects of maternal hormones on the fetus. Other multiperforate sections show more uniform aggregations of tubules, acini, alveoli, sacules, or sinusoids, whose spaces differ in their size, configuration, lining epithelium, content, and supporting stroma.

Taken as a group, a useful first approach to the analysis of multiperforate sections is by the size of the spaces. Some of these are quite large, arbitrarily defined as a space that is at least twice as wide as the height of its lining epithelium. This applies to the inner ear, certain elements in the kidney, the ovary, the male reproductive organs, apocrine sweat glands, thyroid, erectile tissue, and lung. Small spaces, however, predominate in the eccrine sweat glands, lacrimal and salivary glands, breast, pancreas, Brunner's glands, and the accessory sexual glands of Bartholin and Cowper. It is, of course, to be remembered that all exocrine glands have ducts that will appear as larger spaces scattered here and there in what is otherwise a small-space multiperforate section.

In configuration, these spaces may be tubular or spheroidal, again a useful distinction. The former are recognized by slitlike parallel profiles of epithelium, and the latter by circular ringlike contours. However, it is inevitable that some elements in a tubular structure will be cut transversely, so circular profiles will be seen; conversely the round profiles of most exocrine glands may be accompanied by random lengthwise cuts of the duct.

Superimposed on these basic tubular or spheroidal configurations may be irregular expansions, as seen in the rete testis, saccular outpouchings, as in the seminal vesicles, or inward projections, as in the prostate.

Sometimes the content of the space is unique, as with the colloid of the thyroid, the spermatozoa of testicular tubules, the accessory male reproductive organs, and the blood of the sinusoids of erectile tissue.

MULTIPERFORATES WITH LARGE SPACES – EAR

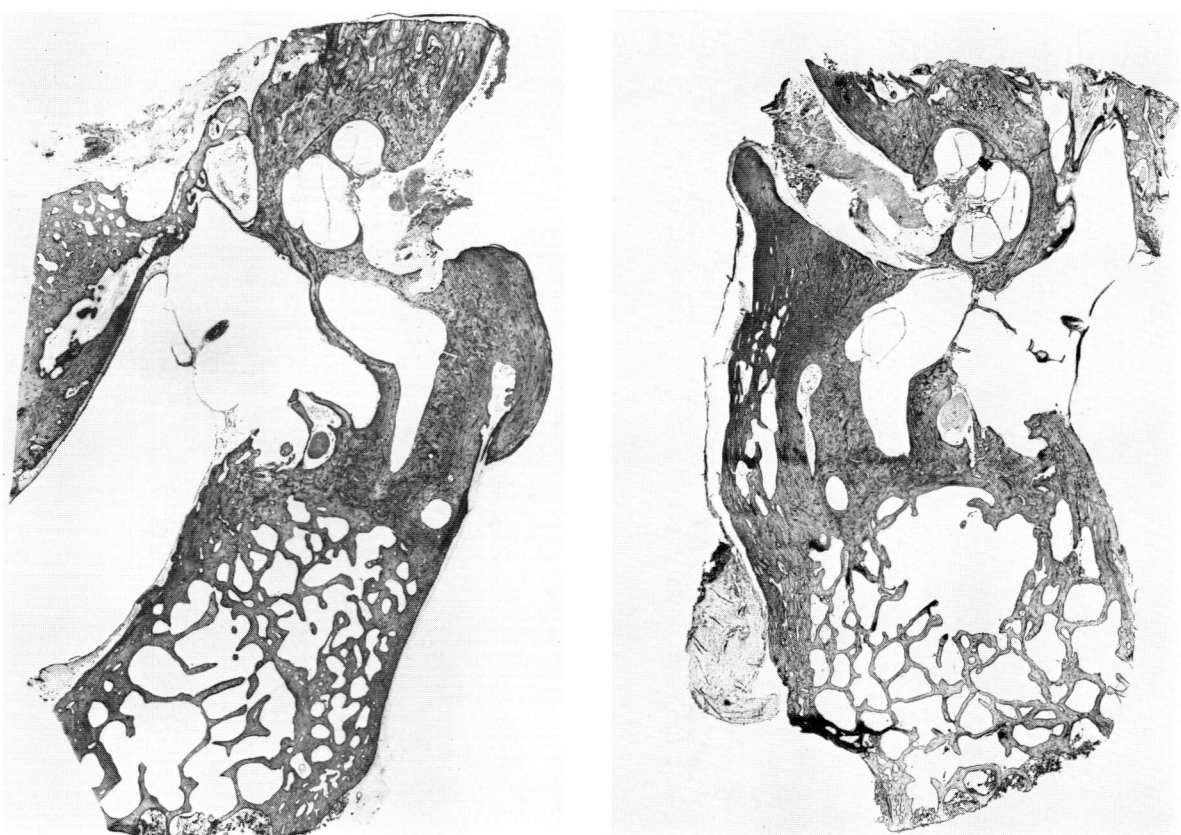

Figure 251. These are horizontal sections at almost the same level and are thus nearly mirror images. The section of the right ear includes most of the stapes and foot plate, and the ductus endolymphaticus lies more deeply than seen in the section of the left ear. The latter, however, shows more of the tensor tympani muscle and more of the stapedius, lying in front of nerve VII. a. *Left ear* (× 3.5) b. *Right ear* (× 4.5)

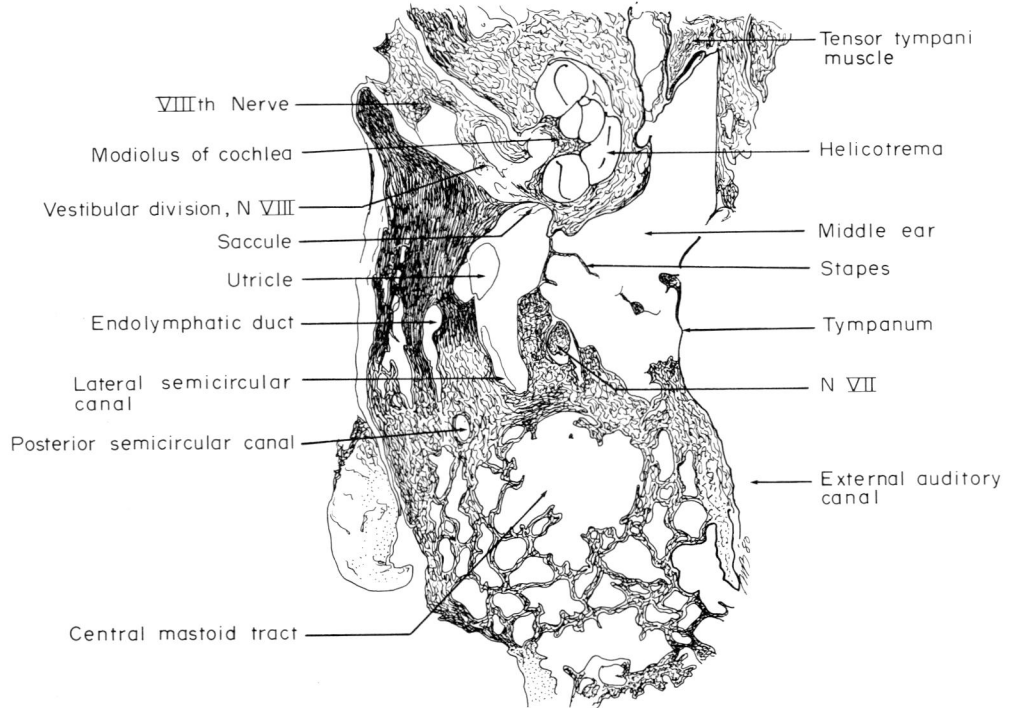

Figure 252. Right ear.

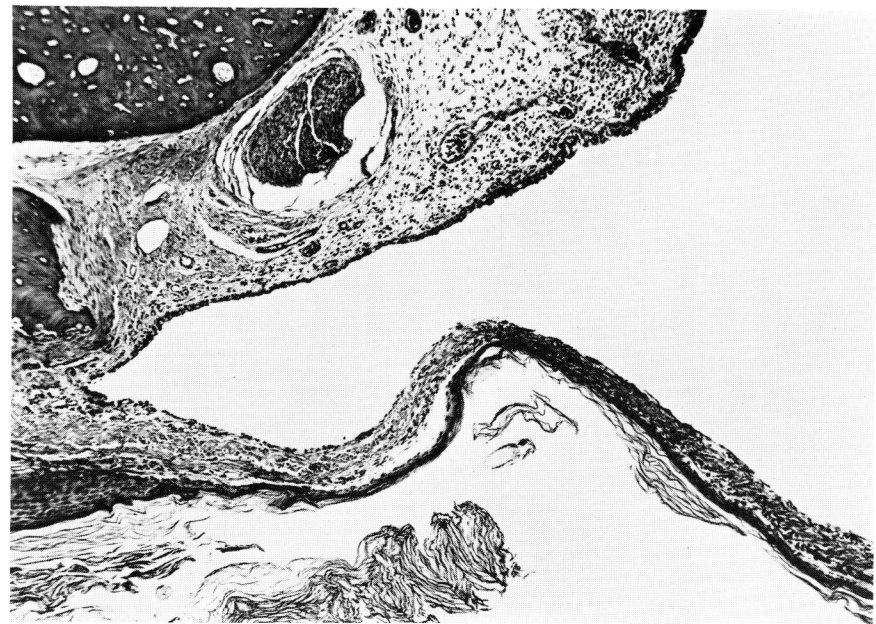

Figure 253. The lower part of this figure shows part of the external auditory canal, which is lined by stratified squamous epithelium with much keratin desquamation (seen as fine lines and flakes). Running across the field is the tympanic membrane, which has a thin fibrous wall and is covered on the deep (middle ear) aspect by a low columnar or cuboidal epithelium, which is a continuation of the partially ciliated epithelium that lines the middle ear above. The large oval structure close to the bone in the left upper quadrant is the seventh nerve. *Middle ear with nerve VII and tympanic membrane, fetus* (×80)

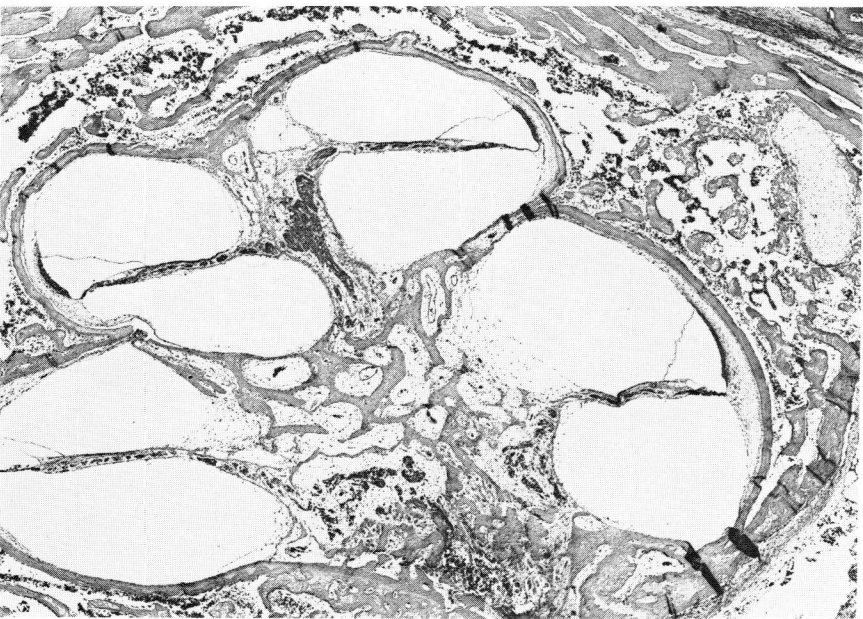

Figure 254. The central bony core seen in the lower center of this figure is the modiolus, with the spiral ganglion. The cochlear spiral is cut across four times, each cut appearing as a reniform space divided across its middle by a thin dark line which includes the osseous spiral centrally and the basilar membrane of the organ of Corti peripherally. In each space the large apical division belongs to the scala vestibuli, and the smaller peripheral wedge-shaped subdivision is the scala media, or cochlear duct. The inferior part is the scala tympani. *Cochlea, fetus* (×22)

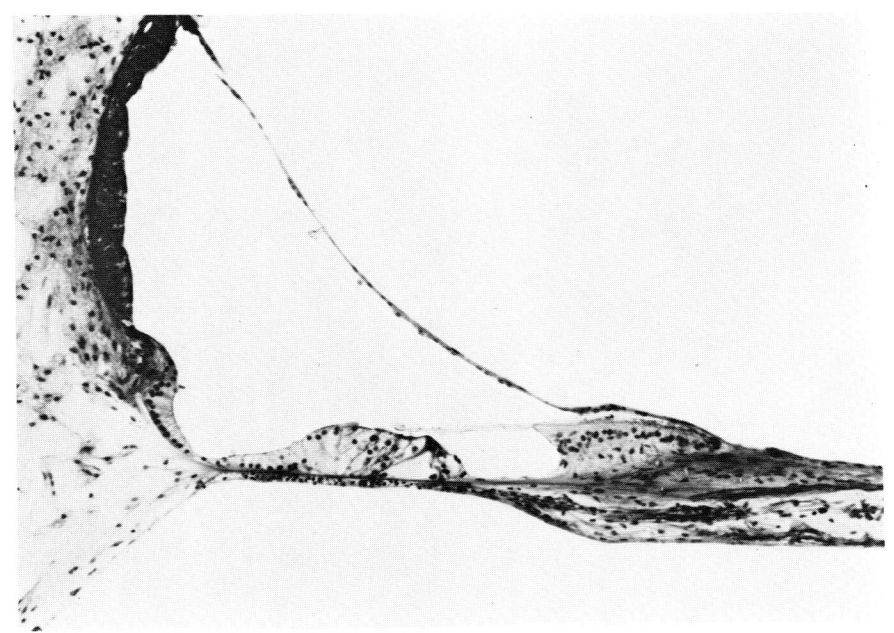

Figure 255. *Cochlear duct* (× 125)

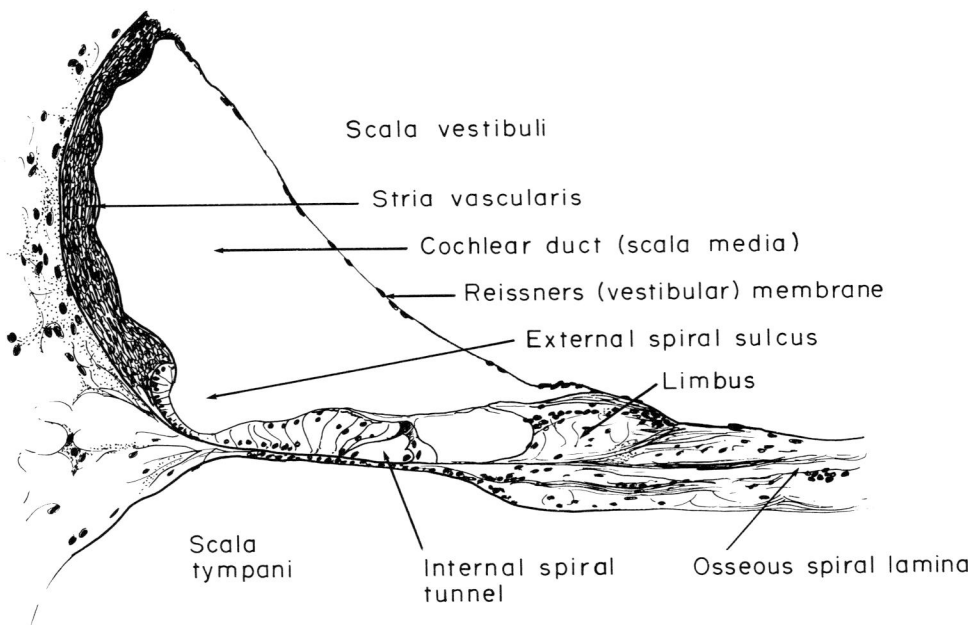

Figure 256. Diagram showing parts of cochlear duct.

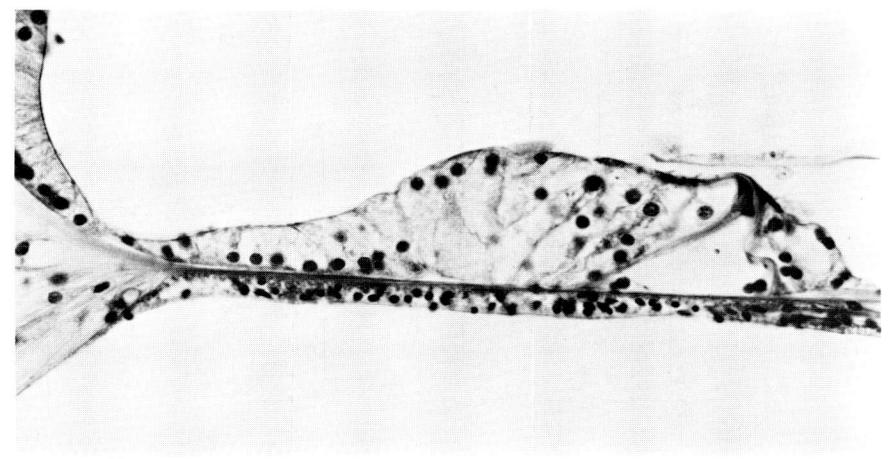

Figure 257. *Organ of Corti* (× 300)

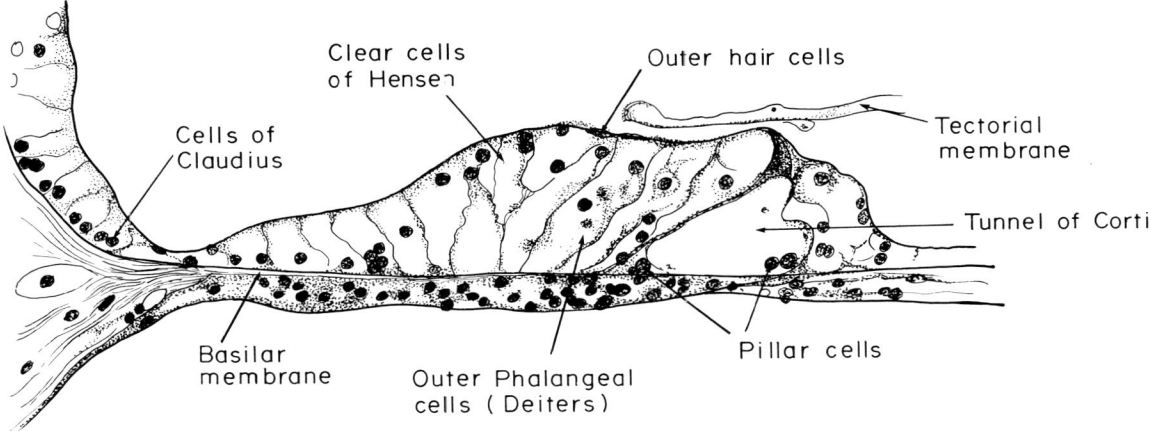

Figure 258. Diagram showing parts of organ of Corti.

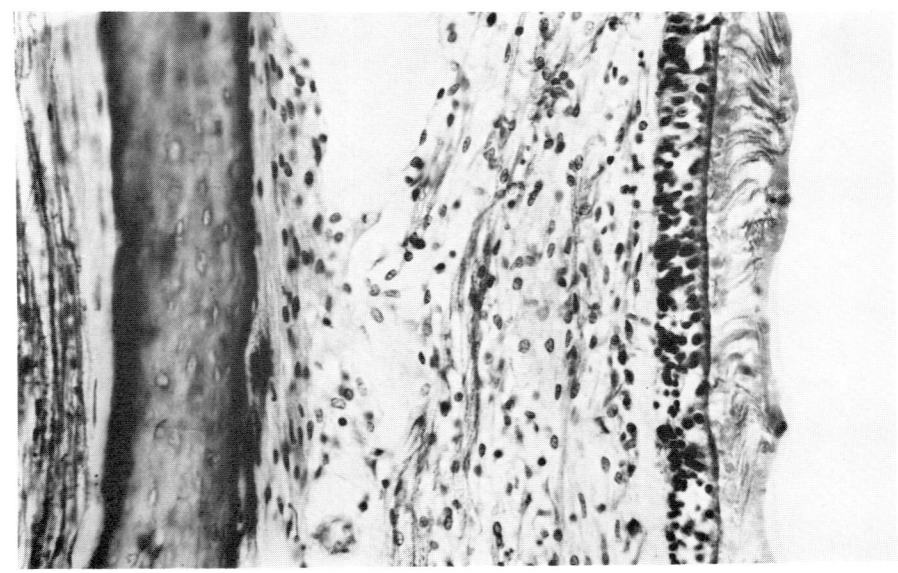

Figure 259. *Macula sacculi* (× 250)

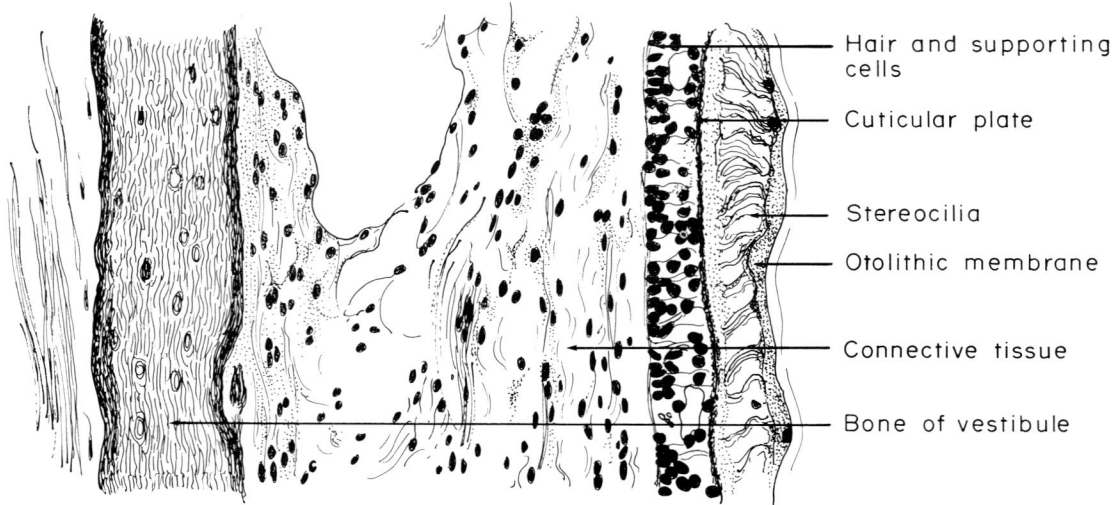

Figure 260. Diagram showing parts of macula sacculi.

MULTIPERFORATES WITH LARGE AND SMALL SPACES – KIDNEY

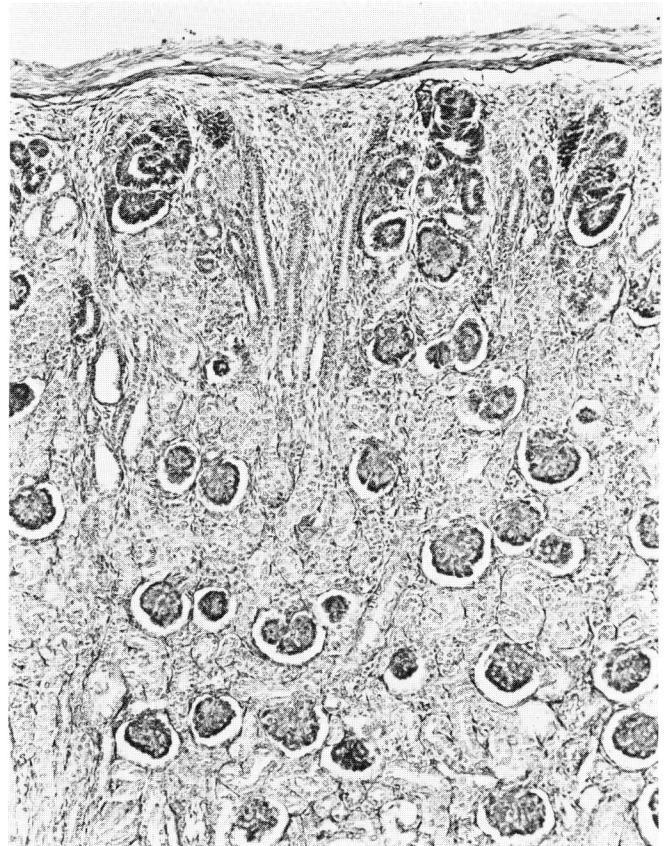

Figure 261. The larger spaces in this preparation are unique because they are almost filled by little balls, or glomeruli, ("Malpighian corpuscles") reducing the cavities to crescentric slits. This is a fetal kidney, and the nephrogenic zone (in which the glomeruli are developing by epithelial projections into the tubules) is seen below the capsule that marks the upper margin. Between the glomeruli are innumerable small spaces representing tubules. Some are cut transversely and appear as small rings; others are cut lengthwise and are seen as parallel slits. Between groups of developing glomeruli in the upper field are collections of long parallel tubules forming the beginning of the medullary rays; they include both collecting tubules and Henle's loops. *Renal cortex* (× 140)

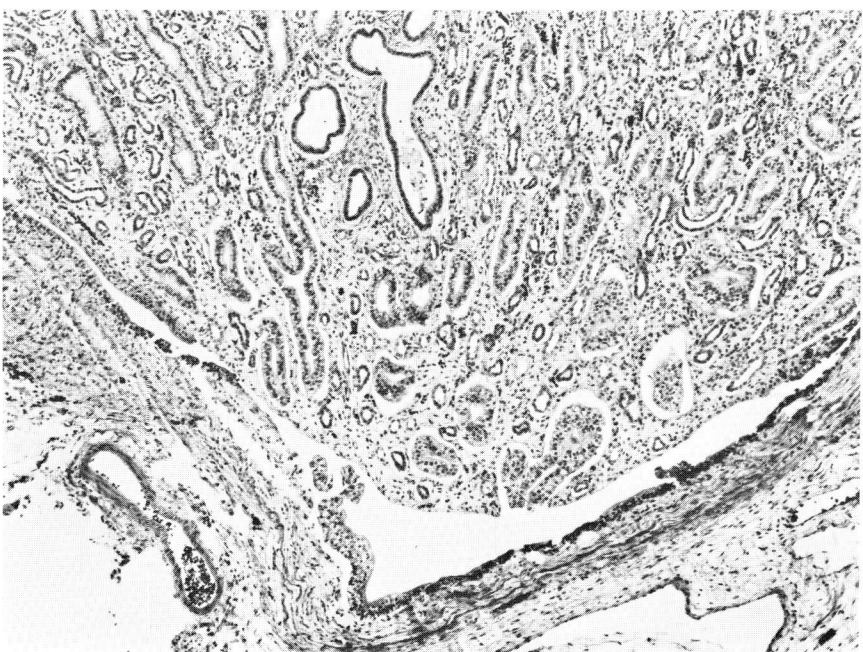

Figure 262. This field shows tubules only. The larger channels with columnar lining cells are collecting ducts; smaller tubules are part of Henle's loops. Some collecting ducts are seen to join and open on the V-shaped space of the calyx below. The renal pelvis has a thin fibrous and muscular wall lined by transitional epithelium. *Renal papilla*, fetal kidney (× 200)

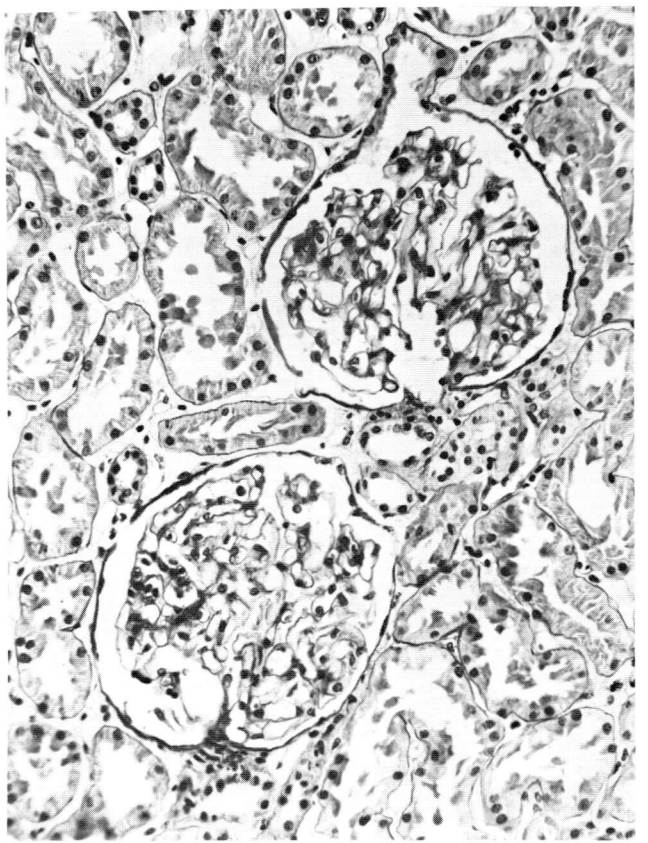

Figure 263. Two glomeruli are seen here. The one in the upper right has an opening through Bowman's capsule, forming the beginning of the proximal convoluted tubule (urinary pole). Immediately opposite, just outside the capsule at the lower pole, are two rings with small cells and closely grouped nuclei; these are distal convoluted tubules. Between the uppermost of these and the glomerulus are four or five nuclei belonging to the granular cells in the wall of the afferent arteriole. The cells of the upper wall of the adjoining tubule are closely compacted together to form the macula densa. This combination of granular cells and macula densa constitutes the juxtaglomerular complex. The same features are visible at the vascular pole of the lower glomerulus, just above the lower edge of the figure. *Renal cortex* (×50)

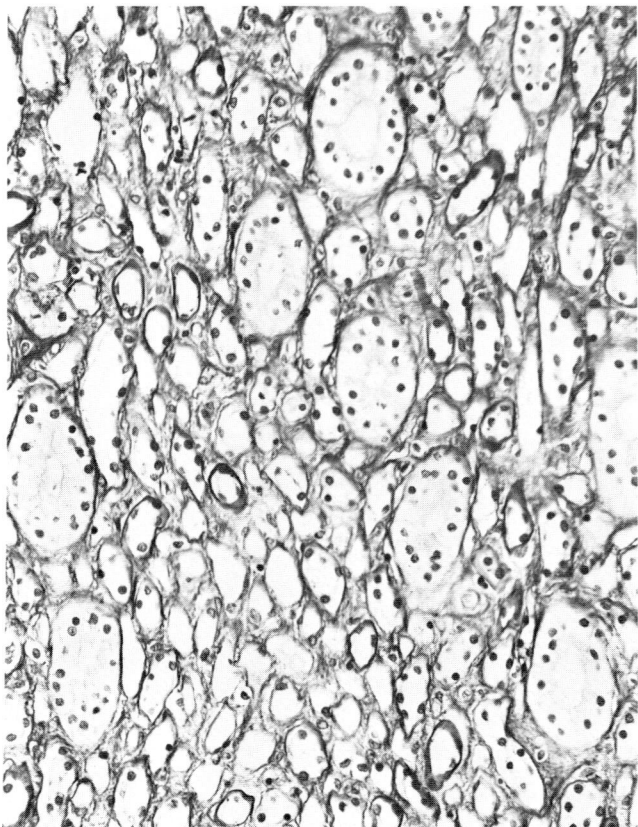

Figure 264. This section has both large and small ovoid spaces. The larger have tall cells with pale cytoplasm and are collecting tubules; smaller tubules with inconspicuous cells, seen mainly as nuclei within a ring of basement membrane, are the thick and thin Henle's loops. Veins are also present but are difficult to recognize unless red cells are identified. One large vein is present in the left upper corner. *Renal medulla*, Jones' silver (×200)

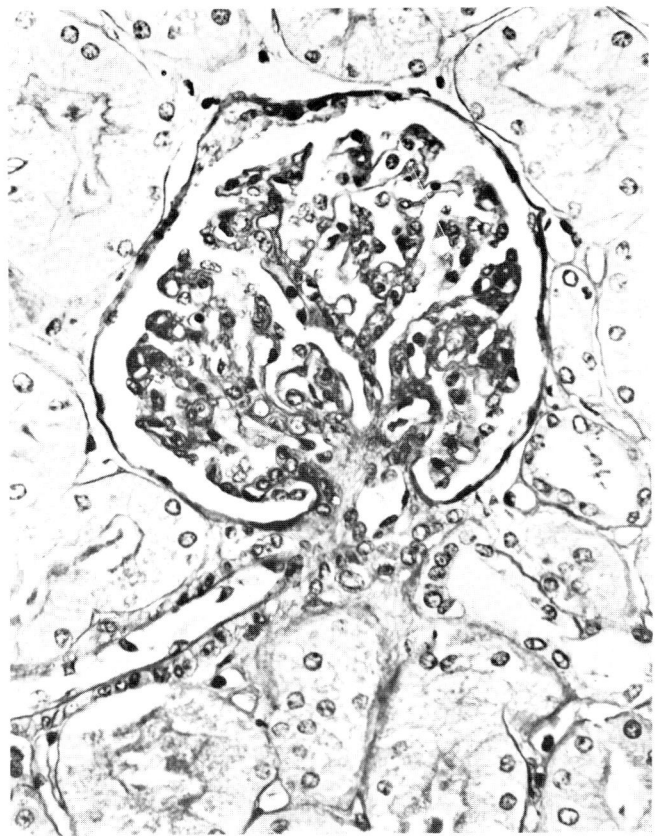

Figure 265. The afferent arteriole to this glomerulus runs obliquely upwards in the left lower quarter. The glomerulus itself is surrounded almost entirely by proximal convoluted tubules with bulky epithelium. The right lower quarter includes two distal convoluted tubules with much flatter epithelium and more numerous cells. The lower tubule runs obliquely, and the macula densa is well seen at its upper end. The dark line marking the inner surface of proximal tubules is the brush border, seen by PAS, in the left lower quarter. The dark circular line around the glomerulus, separating the urinary space from the tubules of the parenchyma, is the basement membrane of Bowman's capsule. *Glomerulus* (×350)

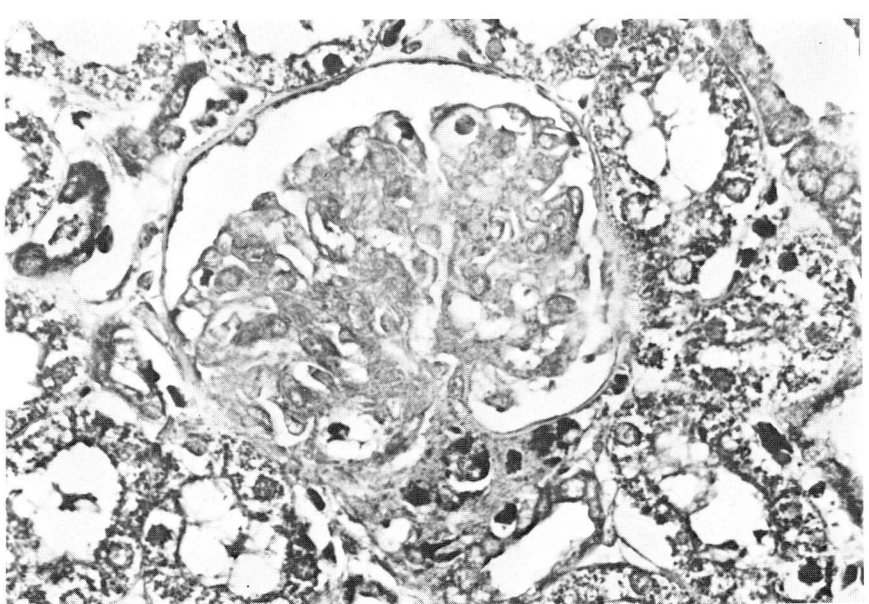

Figure 266. This is a paraffin section stained with crystal violet and mounted in Apathy's aqueous medium to show the granules in the juxtaglomerular (JG) cells, which lie in the triangle between afferent and efferent arterioles and the macula densa. The granules appear here as black material in the cells at the root of the glomerulus; they contain renin. However, this stain is not specific, and some coarse granules may be lipofuscin. The distal tubule with the macula densa lies in the four to five o'clock axis immediately below. In the normal human, JG granules are too few to be photographed; this is from an eight-year-old child with hyperplasia of the JG cells. *JG granules* (×400)

MULTIPERFORATES WITH LARGE SPACES

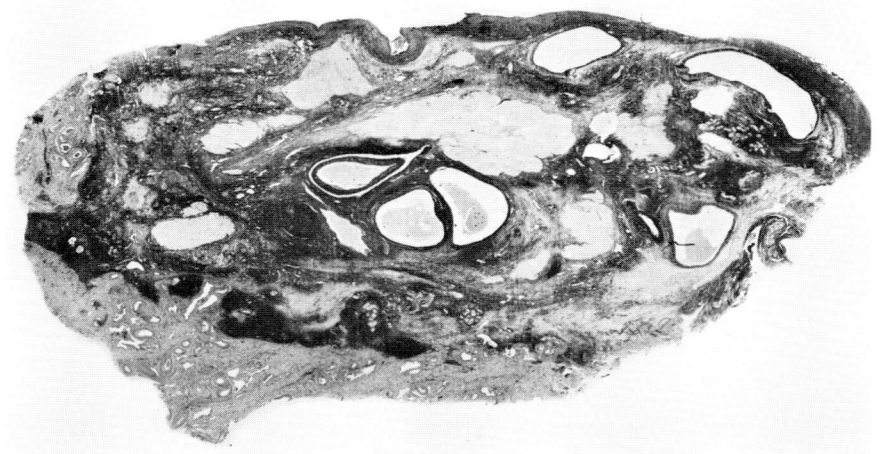

Figure 267. This is an ovoid fibrous structure with small, irregularly placed cysts (atretic follicles) and several large, irregularly shaped, pale, hyalinized solid islands, which are corpora albicantia. This is typical of the ovary in the reproductive age. *Ovary, normal adult female* (×4)

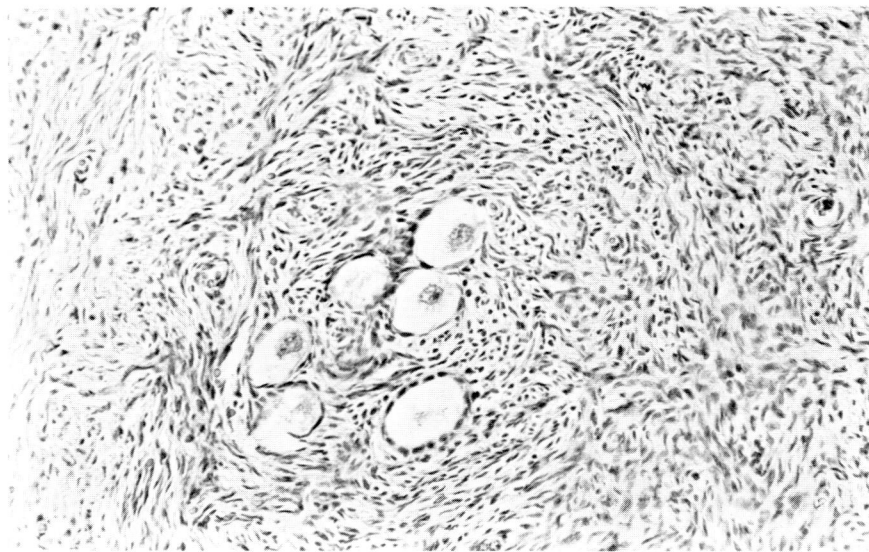

Figure 268. Here there is a fibrillary, curlicued, swirling stroma, in which lies a group of large cells up to 120μ in diameter, with pale cytoplasm. The nuclei have prominent nucleoli. These are ova, each surrounded by a ring of flattened follicle cells. *Ovarian cortex*, primordial follicles (×200)

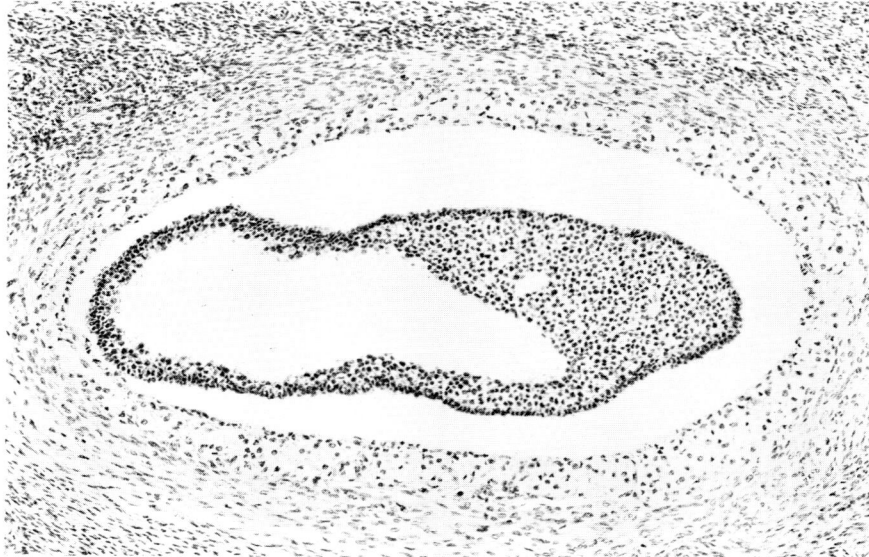

Figure 269. Of the several hundred thousand ova present in the immature ovary, most develop only partially and degenerate to form small atretic follicles, as illustrated here in the mass of granulosa cells (artefactually retracted). The immediate periphery of the larger space is a row of large pale cells, the theca interna. Lying outside this again are the loose spindle cells of the theca externa. *Atretic follicle* (×100)

MULTIPERFORATES WITH LARGE SPACES

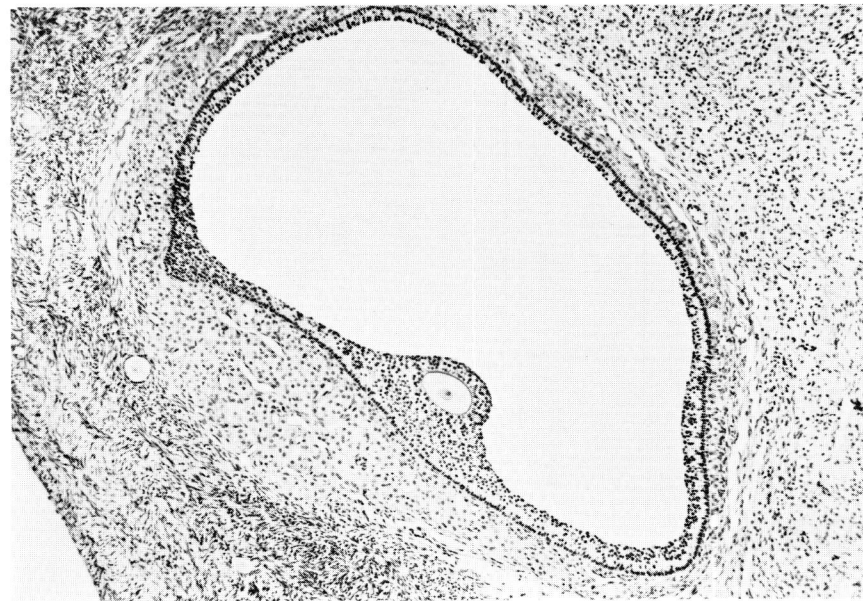

Figure 270. This section of ovary shows the cuboidal germinal epithelium down the left margin with a normal graafian follicle centrally. The stratified lining layer of polygonal cells is the granulosa, with a mound just below center named the discus proligerus, which contains the ovum. *Graafian follicle* (×80)

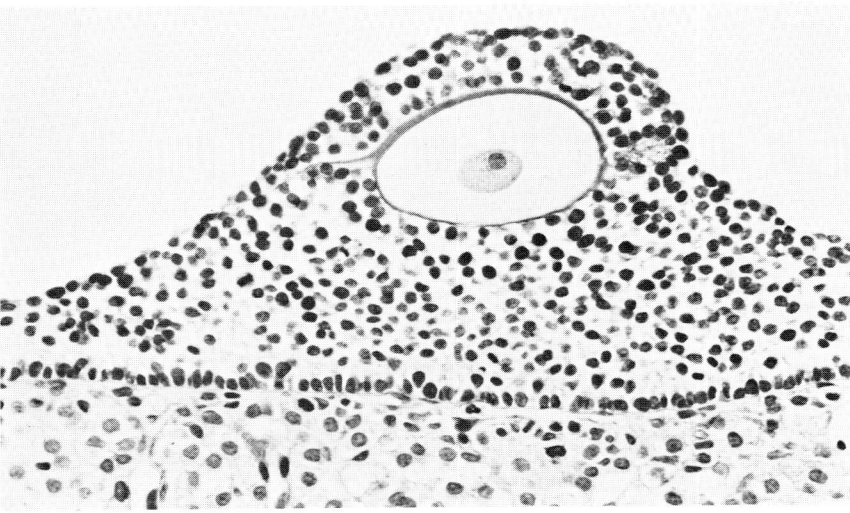

Figure 271. At higher power and stained with PAS, the ovum is surrounded by a glycoprotein membrane known as the zona pellucidum. Theca interna cells are seen across the bottom of the plate. *Ovum*, PAS diastase (×300)

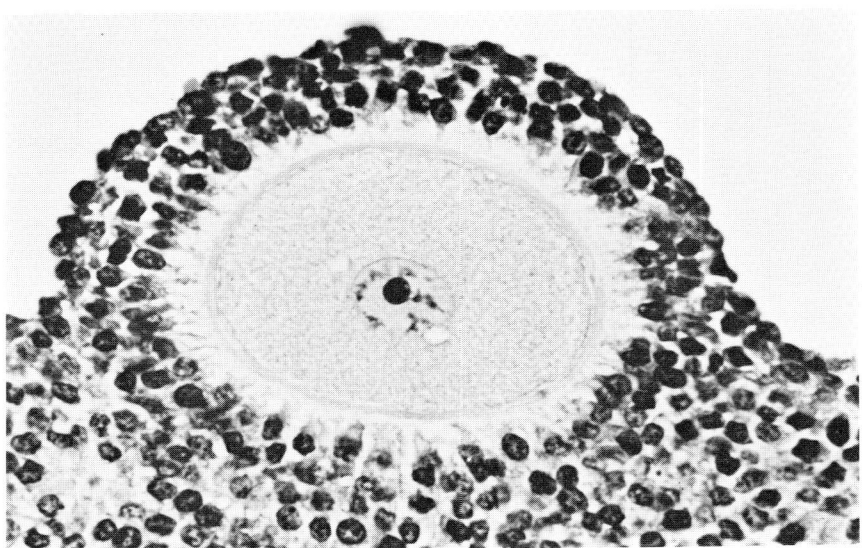

Figure 272. The granulosa cells surrounding the ovum tend to be arranged radially, constituting the corona radiata. The nucleus may be as much as 25µ across, and the nucleolus is equally prominent. *Ovum* (×480)

MULTIPERFORATES WITH LARGE SPACES

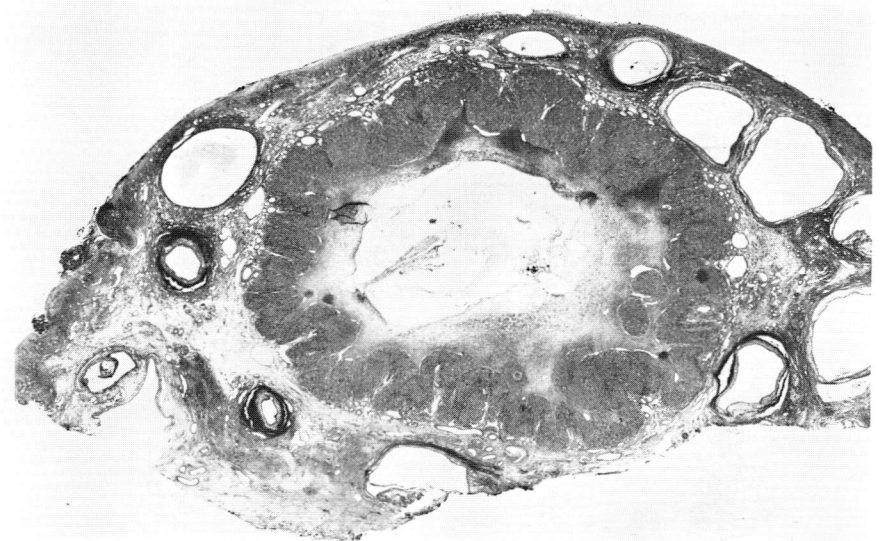

Figure 273. In the late phase of the menstrual cycle, the granulosa cells acquire large amounts of lipid (luteinization). After ovulation the follicle collapses, and its wall becomes convoluted around residual cyst fluid, serum, and blood. The luteinized granulosa cells are invaded by capillaries from the theca interna, and ultimately this structure will be replaced by hyalinized fibrous tissue as a corpus albicans. *Involuting corpus luteum* ($\times 4$)

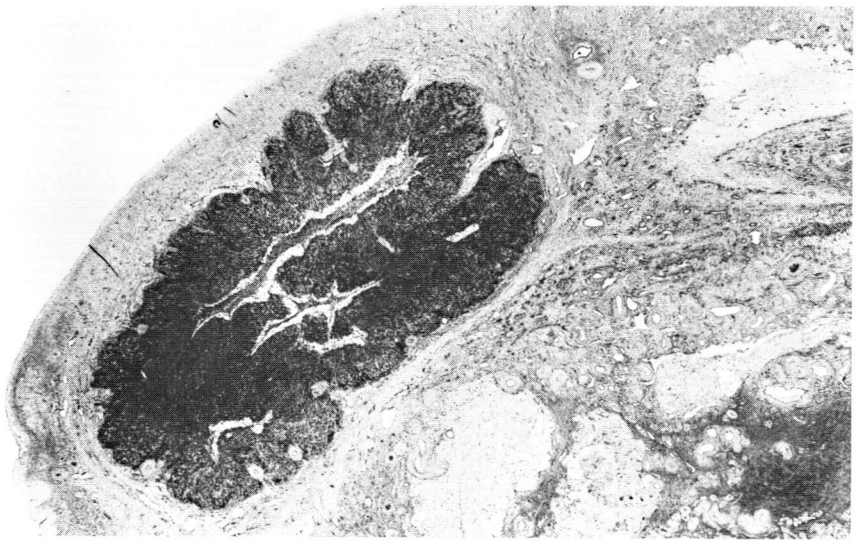

Figure 274. This specimen was processed through Carbowax and colored with oil red O to indicate the lipid content of the luteal cells that form the convoluted black mass to the left of center. The four irregular, pale structures on the right are corpora albicantia. *Ovary, corpus luteum* ($\times 13$)

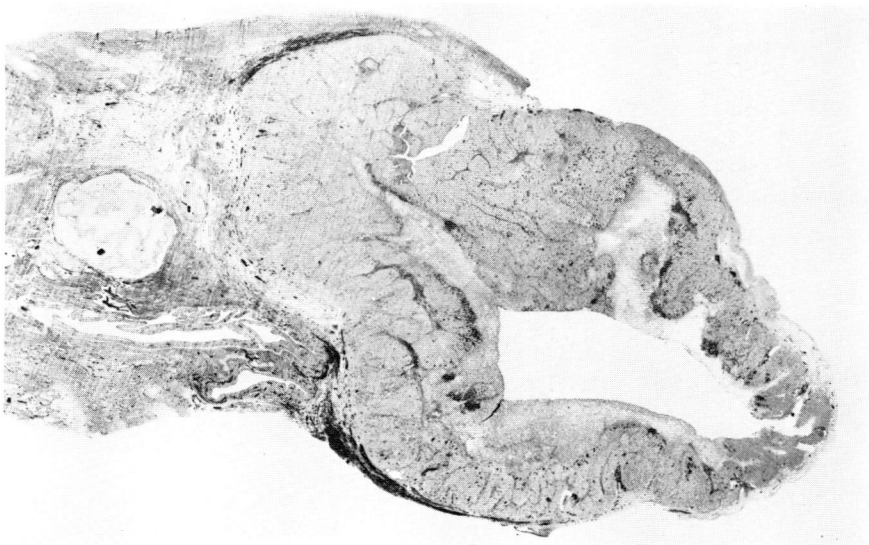

Figure 275. In the event of pregnancy, the follicle persists and enlarges. The granulosa cells and the theca interna cells have become large and pale because of lipid accumulation. Involution and organization are postponed until delivery. *Corpus luteum of pregnancy* ($\times 4.5$)

MULTIPERFORATES WITH LARGE SPACES

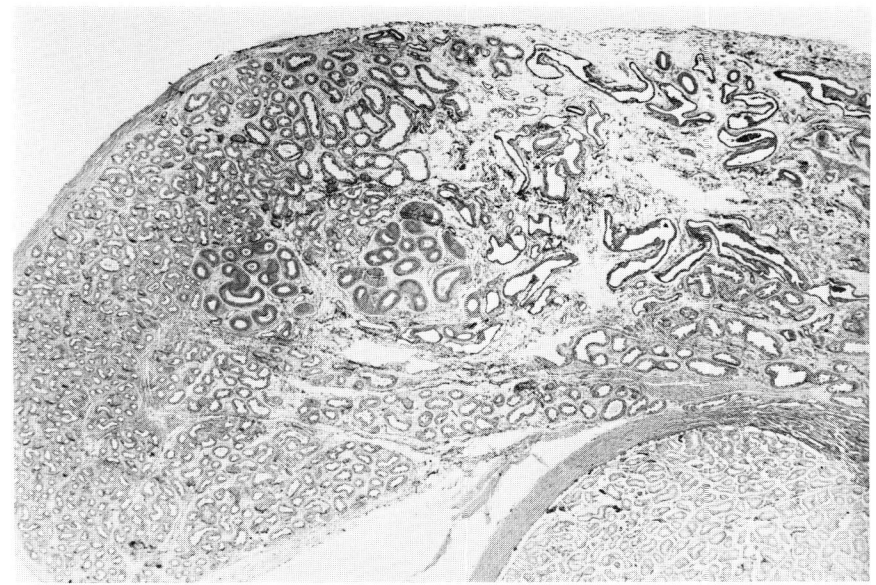

Figure 276. This is a survey picture showing two adjoining tubular structures. In the lower right corner is testis, while the bulk of the plate consists of ductuli efferentes. The small groups of tubules (left of center) with taller epithelium are part of the ductus epididymis. *Testis and epididymis* (× 6.5)

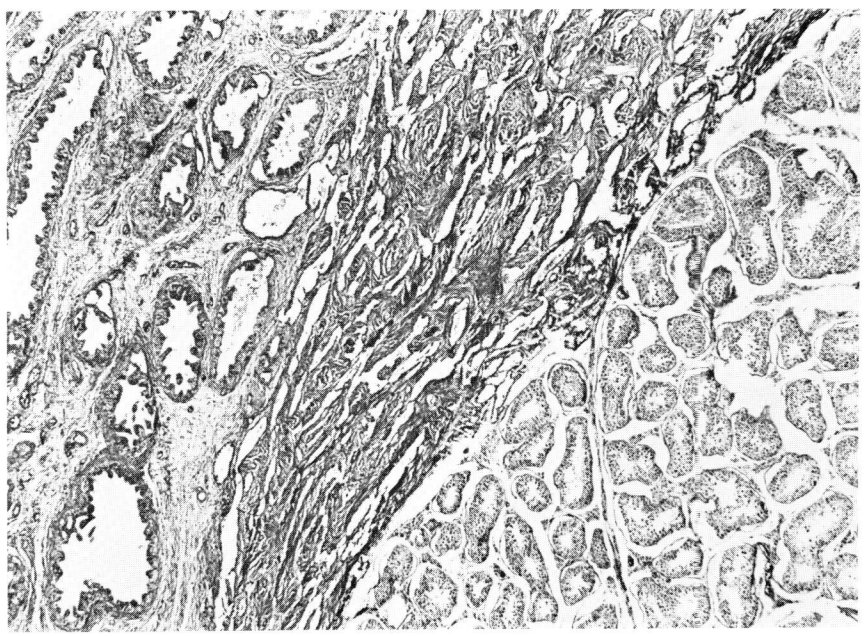

Figure 277. The tubules in the right lower corner are seminiferous; in the middle zone running obliquely is the rete testis; while the left third contains ductuli efferentes. More detail is shown in subsequent plates. *Testis* (× 27)

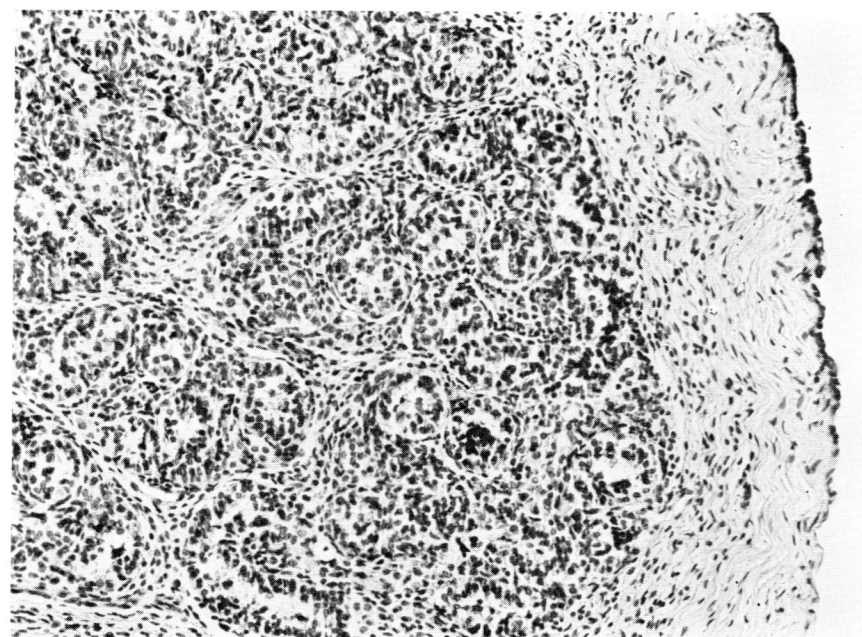

Figure 278. Along the right margin a low cuboidal epithelium overlies fibrous tissue. The bulk of the tissue is tubular with many circular profiles and a highly cellular stroma. This is the embryonic testis without evidence of spermatogenesis. *Fetal testis* (× 140)

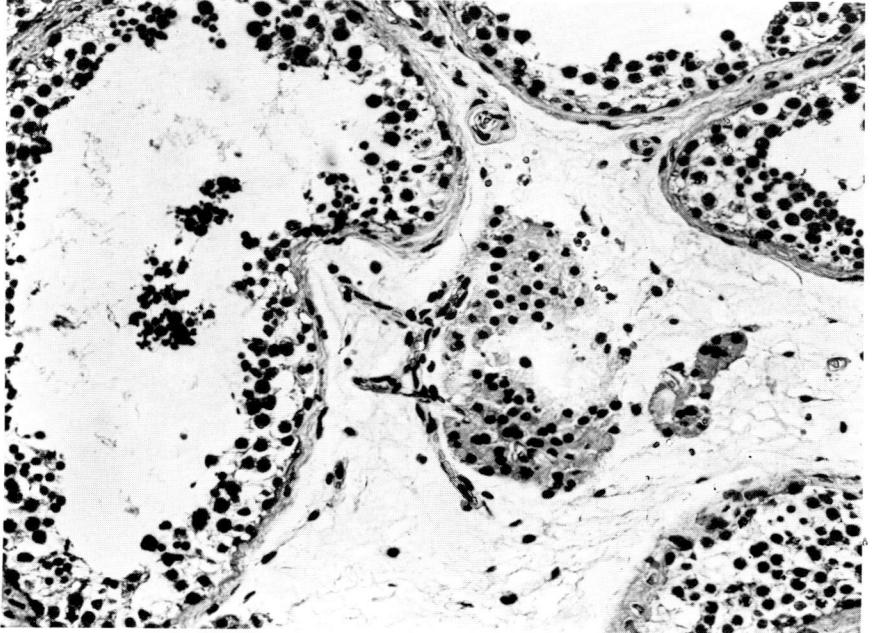

Figure 279. In the adult testis, tubules are much larger and show differentiation of spermatocytes. Each tubule is outlined by basement membrane and surrounded by small amounts of loose connective tissue in which are clusters of large cells in epithelioid arrangement. These have eosinophilic finely granular lipid-containing cytoplasm (lipochrome) and may contain crystalloids of Reinke identifying the interstitial cells of Leydig. *Testis with interstitial cells of Leydig* (× 200)

MULTIPERFORATES WITH LARGE SPACES

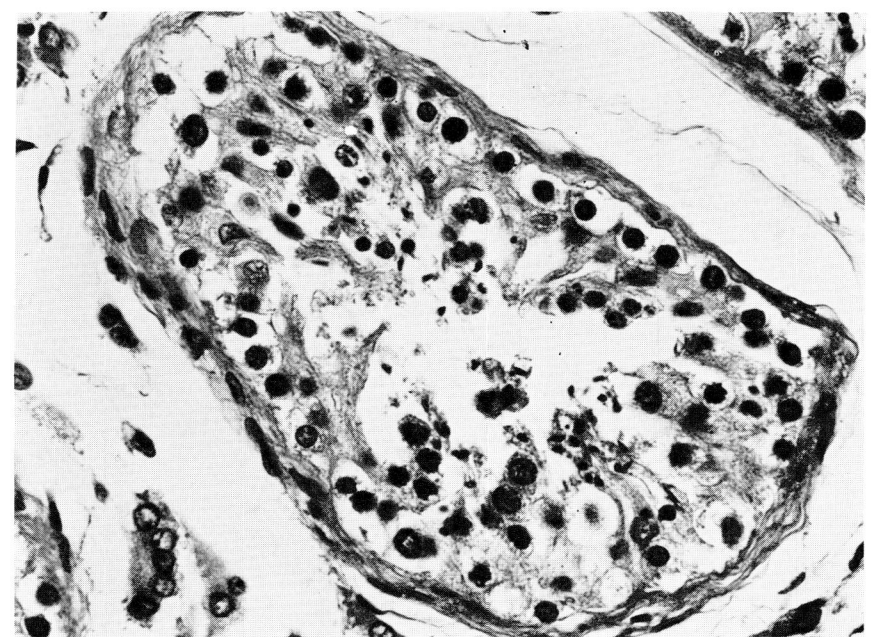

Figure 280. This tubule has a multilayered epithelium with a variety of cell types, including tiny spermatozoa in the center. The periphery is a thin fibrous wall, and below this in the upper part of the figure is a row of clear cells with very round, densely staining nuclei; these are spermatogonia. As seen in the lower part of the tubule, these cells become larger as they mature to primary spermatocytes, then decrease in size with maturation to secondary spermatocytes, spermatids, and sperm. The more irregular-shaped nuclei with paler staining reaction are from Sertoli's cells. *Adult testis, seminiferous tubule* (× 400)

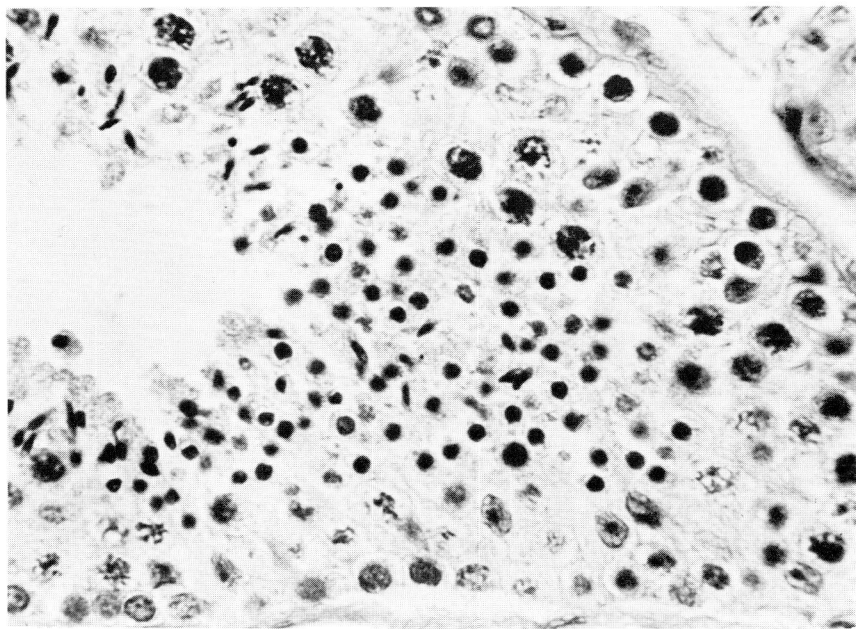

Figure 281. In this particular tubule the different sizes of developing germ cells are more apparent, and a number of Sertoli's cells with large oval irregular nuclei and prominent central nucleoli are seen, particularly just above the lower margin on the right. Sertoli's cells may show tiny crystalloids not easily seen or photographed. *Seminiferous tubule* (× 500)

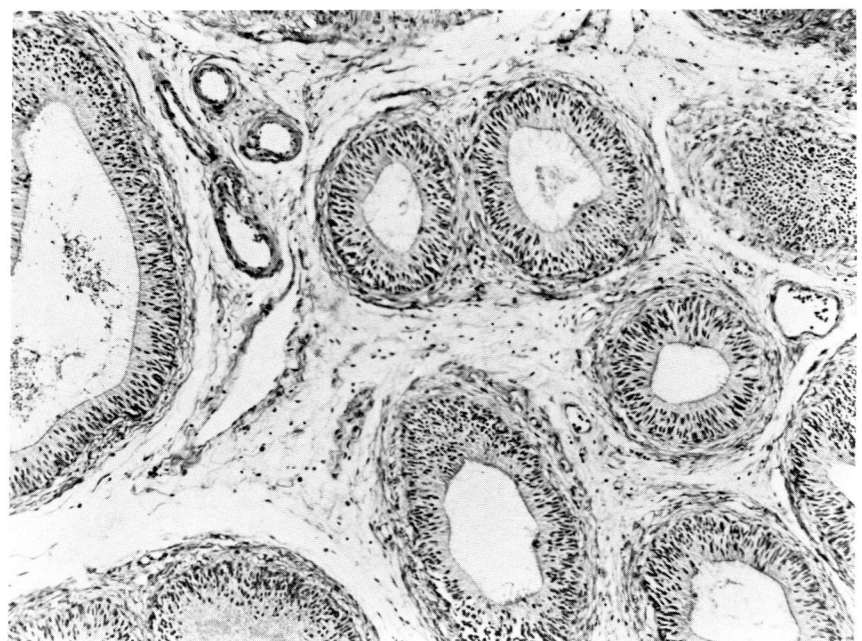

Figure 282. Here there are chiefly smooth circular profiles lined by a very regular, apparently stratified columnar epithelium. The supporting tissue is loose connective tissue, but there is a thin zone of nonstriated muscle arranged circumferentially around each tube. The ductus epididymis runs from the head to the tail of the epididymis, where it joins the vas (ductus) deferens. *Ductus epididymis* (×80)

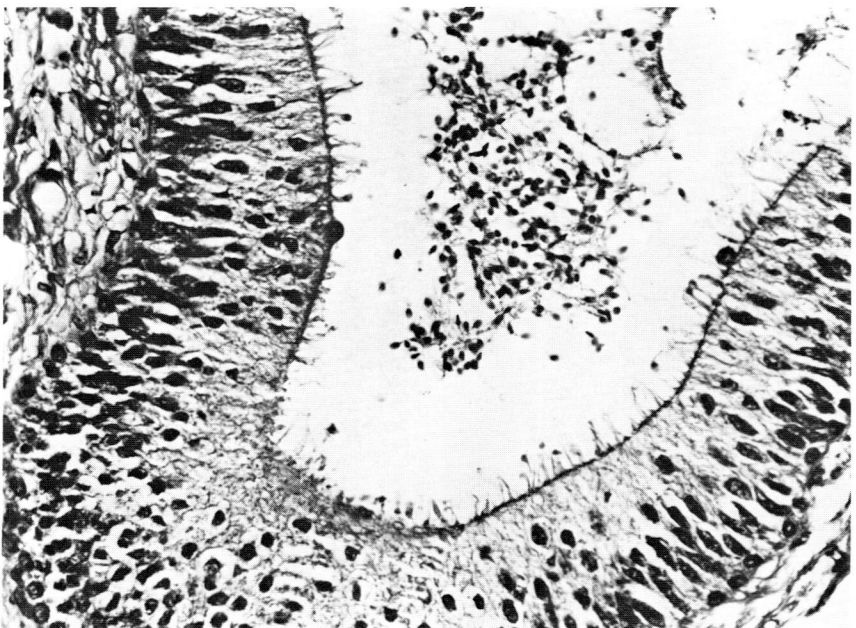

Figure 283. At higher power, the surface of the pseudostratified columnar epithelium bears relatively long, thick processes known as stereocilia; these are nonmotile. The cytoplasm may contain brown lipochrome granules. The lumen contains numerous spermatozoa identifiable by their spear-shaped heads. *Ductus epididymis* (×320)

MULTIPERFORATES WITH LARGE SPACES

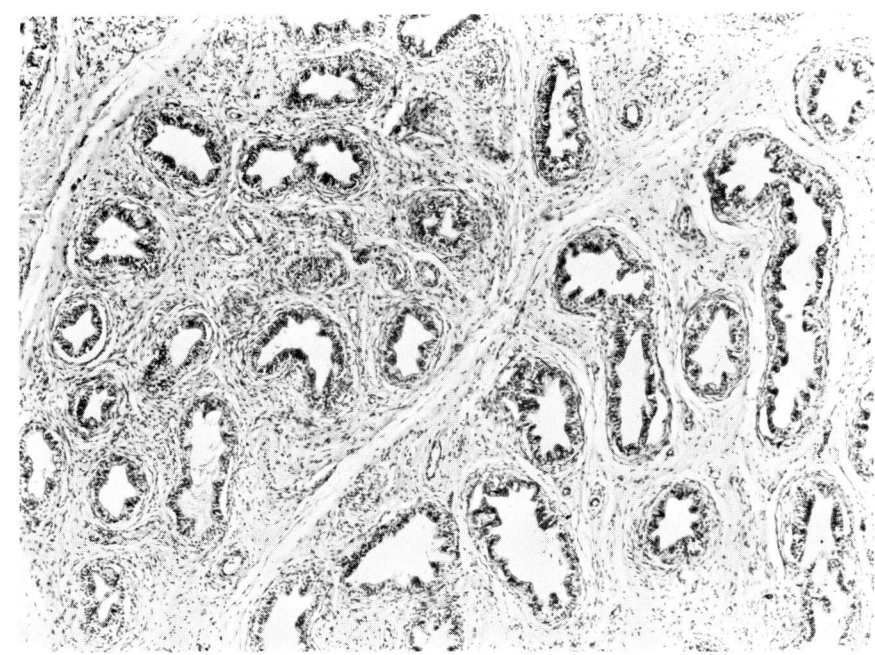

Figure 284. This shows irregular parallel and circular profiles in a fibromuscular stroma. The height of the lining epithelium appears variable. These tubules are smaller and less uniform than those of the ductus epididymis. *Ductuli efferentes* (× 8)

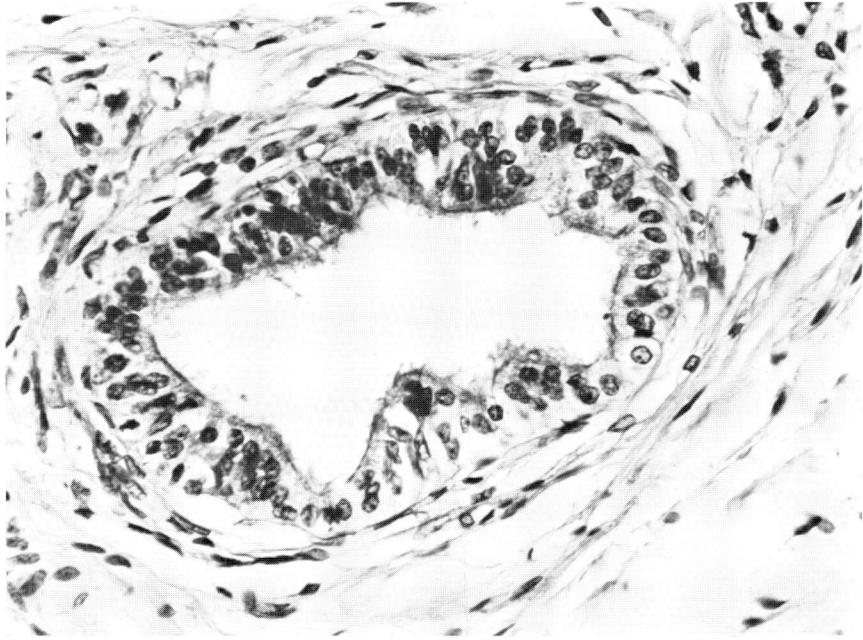

Figure 285. Some of the epithelium appears stratified; in other parts it is of single cell thickness. Some of the cells are ciliated, and yellow-brown pigment may be prominent. *Ductuli efferentes* (× 250)

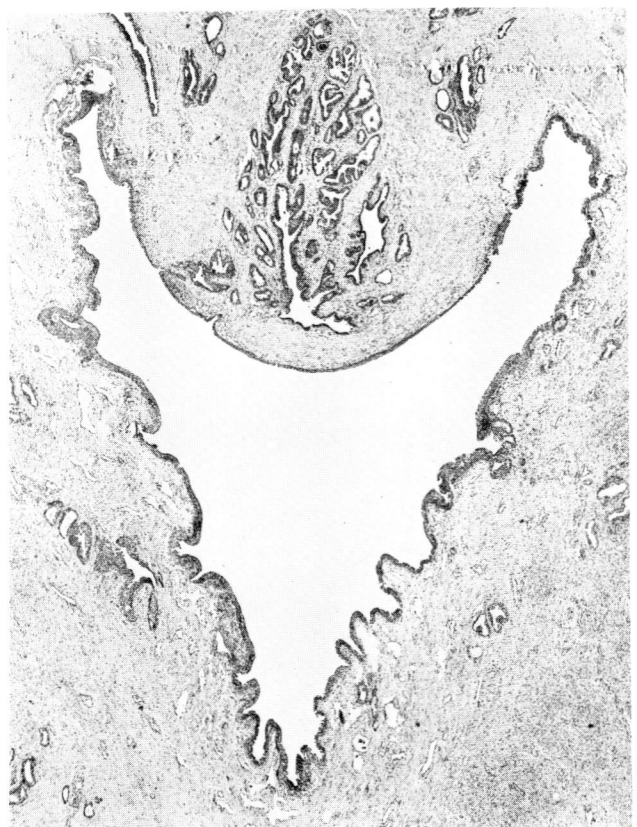 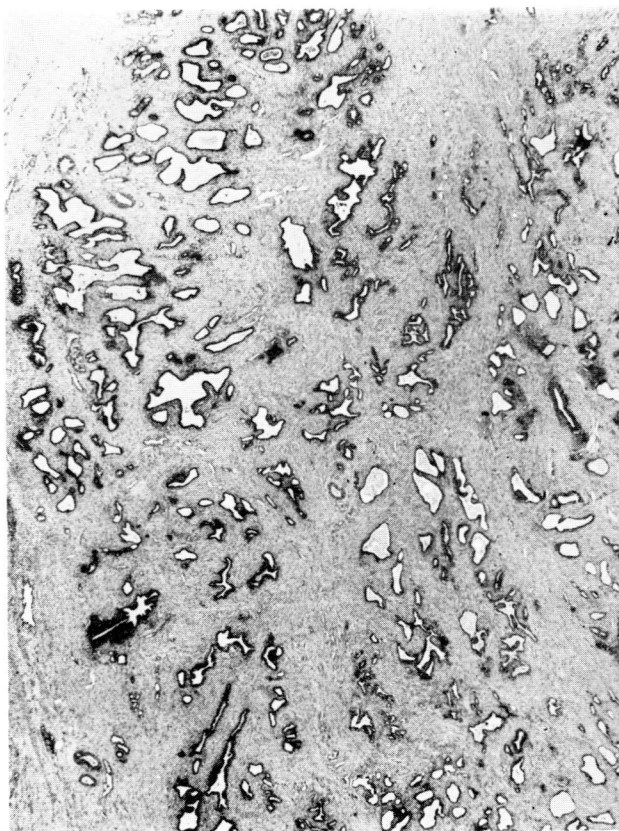

Figure 286. In the center of this figure is a large space invaginated from the top to give it a bicornuate configuration. This is from the prostatic section of the urethra, and the invagination is the verumontanum, or colliculus seminalis, which projects into the posterior wall. Within this hill the collection of ducts and tubular spaces in the upper center is the utriculus masculinus (prostaticus), which is believed to be the male homolog of the uterus. On each side and at a slight distance from the main utricle, like a pair of eyes, are other ducts, some from the prostate proper but including the two ejaculatory ducts, each of which is the termination of a ductus deferens. *Prostate* (× 16)

Figure 287. The body of the prostate is identified by numerous large irregular spaces lying in a dense fibromuscular stroma. Some are clearly tubular in nature. A lobular type of construction is present, although not striking in this plate. *Prostate* (× 10)

MULTIPERFORATES WITH LARGE SPACES

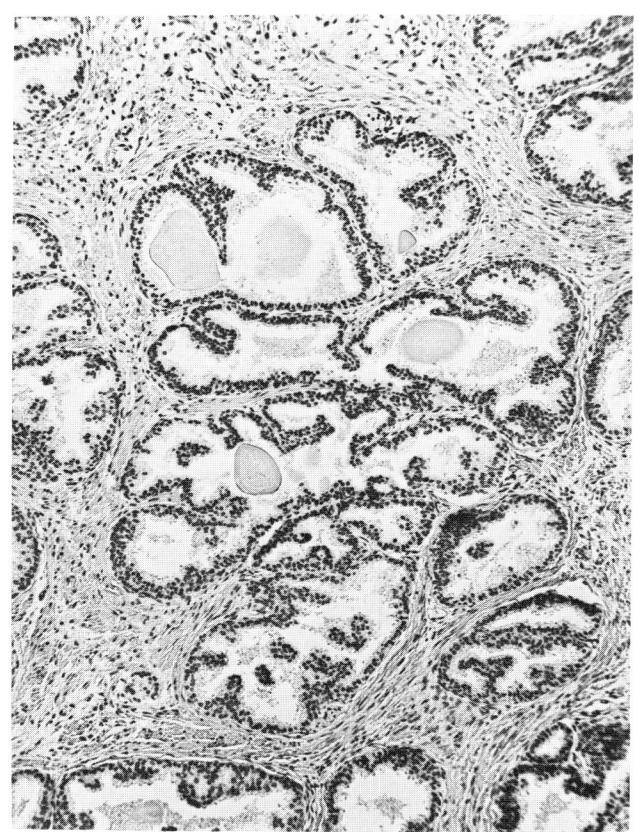

Figure 288. At higher power the fibromuscular stroma is now apparent and within many of the spaces are acellular concretions. *Prostate* (×80)

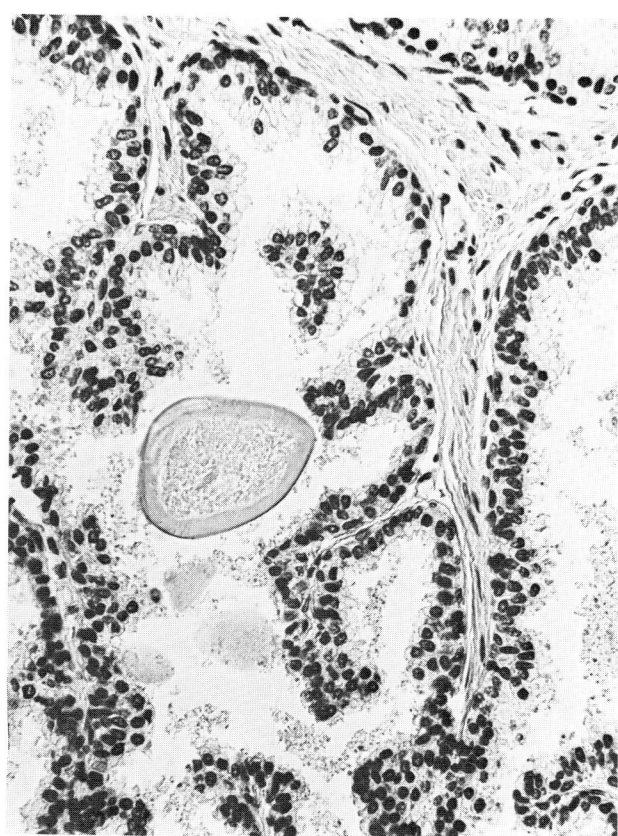

Figure 289. The papillary projections of epithelium with their scanty supporting stroma are now clearly seen. The lining cells in some areas are plainly in a single row, but in others there is a second peripheral row of flat cells. There is even a stratified appearance due to obliquity of sectioning. Lipochrome may be present. The nature of one of the concretions with a thick hyaline capsule and a more granular center is also more apparent. There is a great variation in the structure of these bodies, some being amorphous and ill-defined eosinophilic masses, others basophilic or calcified. *Prostate* (×250)

MULTIPERFORATES WITH LARGE SPACES

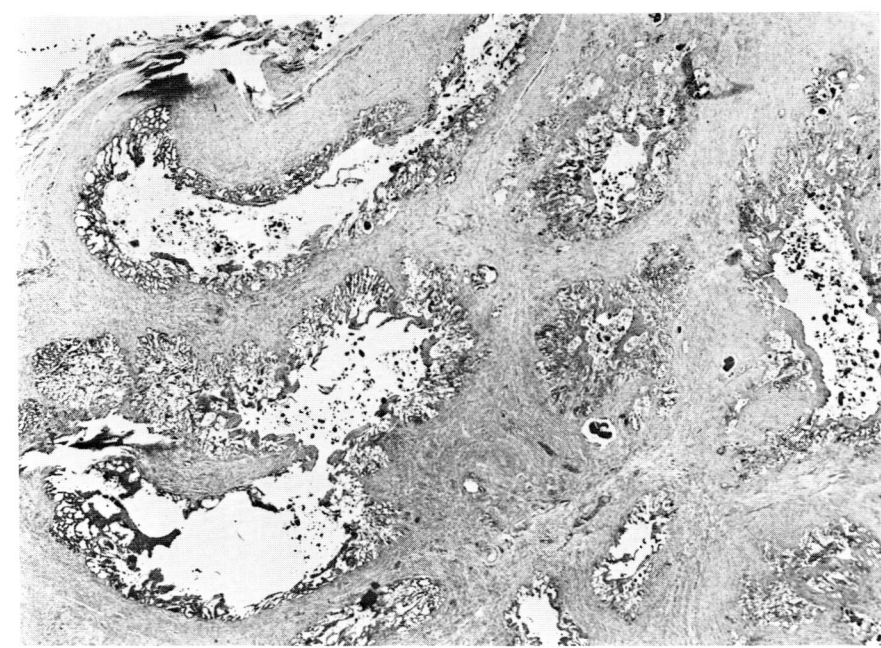

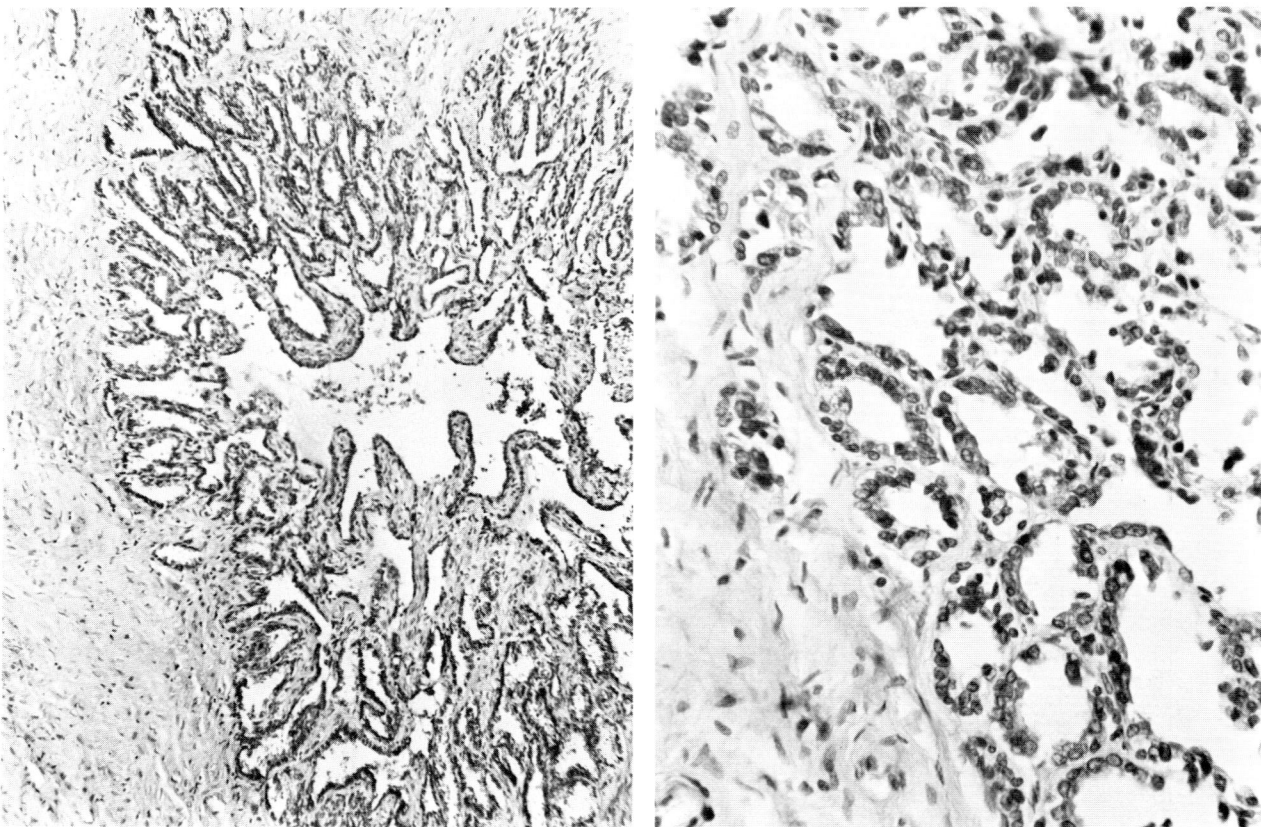

Figure 290. a. The upper low-power plate shows large spaces with scalloped irregular margins supported by rather dense fibrous stroma. (×10) b. Increased magnification shows the saccular outpouchings from the central space. (×80) c. The high power in the lower right reveals that these are lined by a single row of epithelial cells, sometimes appearing double or pseudostratified because of oblique cuts. Many of these cells contain a yellow lipochrome pigment easily seen in H & E sections but not readily demonstrable in a black and white plate. *Seminal vesicle*

MULTIPERFORATES WITH LARGE SPACES

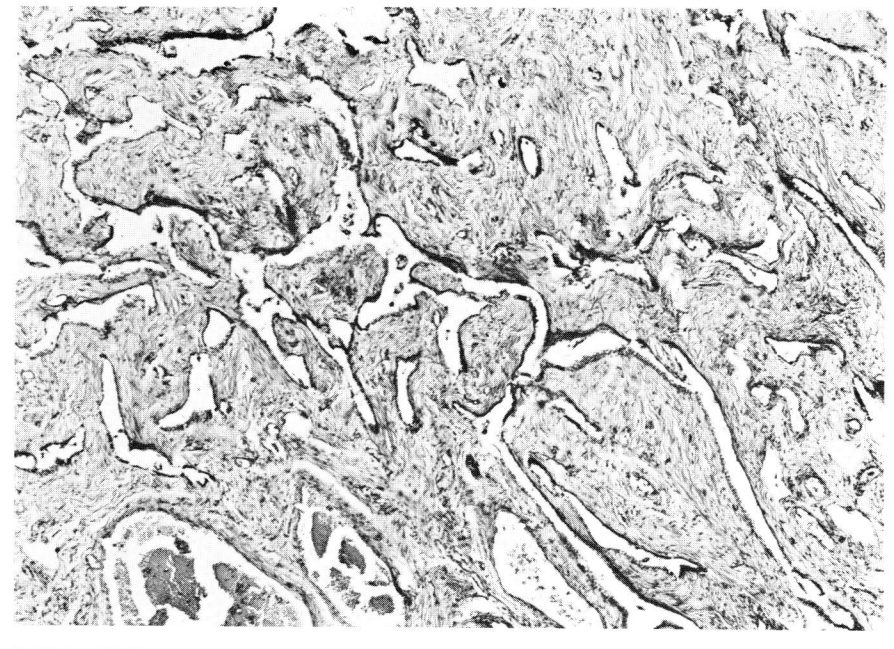

Figure 291. Irregular slitlike intercommunicating spaces found between the testis and the epididymis are the rete testis (already illustrated in the survey picture of this region (Fig. 276). Most of the spaces are empty. The lining epithelium is not particularly conspicuous, and at this power it may be difficult to distinguish rete spaces from blood vessels, of which two (with red cells) are seen in the left lower quadrant. Spermatozoa may be found in these spaces, although not seen in this preparation. *Rete testis* ($\times 44$)

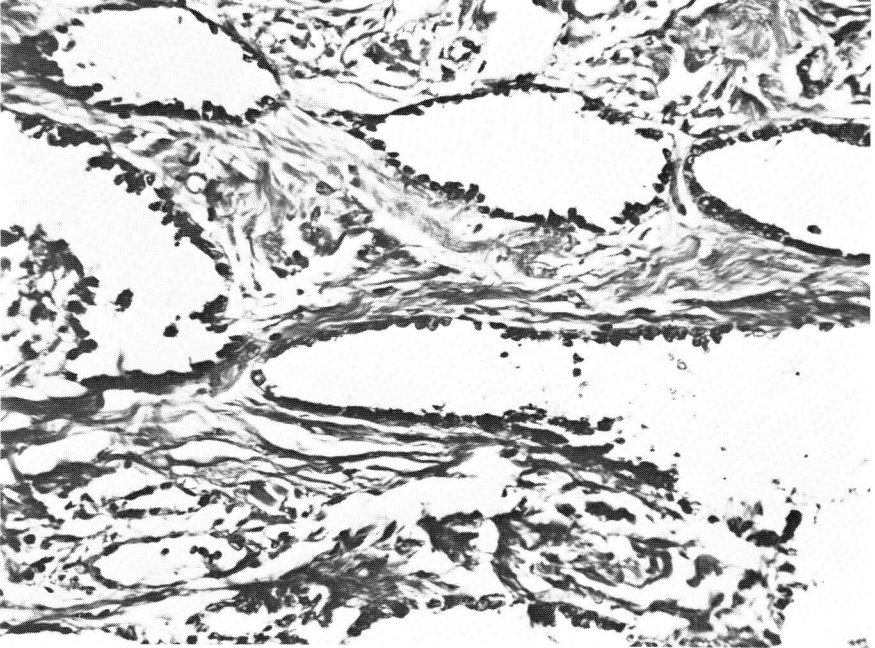

Figure 292. At high power the epithelium is characteristically of variable height, although cells have minimal cytoplasm. Sometimes a double row is seen, sometimes it is stratified in appearance, but in fact it is a single layer of cuboidal or low columnar cells. *Rete testis* ($\times 200$)

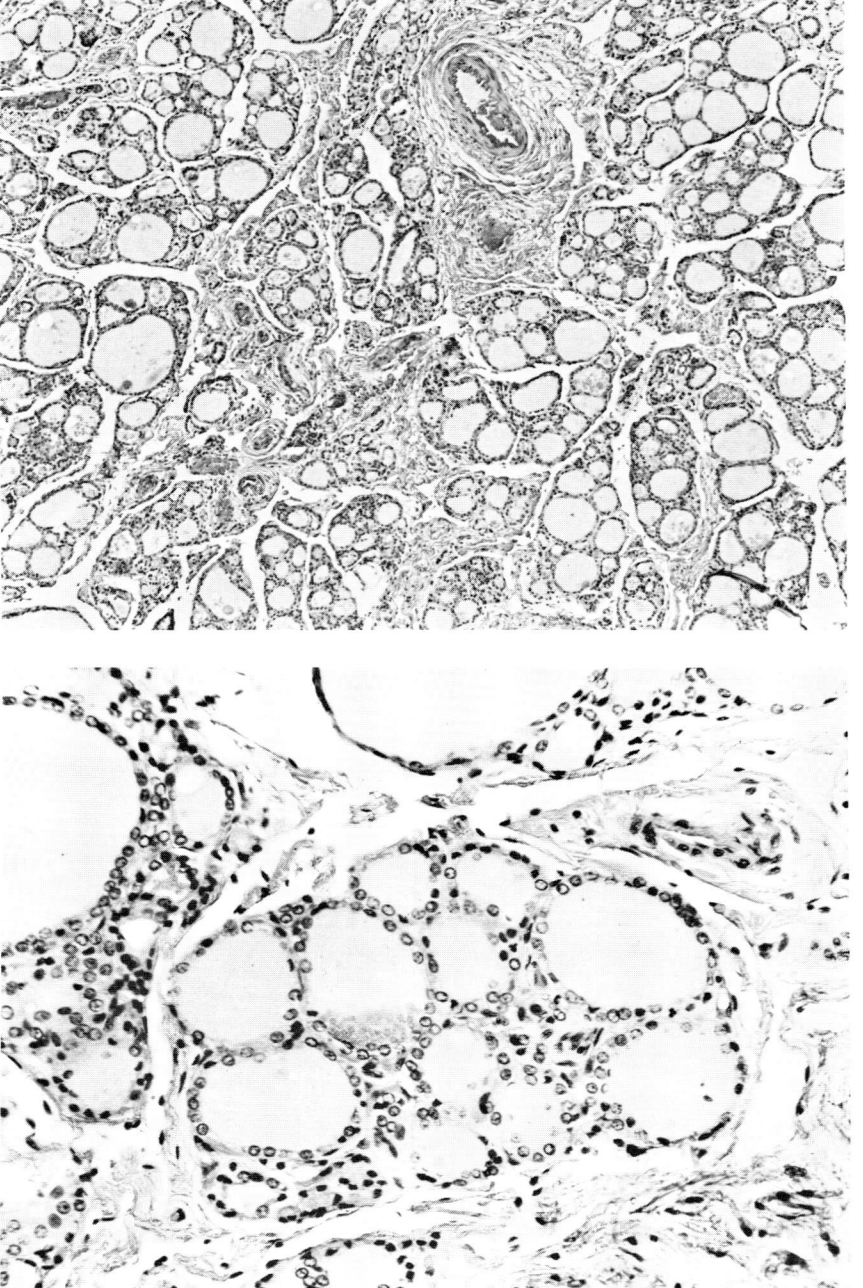

Figure 293. The spaces here are regular with circular profiles and no suggestion of tubule formation (except for the blood vessels in the upper central field). A distinct lobular grouping is apparent, the lobules being separated by scanty fibrous tissue. Each space is occupied by homogeneous grayish material, which in an H & E preparation is eosinophilic. The combination of lobular architecture, circular profiles, colloid content, and absence of ducts is characteristic for the thyroid. *Thyroid* (× 50)

Figure 294. The cells lining the follicles are sometimes square in profile (cuboidal) or more often laterate, resembling a brick lying on its side. Ten to twenty or thirty follicles constitute a lobule. The colloid material is chiefly thyroglobulin, containing iodinated compounds that are metabolically active on release to the blood. Mucoproteins and enzymes are also present. *Thyroid* (× 200)

MULTIPERFORATES WITH LARGE SPACES

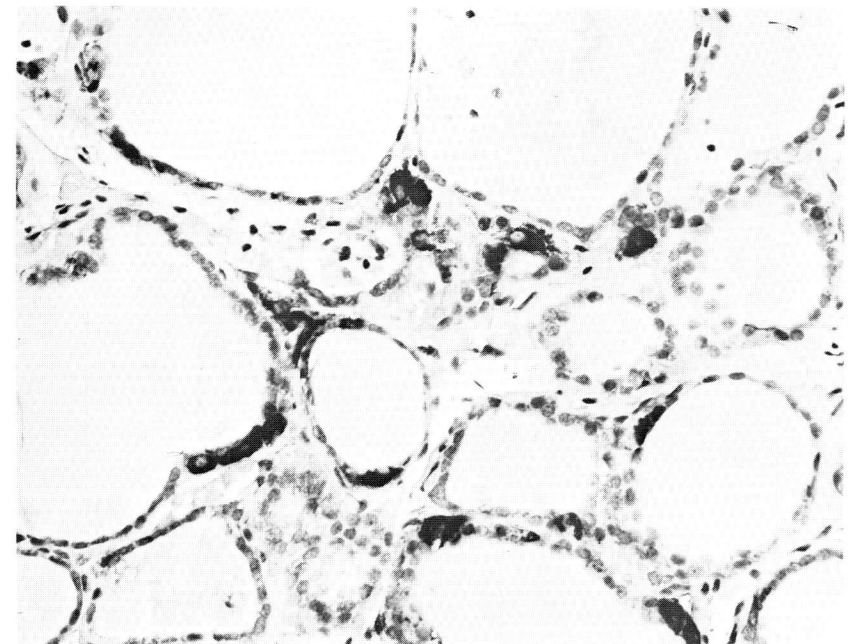

Figure 295. Calcitonin-secreting C cells in the human thyroid are found not only in parafollicular position, outside the follicles, but also beneath or among the cells that line the follicle. They are found chiefly in the upper and middle parts of the lateral lobes of the thyroid and are most apparent in certain hyperplastic conditions associated with endocrine tumor syndromes. They are not seen in ordinary H & E preparations but can be identified by immunoperoxidase techniques using specific antibodies directed against calcitonin. They appear here as black deposits in interstitial position just below center, and in the lining of follicles at upper left center. *Thyroid*, C cells PAP ($\times 250$)

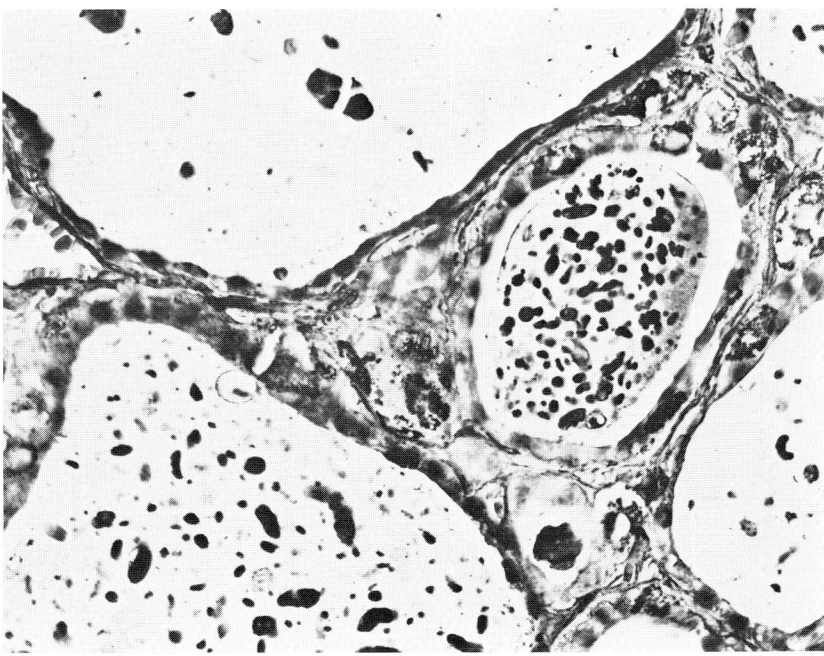

Figure 296. C cells may also be demonstrated by argyrophil techniques when the cytoplasm is rendering black and granular. In this figure, C cells are seen chiefly in the interstitial tissue just below the center of the plate but also in the epithelium lining the follicles, as at eleven o'clock in the follicle on the lower right side. The black bodies seen within the colloid are faintly stained in H & E preparations where they are usually described as colloid degeneration. *Thyroid*, C cells, Fernandez-Pascual (Silver, argyrophil reaction) ($\times 480$)

MULTIPERFORATES WITH LARGE SPACES

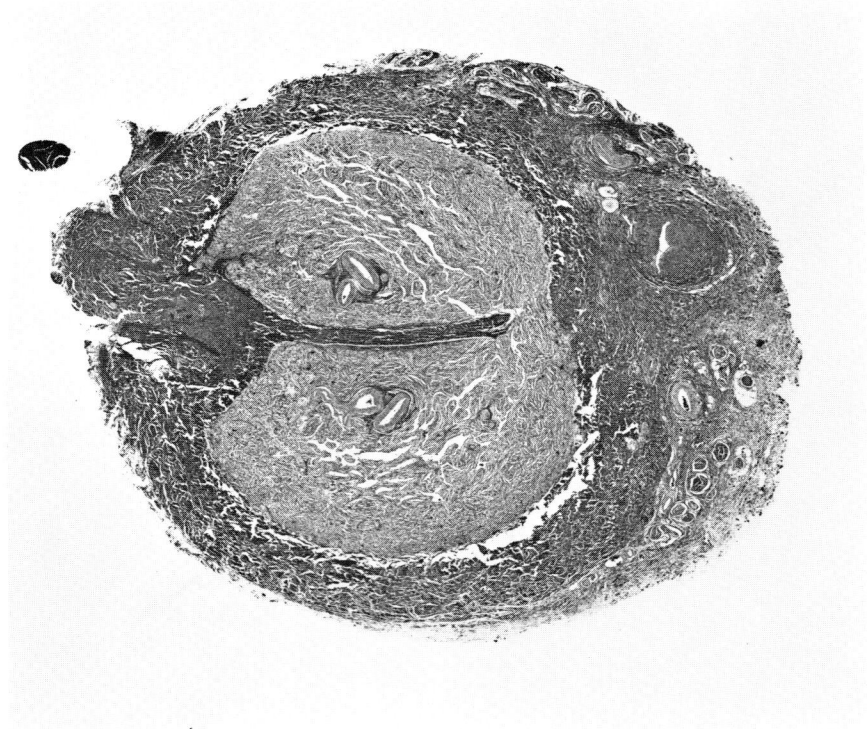

Figure 297. The periphery of this structure is fibrous tissue with vessels, nerves, and nerve endings, and the grayer central part with numerous irregular spaces is erectile tissue, almost completely divided in two by a thin fibrous septum. These are the corpora cavernosa of the clitoris, each with large central artery and vein. They join anteriorly to form the glans. In contradistinction to the male erectile tissue there are only two bodies, and there is no urethra. *Clitoris* (× 10)

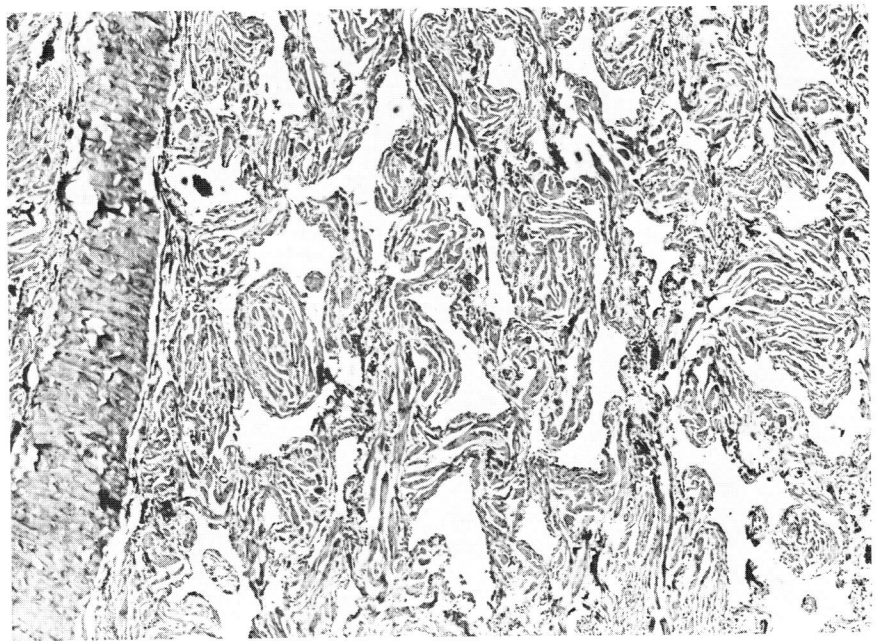

Figure 298. Here there are multiple large irregular and anastomosing vascular spaces (sinusoids), very few containing identifiable red cells despite its being erectile tissue. Along the left margin is thick fascia enclosing one of the corpora cavernosa. The stroma between the vascular spaces is chiefly nonstriated muscle without the laminar arrangement of ordinary vessels. *Erectile tissue* (× 30)

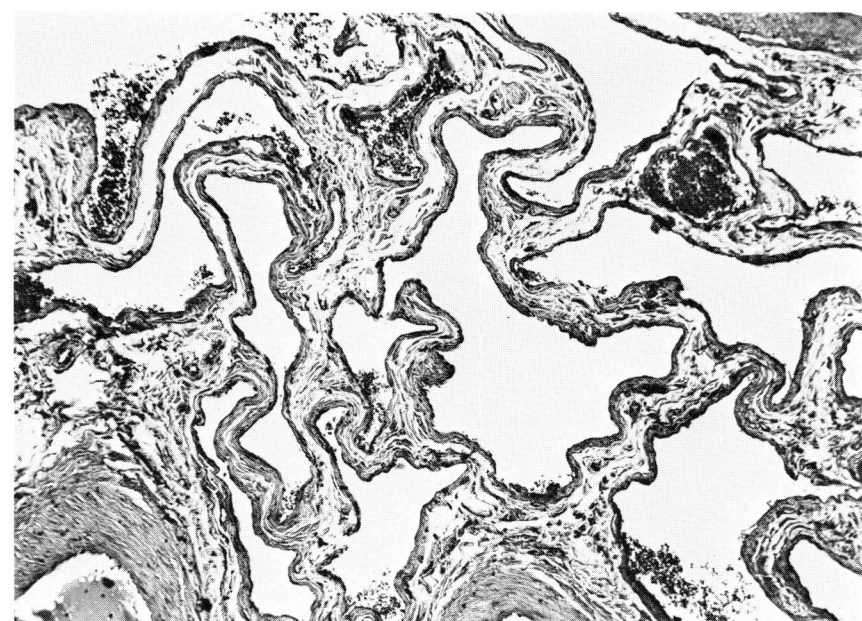

Figure 299. These are large irregular vascular spaces of venous type, lined by endothelium, with some red cells visible in the lumens in the upper left and lower right quadrants. There is a loose intervening fibrous stroma with portions of two large, thick vessels along the lower margin of the plate. This construction is unique for the pampiniform plexus of the spermatic cord. *Pampiniform plexus* (× 80)

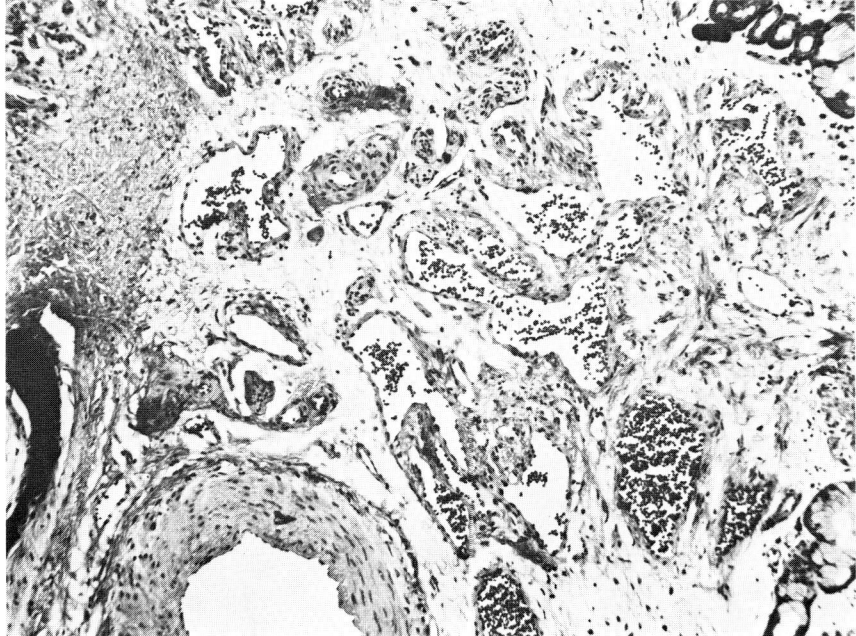

Figure 300. Multiple thin-walled dilated vascular spaces of venous type are found in the lamina propria of the nasal mucosa. Here a fragment of bone is seen in the left margin, a large artery on the lower edge, and minor glands in the right lower corner. *Mucosa over turbinate bones of nose* (× 80)

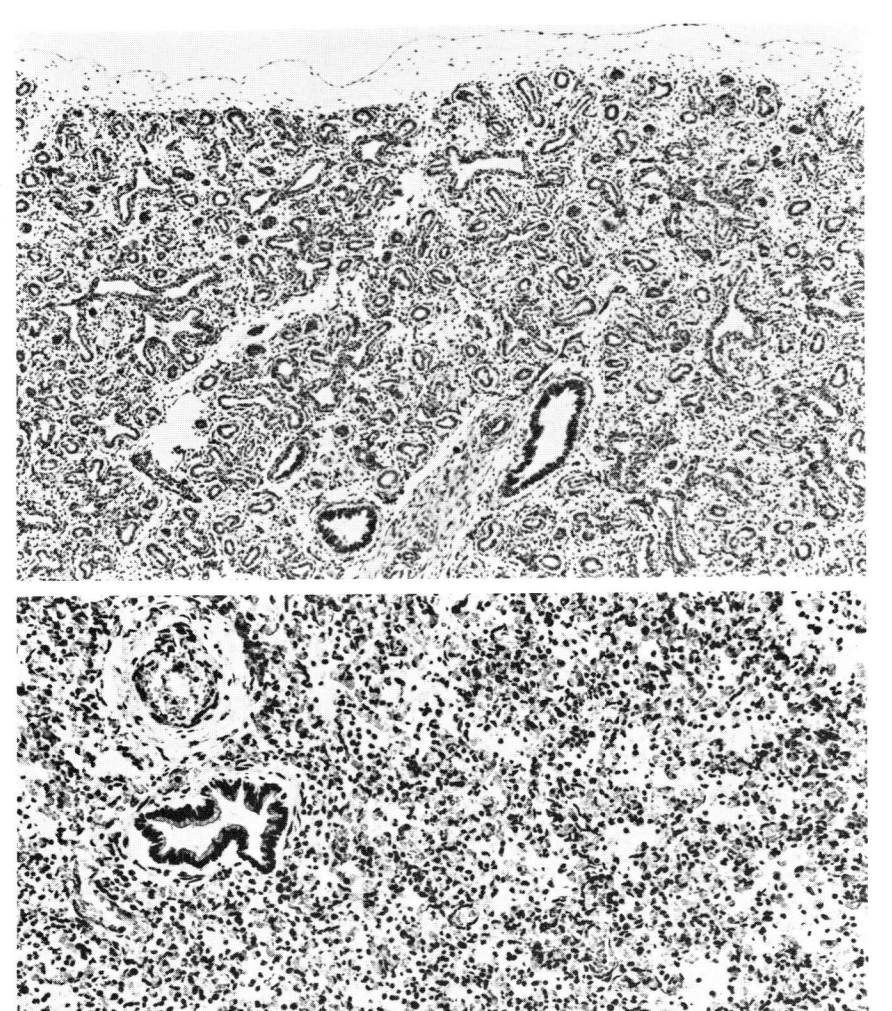

Figure 301. These tubular spaces are separated by considerable amounts of myxoid connective tissue and come from a fetal lung. A bronchus is seen just to the right of center above the lower margin; the upper margin is pleura with loose connective tissue and mesothelial lining. *Fetal lung*, canalicular phase of development, from sixteen-twenty up to twenty-six or thirty weeks of gestation (×60)

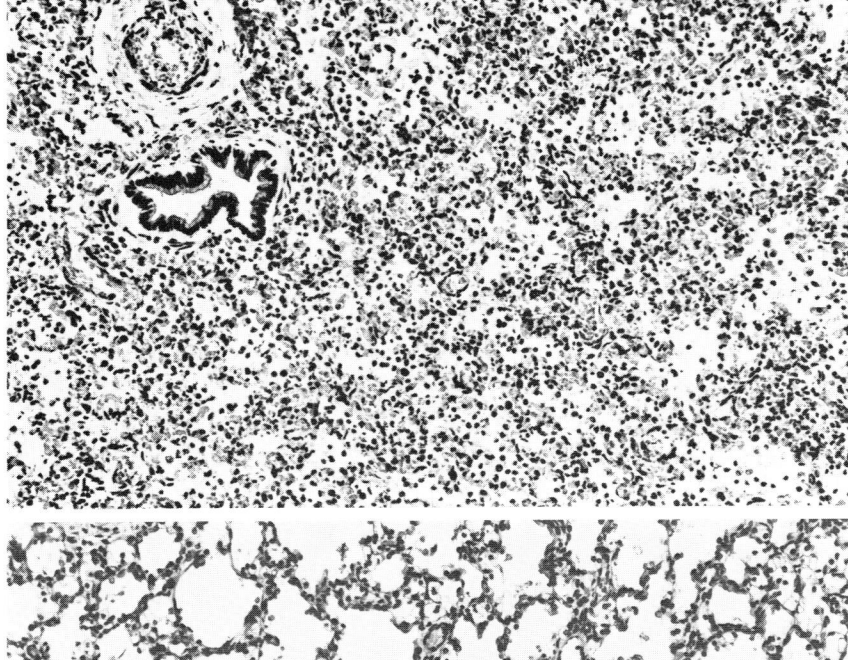

Figure 302. By full term some alveoli are present, but most of the spaces are terminal ducts. The majority of alveoli develop after birth. This specimen comes from a full-term infant delivered by cesarean section after intrauterine death and approximates the normal unexpanded state, with cells and fluid in alveoli. *Fetal lung* (×120)

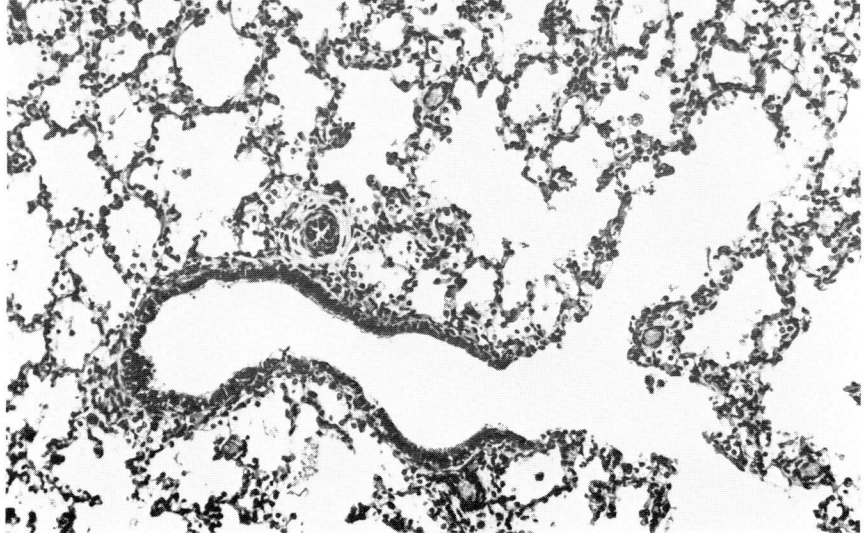

Figure 303. By contrast, this is a lung from a full-term infant in which respiration was established. The air spaces are open and contain air (terminal sac phase). *Infant lung* (×120)

MULTIPERFORATES WITH LARGE SPACES

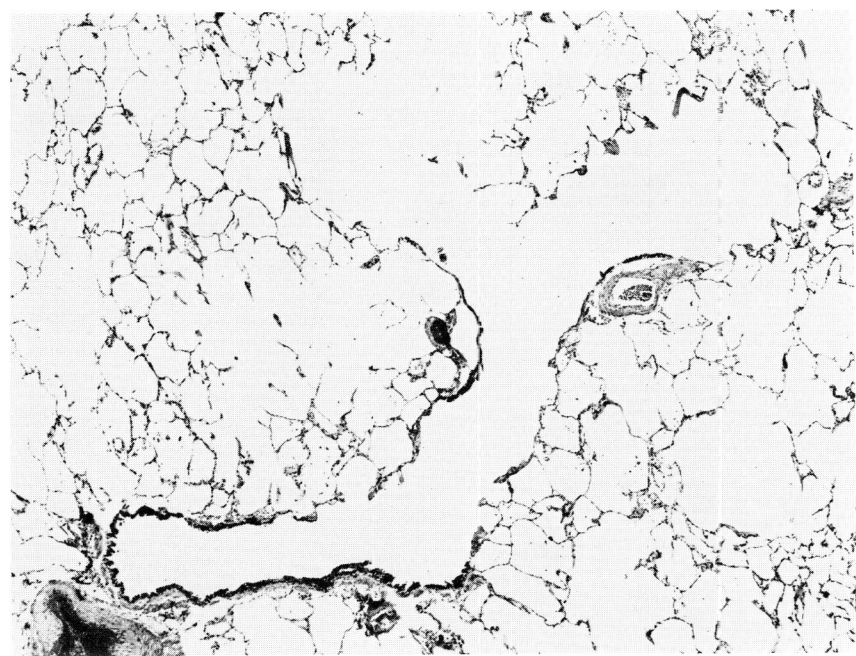

Figure 304. Running across the left lower quadrant is a terminal bronchiole; this turns obliquely upwards as a respiratory bronchiole with alveoli opening directly through its wall. Two alveolar ducts are seen above, their walls showing small nodules of muscle and also giving rise to alveoli. These ducts open into alveolar sacs (atria, or waiting rooms), which give rise to the terminal alveolar spaces. *Lung* (× 31)

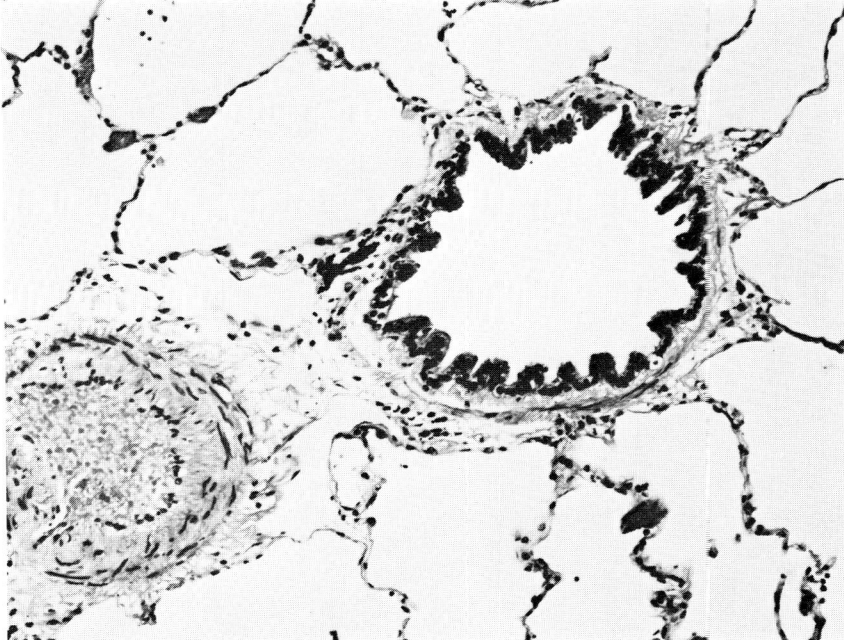

Figure 305. This bronchus is relatively thin walled, without cartilage or glands; it is therefore a terminal bronchiole. Scattered among the ciliated lining cells are peg-shaped nonciliated nonmucous Clara cells. The radiating alveolar walls act as supporting guy ropes to keep the lumens open. Each alveolar wall is a thin plate with collagen and elastin fibers and numerous capillaries faced on each side with an epithelium, which is so thin that it is visible only by electron microscopy. *Terminal bronchiole* and artery with alveolar walls (× 150)

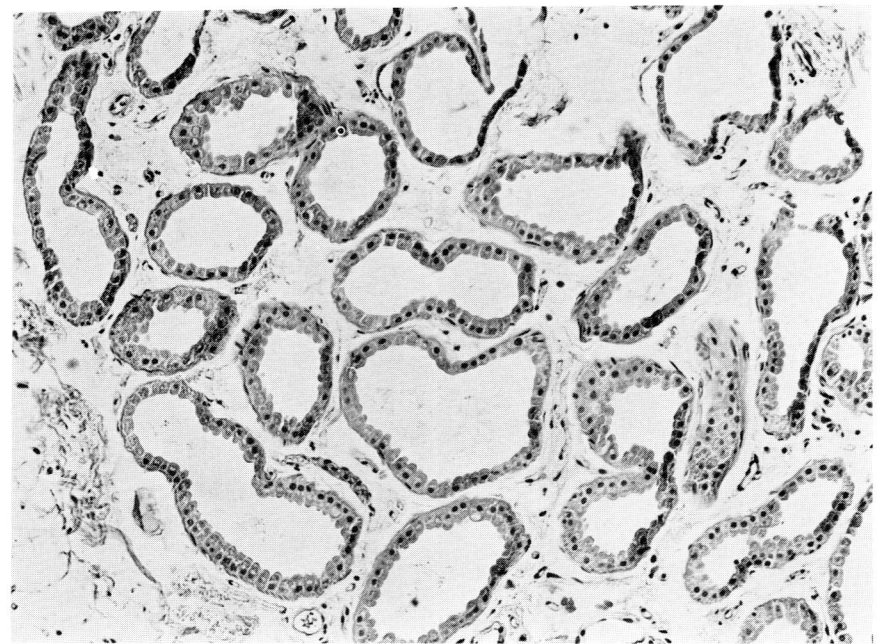

Figure 306. Multiple tubular and circular profiles lined by low columnar cells with distinctive eosinophilic pink cytoplasm, often with nipple-like projections, or snouts, are apocrine glands. A few myoepithelial cells with long nuclei can be seen at intervals beneath the lining epithelium running circumferentially. *Apocrine sweat glands* (× 120)

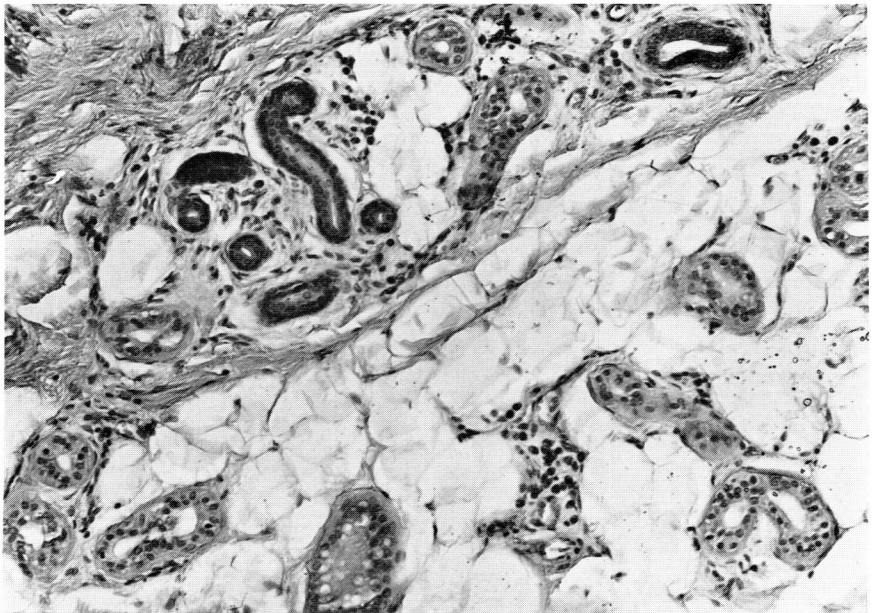

Figure 307. This figure can be divided obliquely into upper left and lower right, the former with a rather dense fibrous stroma, and the latter almost entirely adipose tissue. In both areas there are tubular and circular profiles. The darker staining tubules are ducts; the lighter staining tubules are the secretory glandular portions. Both have myoepithelial cells peripherally, more marked in the ducts. The lining cells are smaller than those of apocrine sweat glands and have pale cytoplasm without nipplelike projections. These glands lie in the lower dermis and upper subcutaneous tissue of the skin. *Eccrine sweat glands* (× 120)

MULTIPERFORATES WITH SMALL SPACES

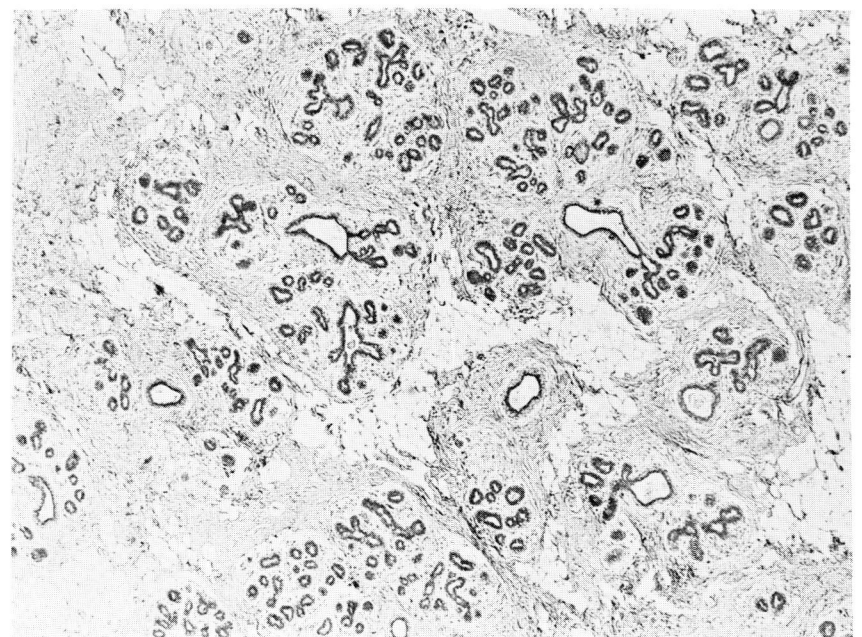

Figure 308. This figure shows numerous lobular collections of small parallel and circular profiles, some communicating with larger spaces, which are more clearly ducts. Within each lobule the connective tissue is rather loose. Around each lobule it is more dense and fibrous, and a considerable amount of adipose tissue may also be seen. This appearance is characteristic of *breast*. (× 27)

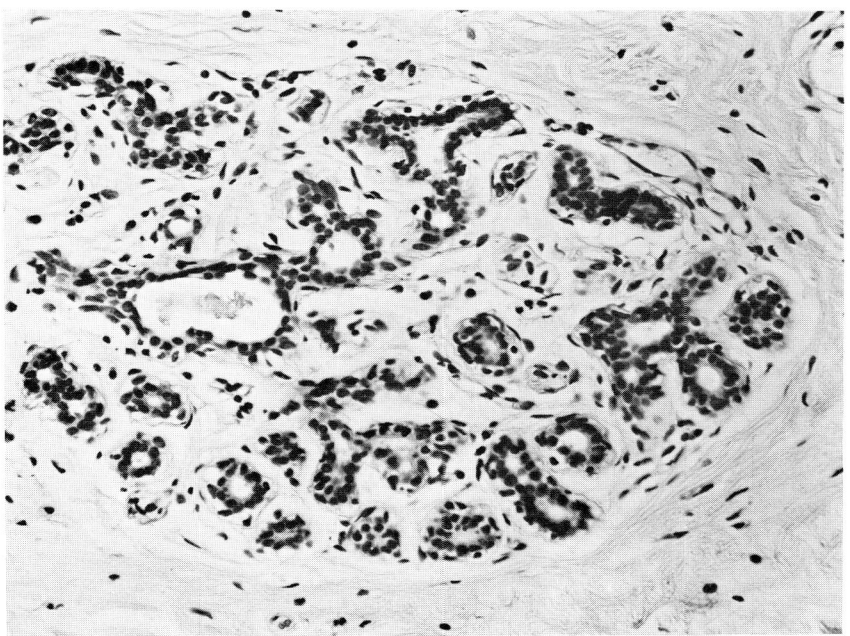

Figure 309. Higher magnification of one lobule shows the difference in stroma outside and within and shows the tubular nature of the glands and the double layer of lining cells with the beginnings of a larger duct in left center. The outer layer of cells (best seen in the center below the upper margin) has clear cytoplasm, and the nuclei are arranged like underlining marks; they are believed to have contractile processes embracing the inner epithelial cells and have thus also been termed basket cells. *Breast* (× 200)

MULTIPERFORATES WITH SMALL SPACES

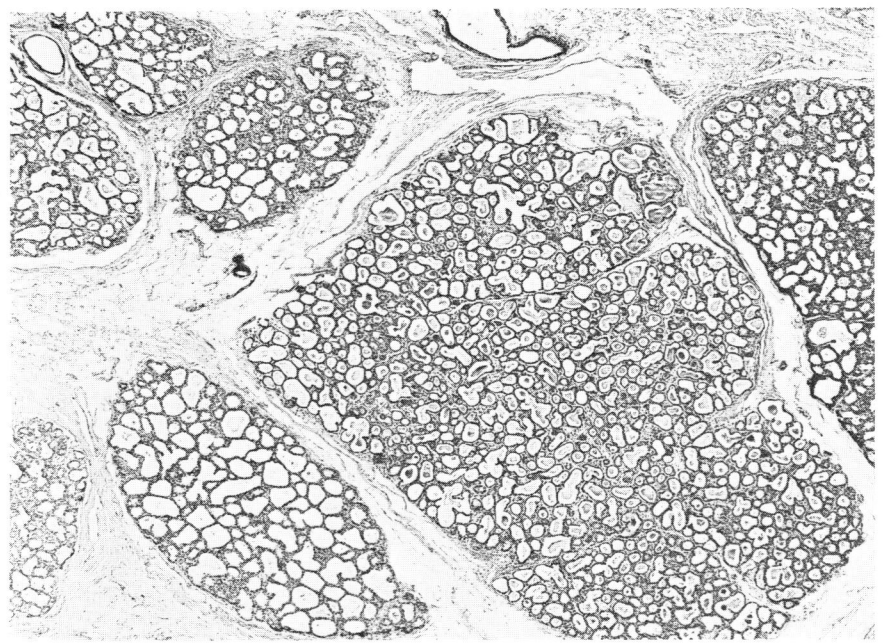

Figure 310. Here the lobules have become very large, and the number of acini in each lobule is enormously increased, so gland elements dominate over stromal components. Secretory material is seen within many of the spaces. The spaces are no longer small, but large. *Breast*, two days post partum (× 27)

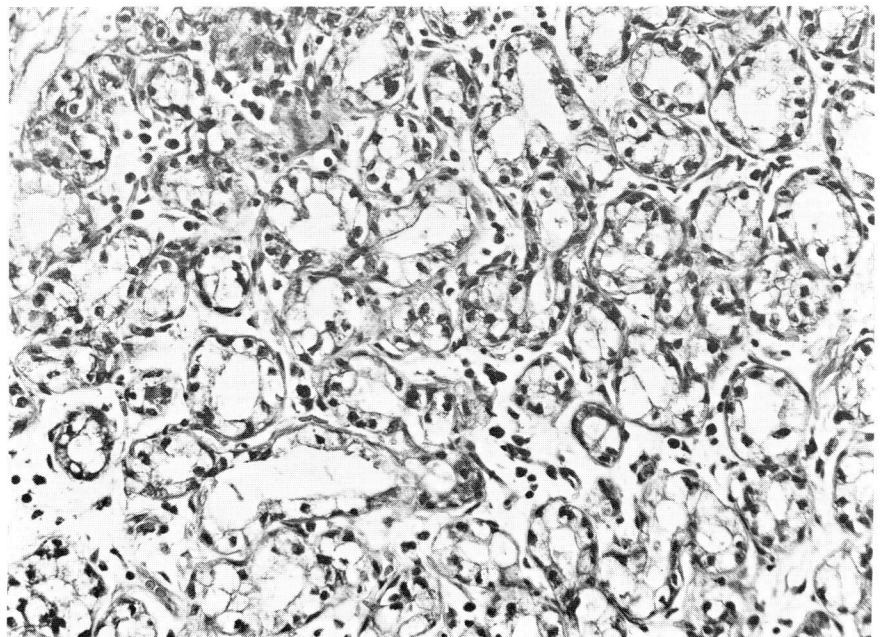

Figure 311. At high power the acini are crowed together, the epithelium is relatively tall, and the cytoplasm is clear because of the active secretion of milk. *Lactating breast*, nine days post partum (× 200)

MULTIPERFORATES WITH SMALL SPACES

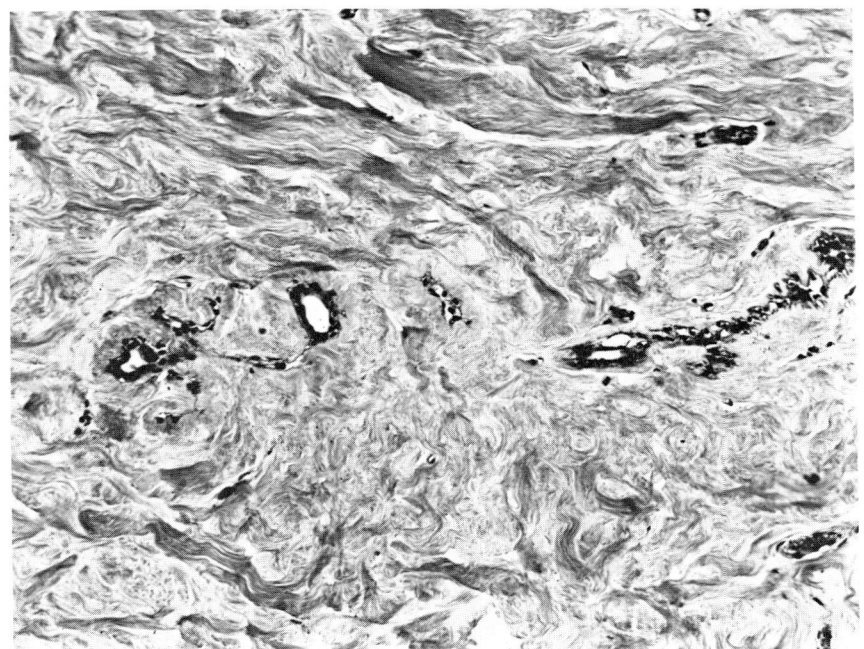

Figure 312. For convenience, other examples of breast tissue are shown here, even if they appear different and more like sweat glands. The stromal fibrous tissue here is dense and hyaline, while the epithelial components are few and reduced to occasional ducts. However, these still have the double epithelial lining of mammary glands. This appearance is normal for the atrophic breast of elderly women. *Atrophic breast* (×120)

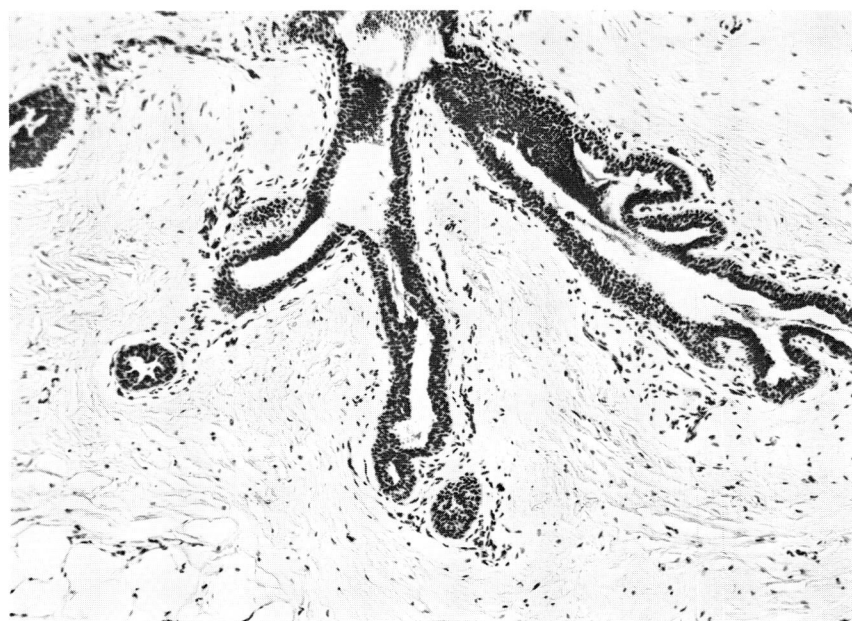

Figure 313. In males, the ducts fail to develop their terminal divisions and lobules, remaining more comparable to the prepubertal female breast. At puberty the epithelium may become heightened and papillary, while the surrounding stroma becomes edematous. This is a hormonal alteration, which in its extreme form may cause breast enlargement known as gynecomastia. *Young adult male breast* (×80)

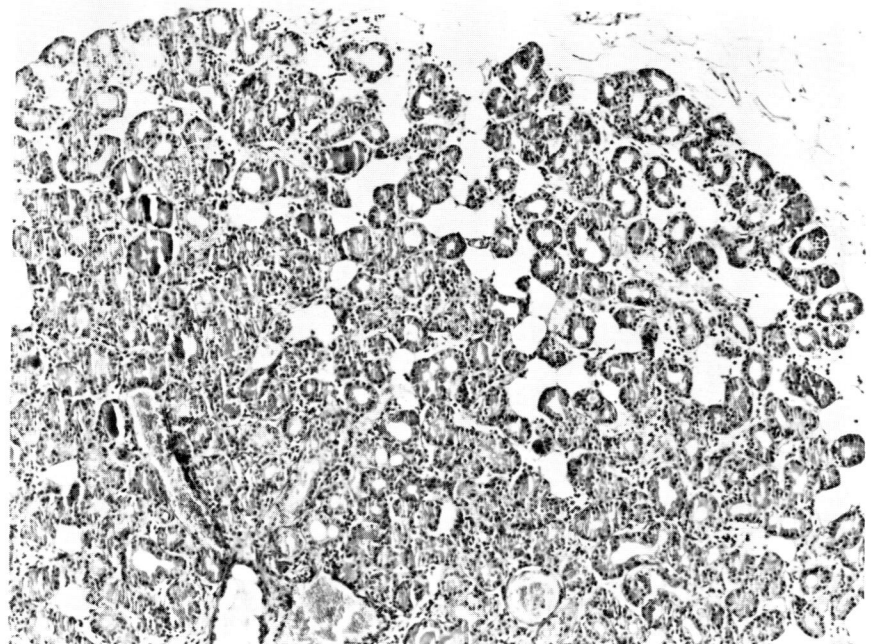

Figure 314. Here small circular profiles predominate with an ovoid duct on the left lower edge of the figure. The acini are open, with readily visible lumens; the lining cells are of a single type with a gray, finely granular (serous) cytoplasm. A small amount of fat is seen, not only outside the gland but also within, most easily identified as two pale tracts running almost vertically downward from the upper margin at the center. *Serous glands, lacrimal* (× 120)

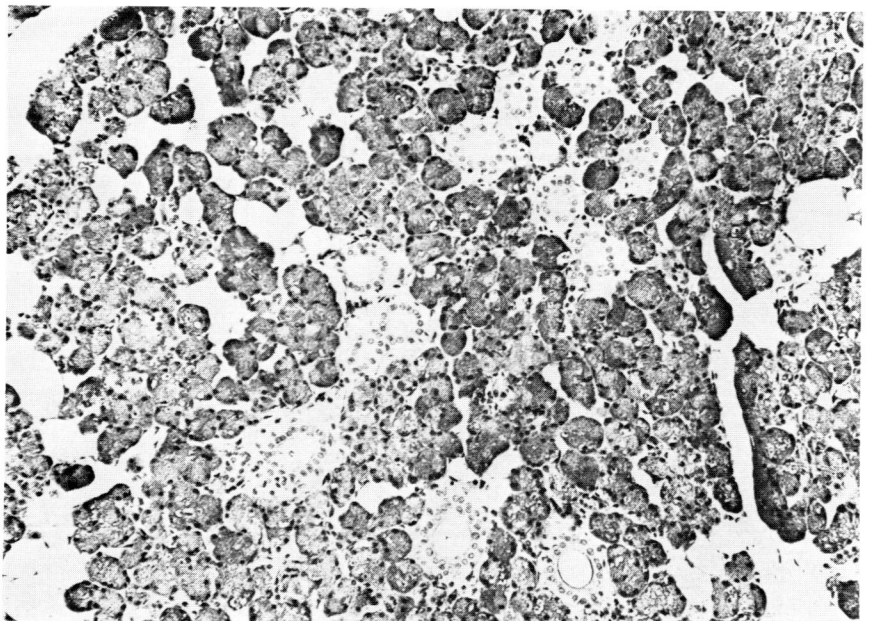

Figure 315. Here there are multiple small closed circular profiles whose cells have dark, finely granular cytoplasm. There are also a number of larger circular profiles, which are ducts lined by cells with bright eosinophilic cytoplasm. The epithelium of the small acinar spaces is uniformly serous in character, which identifies the parotid. A small amount of fat is included between acini. *Parotid* (× 100)

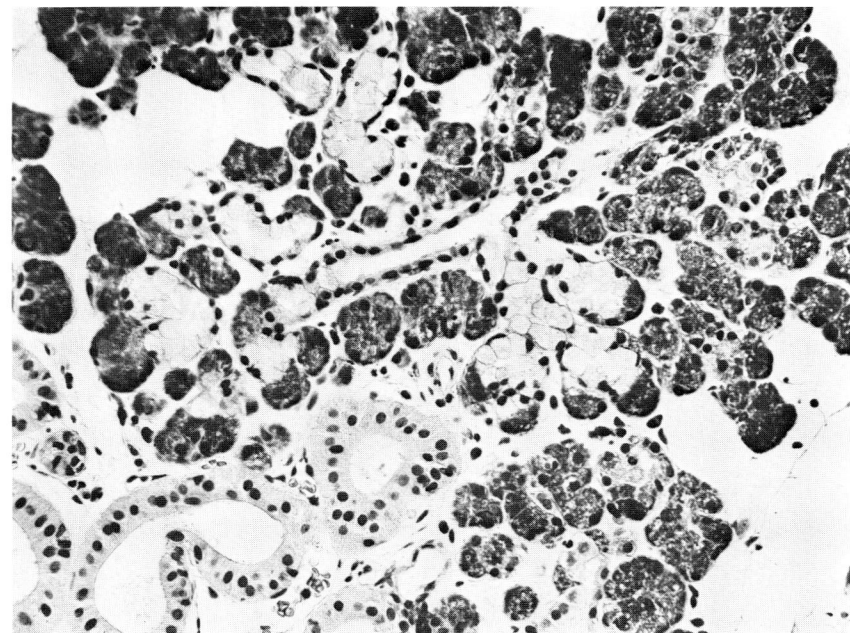

Figure 316. In this figure, ducts with double rows of lining cells are seen in the left lower quadrant. Most of the acini in the upper right are serous in nature, but around the center there are also clear mucous cells, some embraced by dark serous cells to constitute the crescents (demilunes) of Giannuzzi. This is a mixed type of gland and therefore can be identified as the *mandibular,* or submaxillary. (×200)

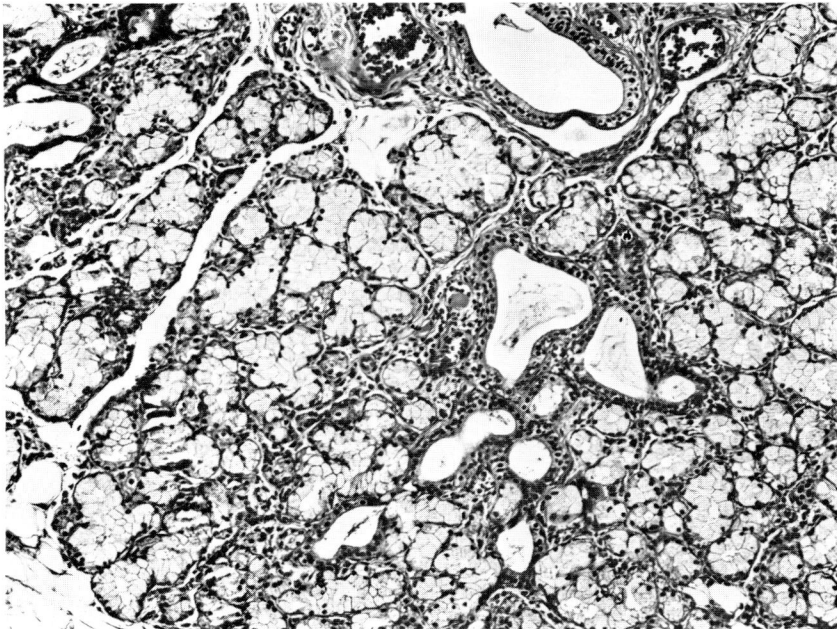

Figure 317. By contrast, the great majority of acini here are lined by uniformly clear mucous cells. Ducts are seen in the center of the field. Occasional serous cells may be found (although not shown here), but the predominance of mucous cells identifies the *sublingual gland.* (×100)

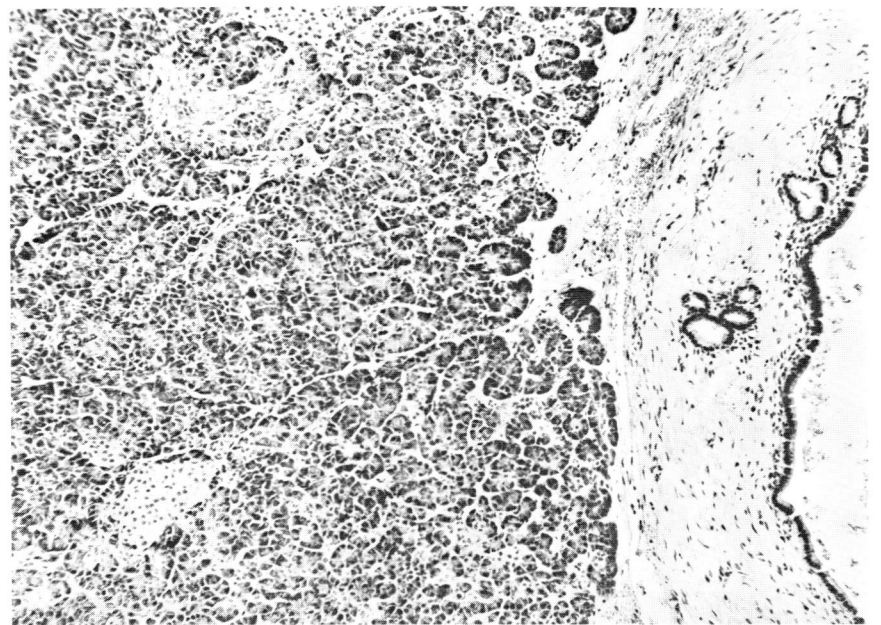

Figure 318. The left two-thirds of this figure contain innumerable small acini, closed, and barely recognizable as spaces. In the left lower quadrant is a small island of paler cells, an even smaller example lying immediately above it. These are islets of Langerhans. Across the right margin of the figure is a duct lined by a single layer of columnar cells with a few minor ducts and gland spaces in its wall. *Pancreas* ($\times 80$)

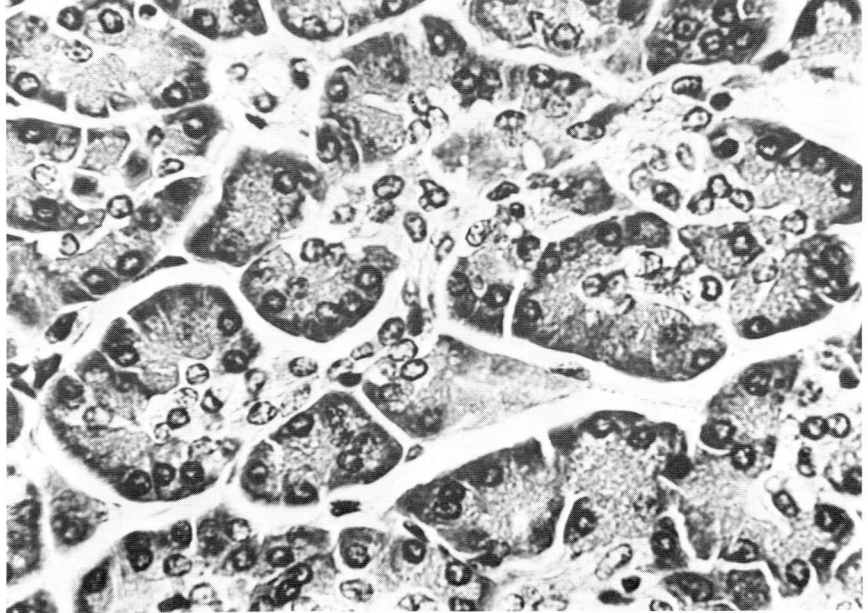

Figure 319. The zymogenic cells of the pancreas are bichromic, with dark-staining basal areas due to content of mitochondria and eosinophilic apices due to secretory granules. Normally the acini are essentially closed. Running downwards in the center of the field then turning obliquely to the left lower quadrant is a double row of nuclei, which represents a small duct. This extends into the concavity of the C-shaped group of parenchymal (zymogen) cells on the left, the enfolded terminal portion of the duct constituting the centroacinar cells. *Pancreas* ($\times 504$)

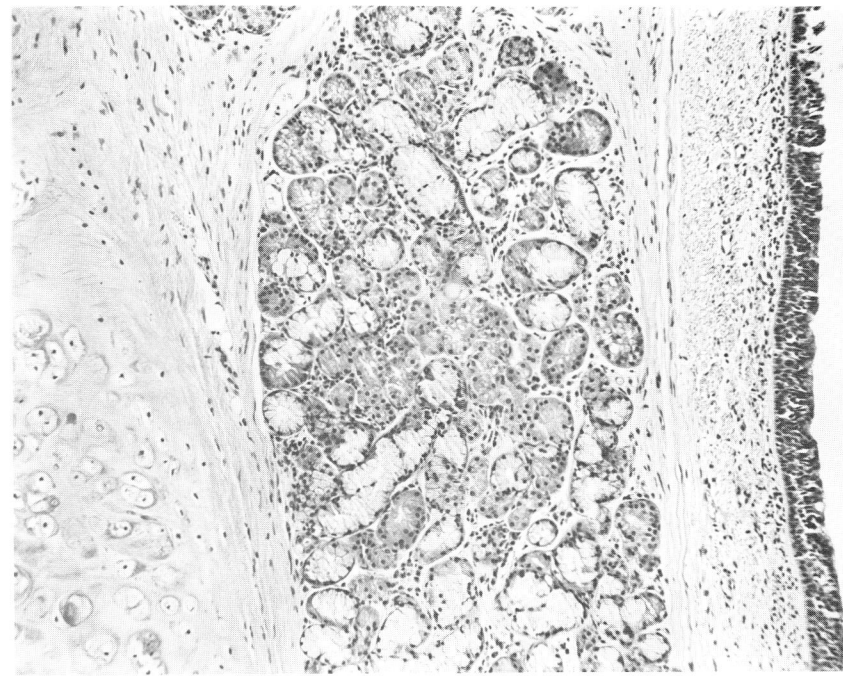

Figure 320. Down the right margin is a pseudostratified ciliated epithelium, in the left lower quarter is cartilage, and between is a collection of glands of mixed type. Some of the acini are serous, some are purely mucous, and some have demilunes with peripheral serous cells and central mucous cells. This mixture is a feature of many minor salivary glands. *Minor glands, trachea* (×110)

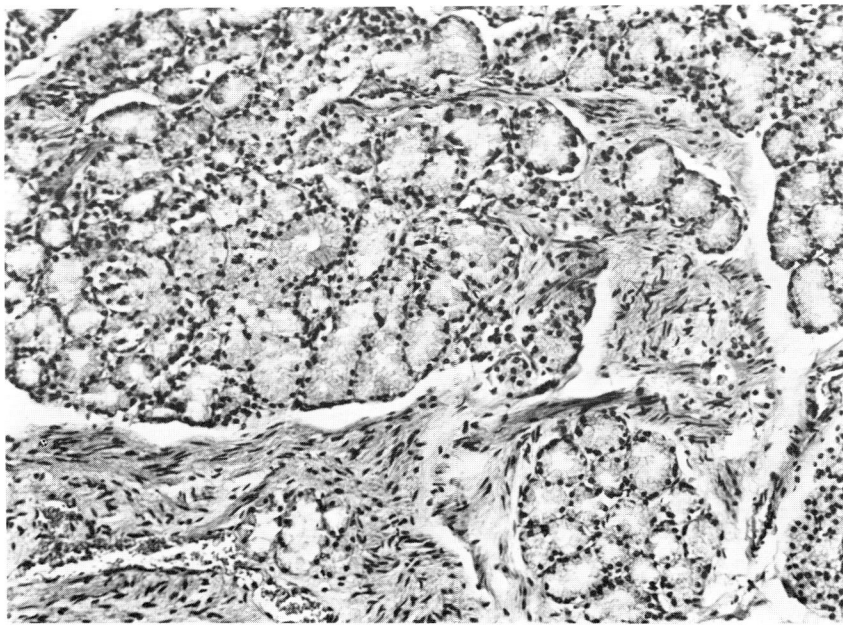

Figure 321. These lobules are separated by strands of nonstriated muscle, which are most obvious in the left lower quarter. The acini are small and are lined by cells with opalescent or clear mucus-secreting cytoplasm. Such glands are found in the duodenum, chiefly in the first part, but extending to the third part and are known as *Brunner's glands.* (×100)

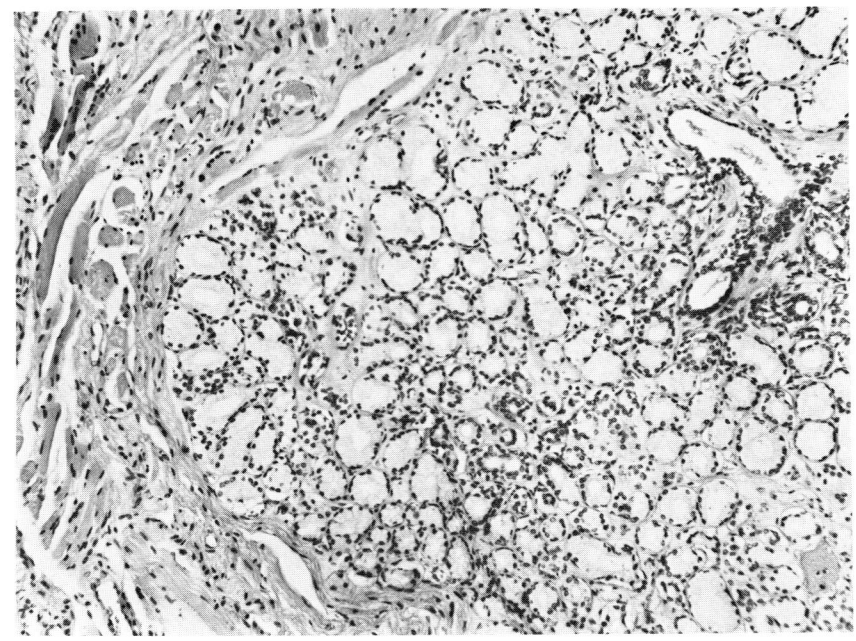

Figure 322. This gland is composed of acini lined by tall, clear mucus-secreting cells. Capsule is seen on the left with nonstriated muscle fibers, which may penetrate within the gland as septa. This is the bulbourethral gland of Cowper, which lies in close relation to the male urethra just below the perineal membrane. *Cowper's gland* (×80)

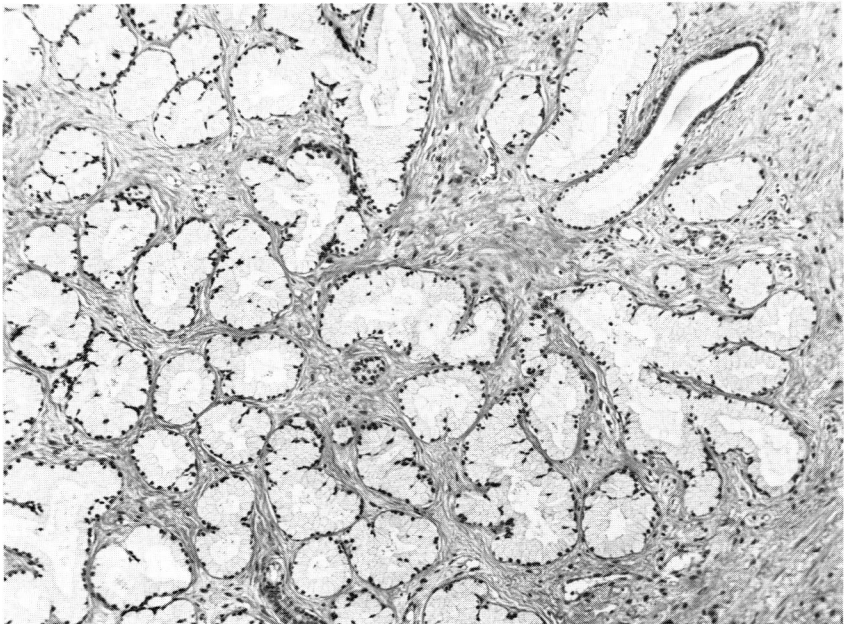

Figure 323. Tubular and circular profiles seen here within dense fibrous tissue and lined by very tall, columnar, clear, mucus-secreting cells are found in Bartholin's glands, which open in the groove between the labia minora and hymen. In the right upper quadrant is the beginning of a duct. Ducts are lined by variable types of epithelium, often transitional or stratified columnar in type, with small glands opening directly through their walls. *Bartholin's gland,* major vestibular or vulvovaginal gland (×80)

Practical Identification

Solid Sections

Many solids are dominated by a single tissue family, which can be immediately recognized as epithelial, neural, muscle, or connective tissue. Within the one family, however, there may be different types of tissues. In the central nervous system, neurones can be regarded as forming a different tissue than the glial tissues of supporting astrocytes, although there is such an intimate admixture that they must be treated together. In the bones, there is an intermingling of osseous elements, adipose tissue, and myeloid tissue, all in the connective tissue family.

In other types of construction, different tissue families are involved. Strictly speaking, all epithelial, neural, and muscle solids include connective tissue elements either as stroma, as wrappings, or at least in blood vessels. Conversely, solids that are preponderantly connective tissues may have an epithelial covering when they project into cavities. Thus, the umbilical cord is covered with amniotic epithelium, and the appendices epiploicae are covered by the mesothelium of the peritoneal cavity. The ossicles of the middle ear have an epithelial surface, a unique combination. Certain lymphoid parts are partly covered by epithelium, as with the adenoid and tonsil. In the thymus, a predominant lymphocytic background includes Hassall's corpuscles of epithelial nature and a less conspicuous network of epithelial cells.

Epithelial Solids

Epithelial solids include the endocrine glands, the liver, and the skin appendages. A useful subdivision is to distinguish those with large cells from those with small cells. An epithelial solid with large cells may be liver, adrenal, sebaceous gland, or hair follicle. The radiating plates of hepatic cells, almost invariably accompanied by at least one triad or central vein, however small the section, are distinctive. Large epithelial cells in double cell plates lying in parallel, the cells containing cholesterol, identify the adrenal, which may appear as an island with distinctive contour. Microparts encountered within the dermis or subcutaneous tissue are sebaceous glands and hair follicles. In the former, the cells are large and vacuolated with lipid content, while the latter is associated with the keratin of the developing hair.

Solid tissue formed of small epithelial cells includes the islets of Langerhans, seen among pancreatic acini, and the parathyroid. The latter is usually a free-standing island, which has been dissected out of connective tissue bed and is recognized by its intermingling sheets and cords of small epithelial cells, among which are clusters and cords of fat cells. A mixture of small, intermediate, and large epithelial cells is characteristic of the pituitary.

Neural Solids

While neuroanatomists have justifiably studied not only serial blocks but serial sections of brain and cord, this is not practical as a routine, and a compromise is usually made. Most of the important structures of the brain can be seen in blocks taken from areas identified by naked eye to include the frontal and occipital poles, the diencephalon at the level of the mammillary bodies, the midbrain at the levels of the superior and inferior colliculi, the mid and lower pons, the medulla above and below the olives, and the cerebellar vermis and hemisphere.

With very large parts, the block is cut to include some distinctive external configuration or part of the ventricular system, whenever possible, to assist in orientation at microscopic level. This is because so many structures that are highly important and that are functionally different are not particularly distinctive morphologically, being combinations of neuron groups and fiber tracts. Identification becomes largely a matter of recognizing gray and white matter in particular positions and arrangements.

A solid neural section may have definable size and contour, as when larger nerves, the spinal cord, and brain stem are cut across. If large glass slides are used, the frontal and occipital poles may also appear in this form. Neural enclaves include the cylindrical nuclear tracts of the spinal cord and some of the nuclei of the brain itself. Peripheral nerve enclaves are the small nerves and nerve endings in connective tissues.

Muscle Solids

With muscle solids the size and shape of the section is little help in identification, and they are thus seldom recognizable as to origin. The large skeletal muscles appear as cutout sections, and small bundles as islands. Muscle spindles are solid microparts found within skeletal muscle. The walls of the heart can usually be examined by through-and-through sections, with endothelium on one surface and serosa on the other; they have been described with lineate sections. The sinuatrial and atrioventricular nodes appear as enclaves within cardiac muscle fibers of larger size, and the general shape of the section may enable them to be localised with confidence. Structures that include visceral muscle are essentially hollow parts, of which only the uterus is so thick that a full-sized cutout solid section is ordinarily obtained, rather than a lineate or annulate type of preparation.

Connective Tissue Solids

Connective tissue solids are divided into two categories — segregated connective tissues in which collagen, elastin, reticulin, or acid mucopolysaccharide separates the cells, and tissues constructed of myeloid and lymphatic tissues. In the first category, large parts seen by cutout sections may be derived from bone or fat but are not further identifiable. Insular sections include the umbilical cord, the round ligament of the uterus, the meniscus of a knee joint, the ossicles of the middle ear, and the appendices epiploicae. Very small islands seen as multiple repeating units projecting into large open spaces are found in the choroid plexuses, the arachnoid villi, and the chorionic villi. Tendons, ligaments, and small bones such as ribs and phalanges, when dissected out, appear as islands, but if small, they may also be seen as enclaves within other connective tissues.

Myeloid tissue, although functionally an organ, is morphologically one of the tissues found within bone. On the other hand, lymphoid solids include large parts such as the thymus and spleen (from which cutout sections are obtained), smaller macroparts such as the tonsils, adenoids, and lymph nodes (from which insular sections are derived), and microscopic nodules of lymphocytes (found as enclaves) in the wall of the intestine in Peyer's patches, in the lymphoid follicles of the appendix, and elsewhere.

EPITHELIAL SOLIDS

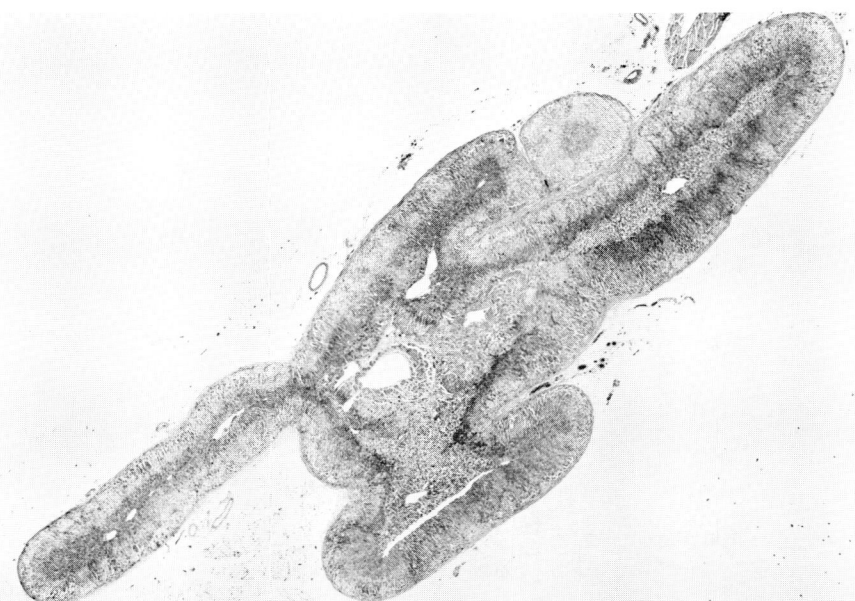

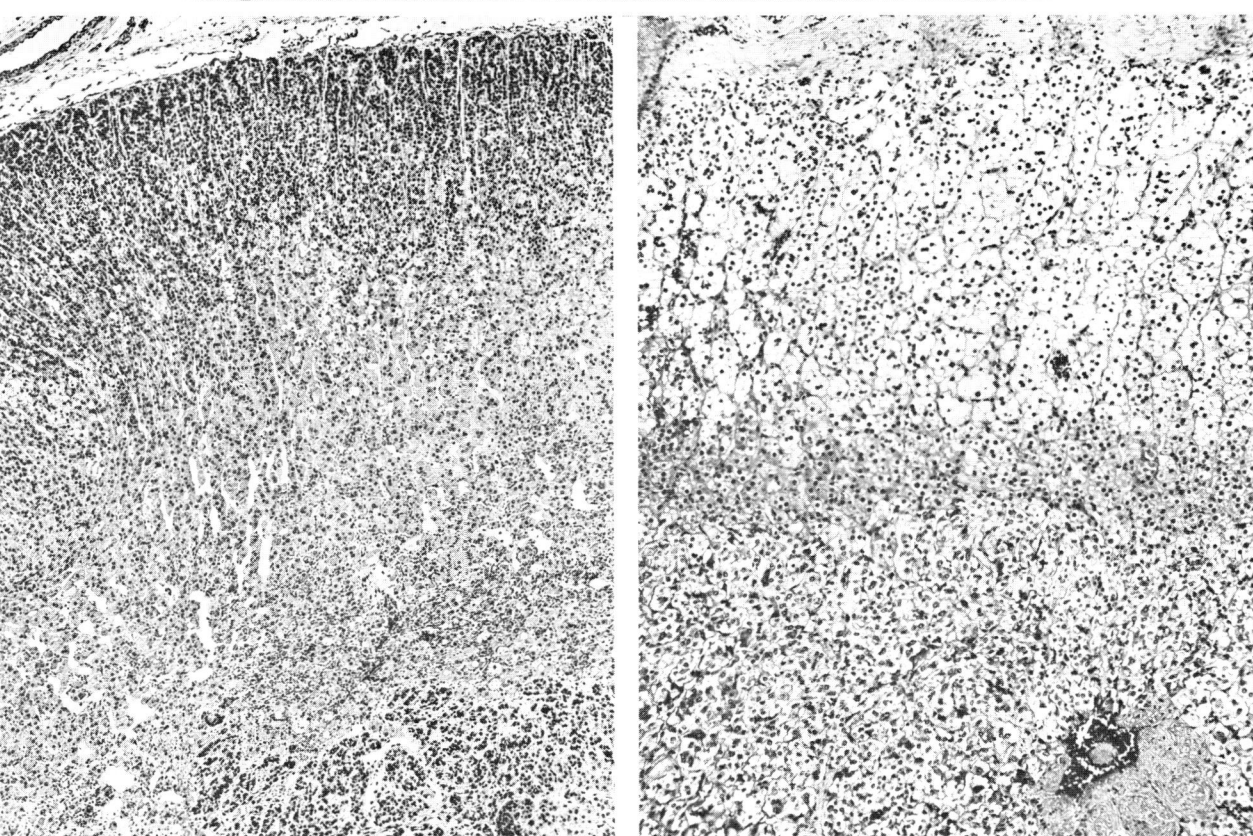

Figure 324. A large irregular island separable into cortex and medulla and composed of large epithelial cells is the adrenal. A flat adrenal, as shown here, comes from the right side; a more triangular contour indicates the left side. In the fetus, there is a very broad zone of provisional cortex that begins to atrophy shortly after birth. In the adult cortex there are three distinct zones: (from outside in) the glomerulosa, fasciculata, and reticularis. The zona reticularis differentiates at about three months of age and is the dark band seen in part a. It runs across the center of part c. The fasciculata has double cell plates, arranged perpendicular to the surface. The adrenal vein seen in the right lower corner of part c has a characteristic variation in the thickness of the muscle in the wall.
a. *Adrenal* (×6.5) b. *Fetal adrenal,* provisional cortex (×50) c. *Adult adrenal* (×80)

EPITHELIAL SOLIDS

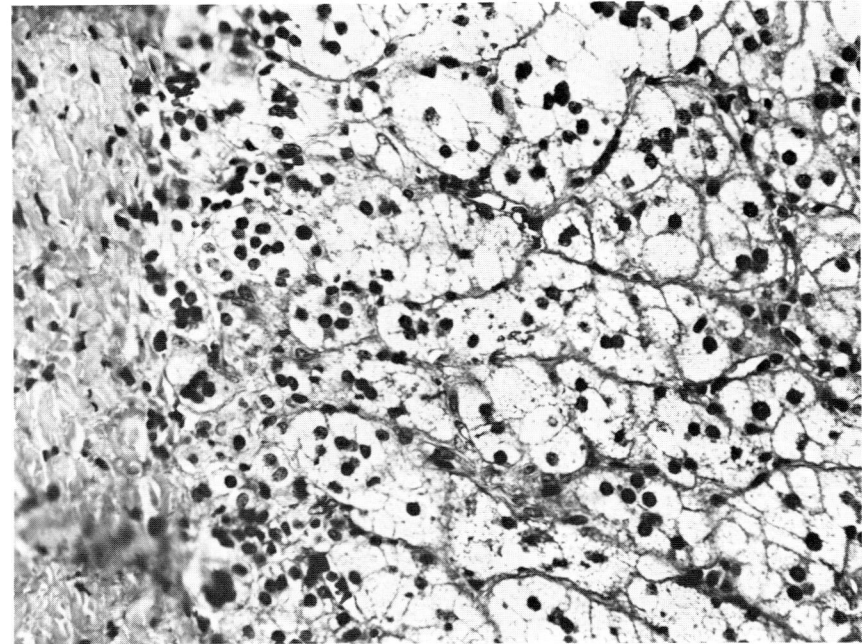

Figure 325. The fibrous band seen down the left margin is the adrenal capsule with the rounded cell clusters of the zona glomerulosa immediately adjacent to it. The center of the figure is the zona fasciculata, with rows of very large vacuolated cells; the darker brown cells of the reticularis containing brown lipofuscin granules are just appearing at the right edge. *Adrenal cortex* (×250)

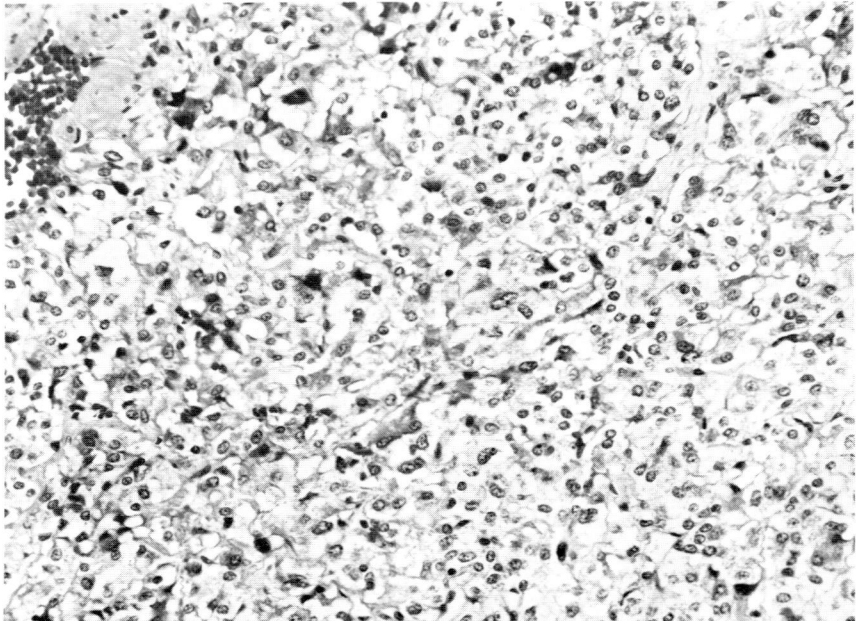

Figure 326. This is also from adrenal. Here the cells are large but show no particular arrangement. Some have a dark cytoplasm, while others are light or gray. After fixation in dichromate, medullary cells appear brown. Cells producing noradrenalin can be selectively stained after formalin fixation as argyrophil. Others are associated with adrenalin formation and will react with lead hematoxylin. The central vein is seen in the left upper corner. *Adrenal medulla* (×250)

EPITHELIAL SOLIDS

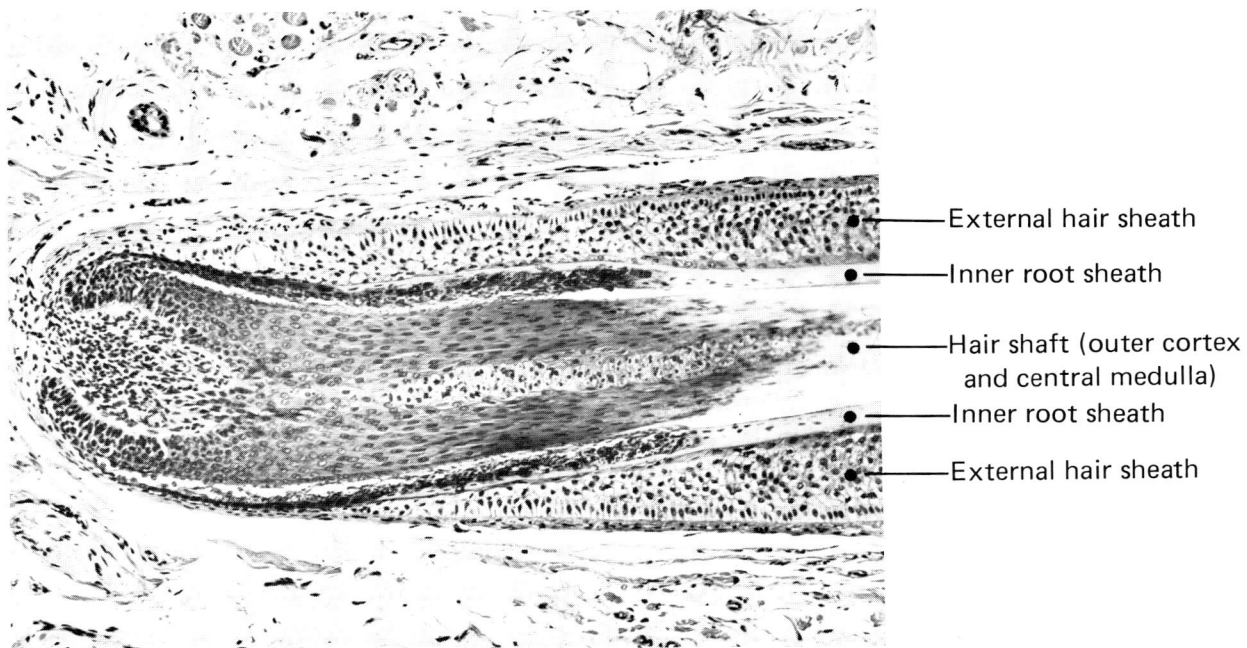

Figure 327. On the left is the root of a hair follicle, with curving epithelial pincers embracing a vascular papilla and extending to the right (outwards) as cellular bands, which become hyalinized at the right margin to form the hair shaft. The hair itself may be fine (lanugo hair of infants, and the "down," or vellus hair of adults) or coarse (terminal hairs, as in the beard, eyelashes, and scalp.) *Hair follicle* (×100)

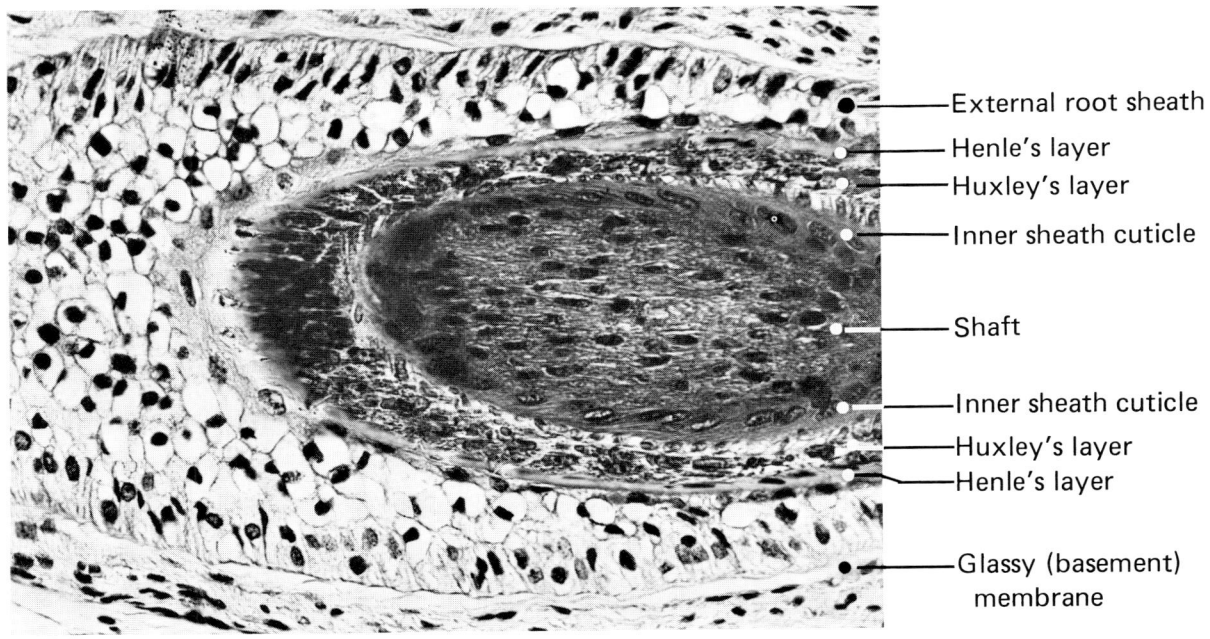

Figure 328. As can be seen at high power, the inner root sheath has three layers. The outer is known as Henle's layer and is recognized as a single narrow row of flat, elongated nuclei, here associated with dense hyalinized cytoplasm. Central to this is a thicker zone two to three cells deep with brightly eosinophilic, coarse keratohyaline granules (Huxley's layer). Between this and the hair shaft is a row of more cuboidal clear cells, which constitute the inner sheath cuticle. *Hair* (×300)

EPITHELIAL SOLIDS

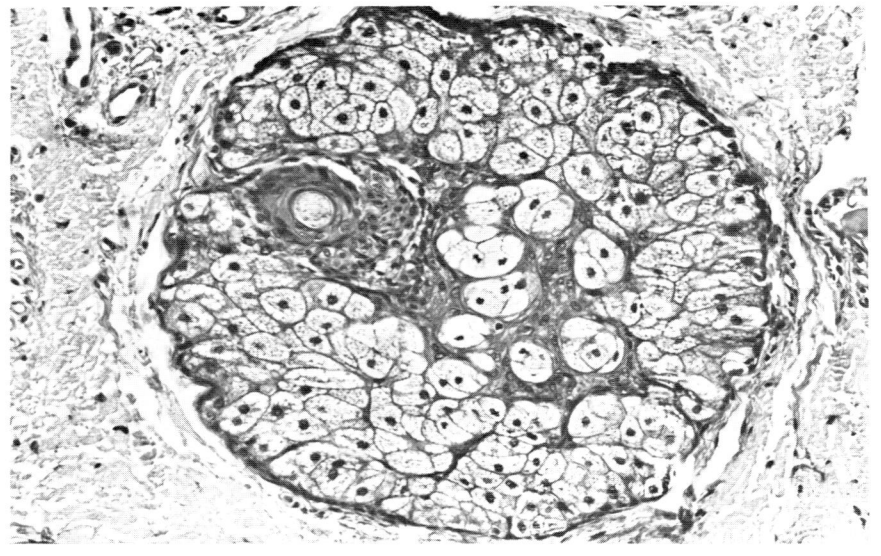

Figure 329. This is an enclave of solid appearance, with large foamy cells in tessellated arrangement. On the left side is a small hair follicle, into which cells desquamate in holocrine fashion. Frozen sections would show lipid cytoplasmic content. *Sebaceous gland* (×160)

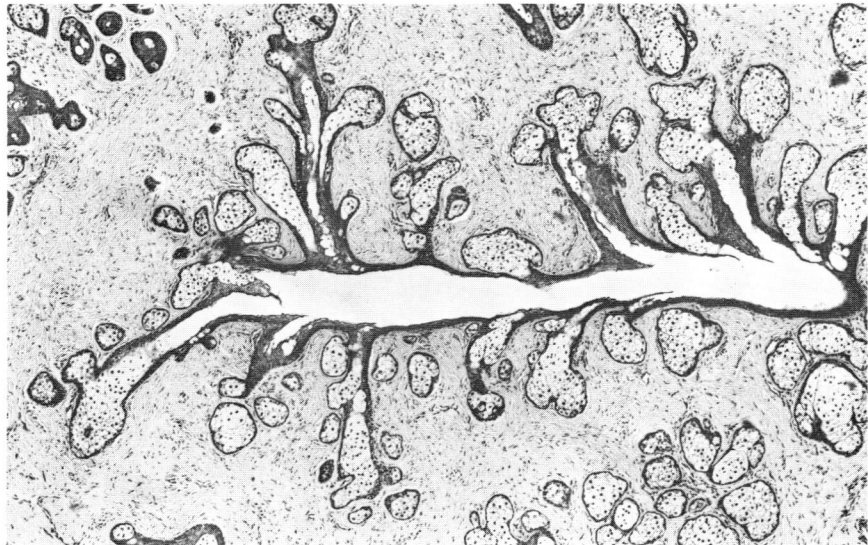

Figure 330. Multiple small sebaceous glands are here seen in a unique arrangement, strung along and communicating with a large horizontal duct. They lie within an unusually dense fibrous tissue, the tarsal plate. The duct opens on the margin of the eyelid. *Meibomian gland* (×50)

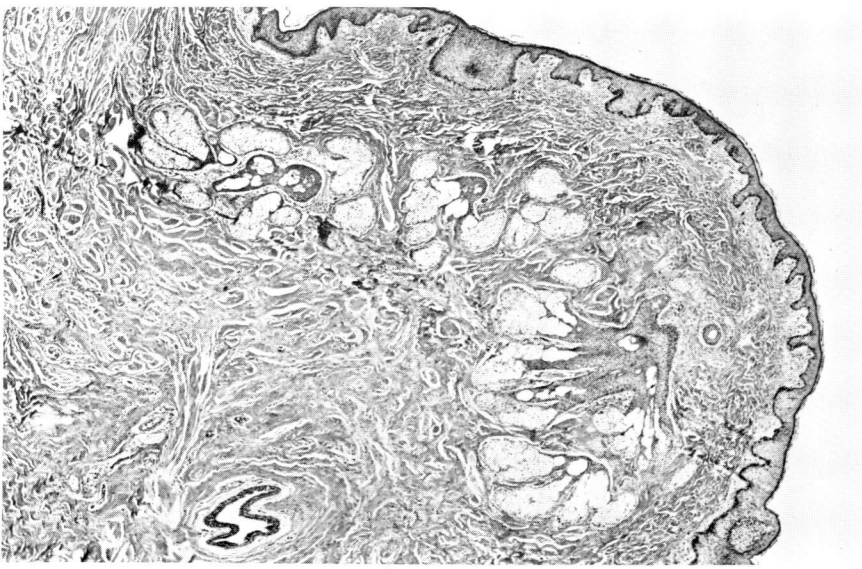

Figure 331. This is a nodular elevation of skin with numerous sebaceous glands, most of which on serial sectioning could be found opening directly on the skin and relatively few into small hair follicles (of which only one is seen). A large duct is present along the lower margin, and there is an unusual amount of nonstriated muscle. This combination is unique for the *Montgomery's tubercles* of the areola of the breast. (×22)

EPITHELIAL SOLIDS

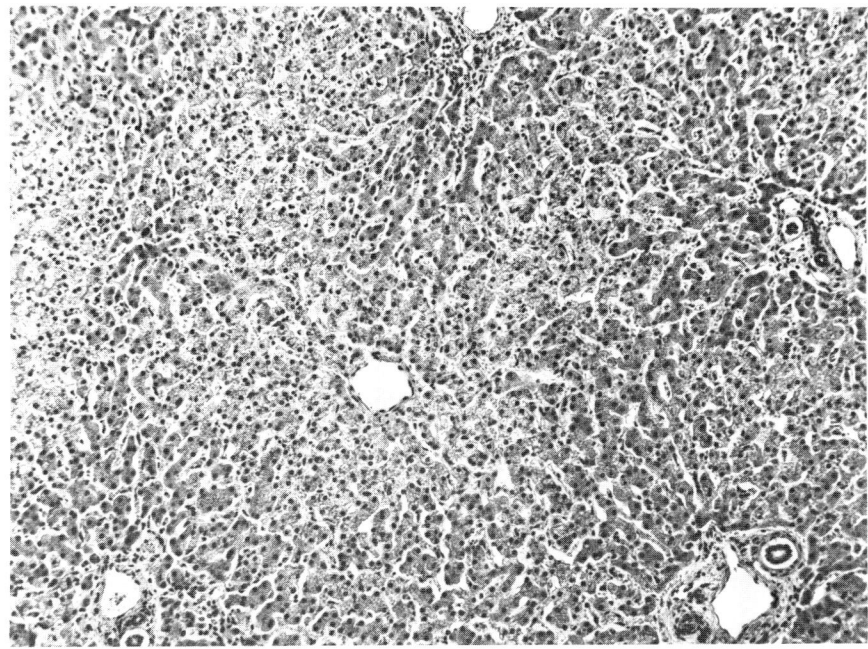

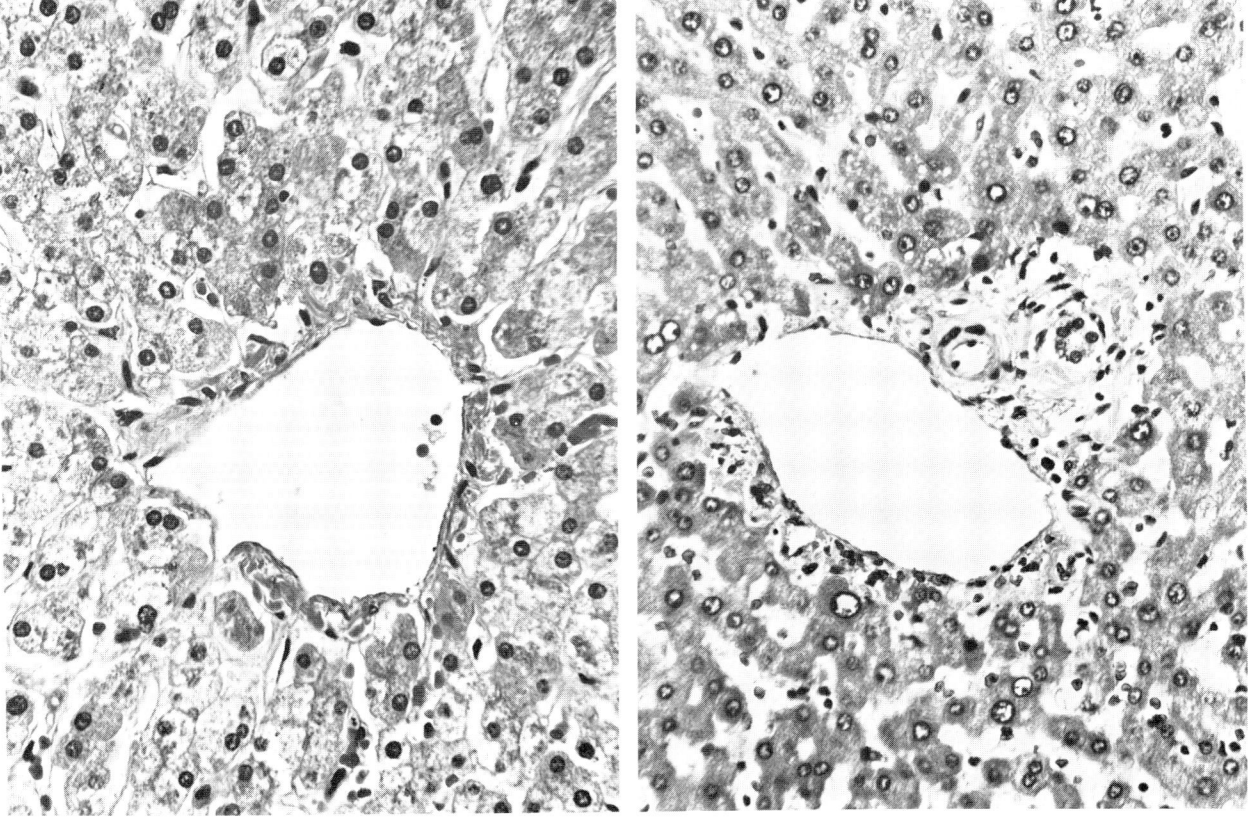

Figure 332. Single cell plates (double in infants) of large epithelial cells in radiating arrangement identify the liver. Slits between the plates contain the venous sinusoids, separated from the hepatic cells by Disse's spaces. a. Close to center is a central vein; the other spaces are triads, each with duct, artery, and portal vein. Low power survey. *Liver* (×80) b. A central vein is seen at higher power with sinusoids lined by flattened nuclei of endothelial and Kupffer's cells. *Central vein area* (×250) c. A triad is shown, the artery lying between the large vein and the small duct with its cuboidal epithelium. *Portal triad* (×250)

EPITHELIAL SOLIDS

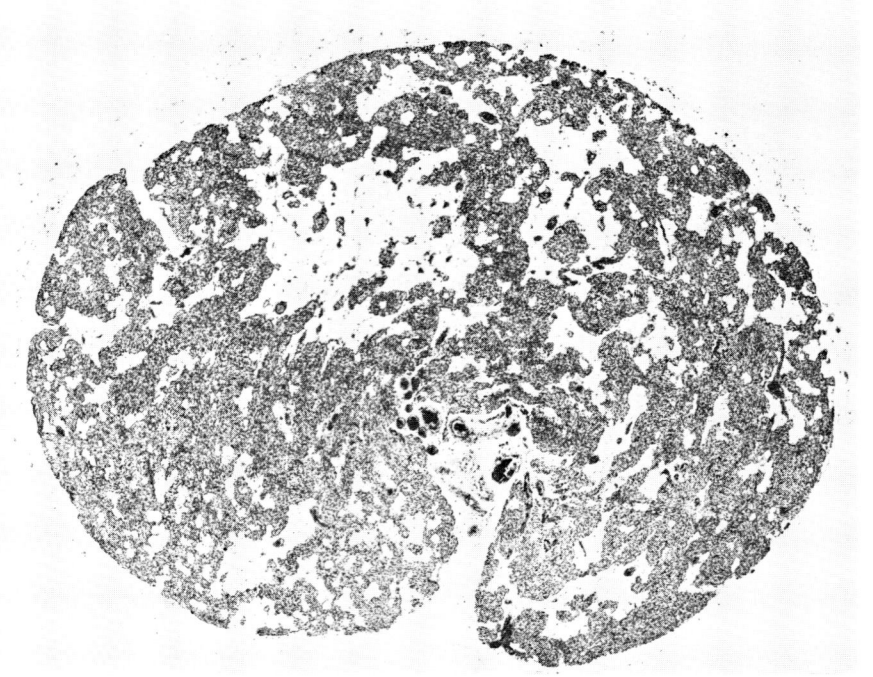

Figure 333. This is a small insular solid surrounded by loose fibrous tissue and poorly encapsulated. It is composed of small cells in irregular anastomosing bands and broader sheets, with considerable numbers of interspersed fat cells. *Parathyroid* (× 23)

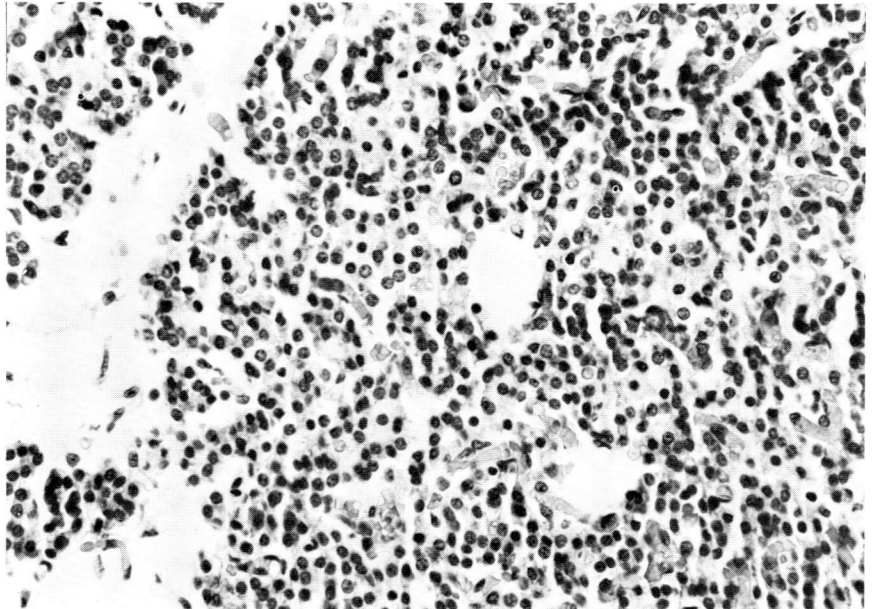

Figure 334. Higher power shows small epithelial cells without definite arrangement, the nuclei uniform and round. Cell walls are not particularly distinct. These are chief cells, which contain small amounts of glycogen. Most adult glands include small groups of eosinophilic cells, and occasional cells may have abundant clear cytoplasm. *Parathyroid* (× 300)

EPITHELIAL SOLIDS

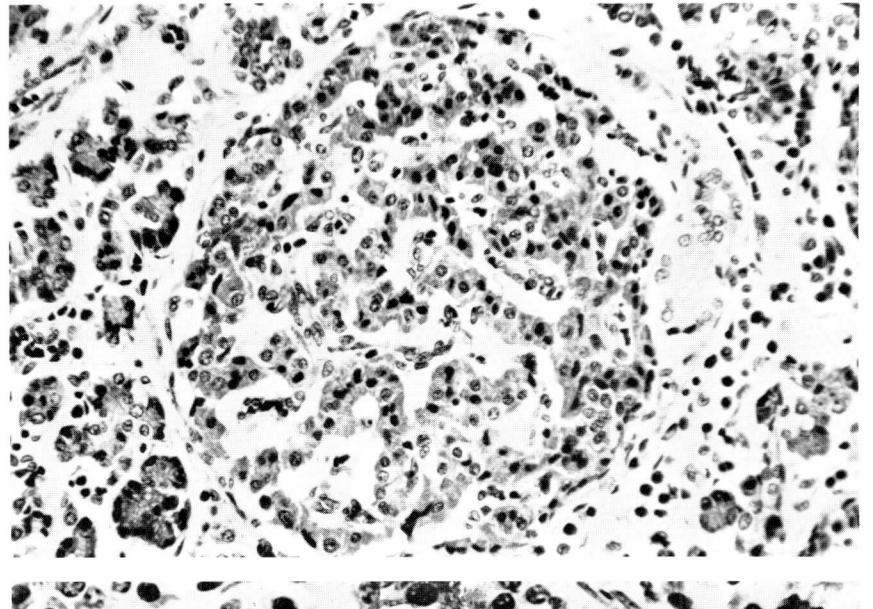

Figure 335. A round or oval group of small epithelial cells enclosed in pancreatic acinar tissue is an islet of Langerhans. In a Gomori preparation, as here, most cells have blue granules and are beta cells. Some smaller yellow staining cells around the periphery (not distinguishable in this plate) represent alpha cells (glucagon). *Pancreatic islet* (× 250)

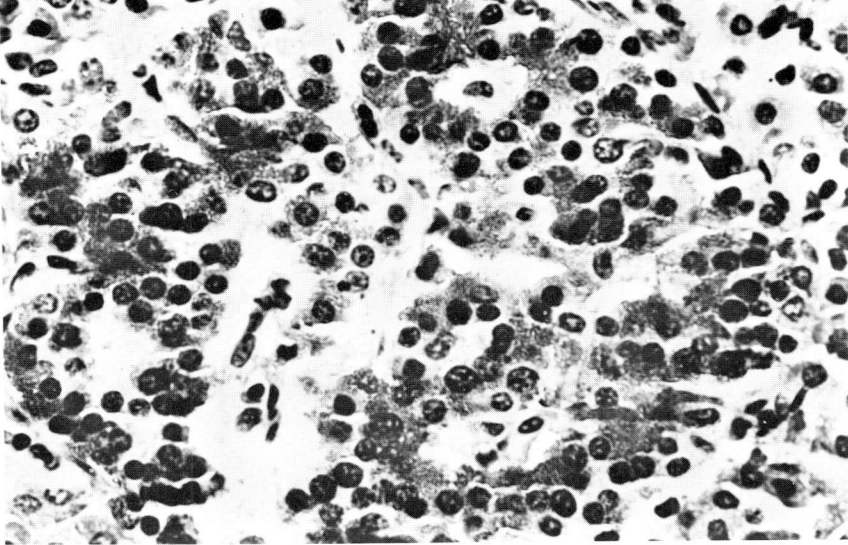

Figure 336. By immunocytochemistry using insulin antibody and the peroxidase-antiperoxidase technique, the beta cells have dark granules and constitute the majority. *Islets* (× 480)

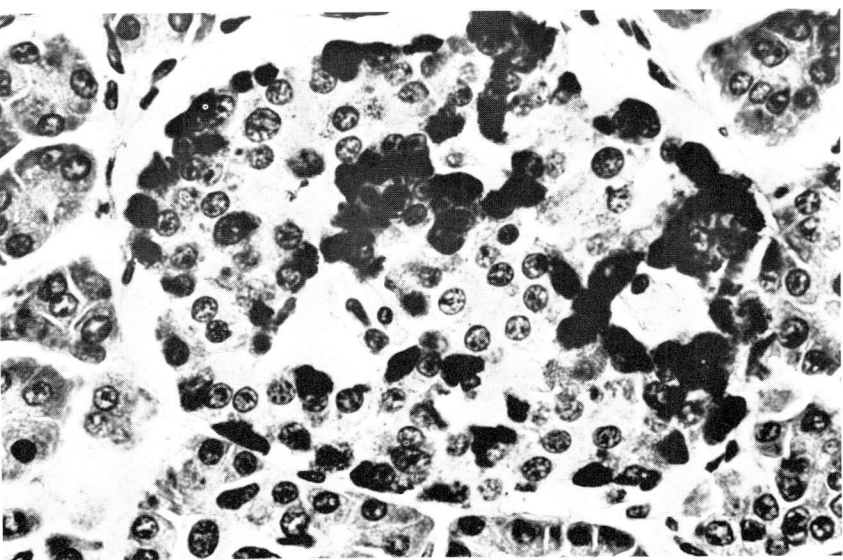

Figure 337. Here the antibody was directed against glucagon using the same PAP technique with diaminobenzidene as chromogen and H & E counterstain. Relatively few cells, chiefly around the periphery, have a black precipitate identifying alpha cells. *Islet*, glucagon containing cells (× 480)

EPITHELIAL SOLIDS

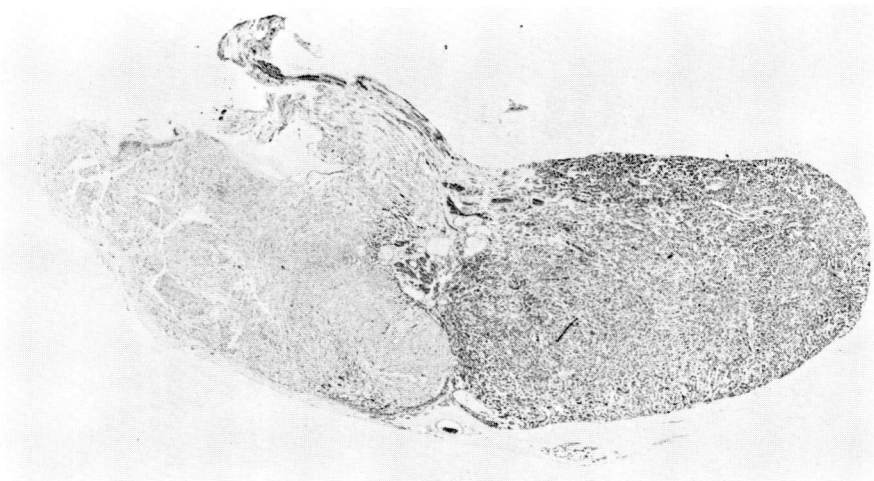

Figure 338. There are two distinct parts to this solid ovoid structure — the darker half proves to be epithelial, and the gray, left half proves to be neural, a combination unique to the pituitary gland. The slightly concavoconvex shape reflects the concavity of the bone of the sella turcica. Running from the center upwards and to the left is an irregular stalk, which is chiefly neural tissue but also contains some epithelial elements. This indicates that the section was cut in the sagittal plane. The neural part is posterior, and the epithelial part anterior. *Pituitary gland* (× 8.5)

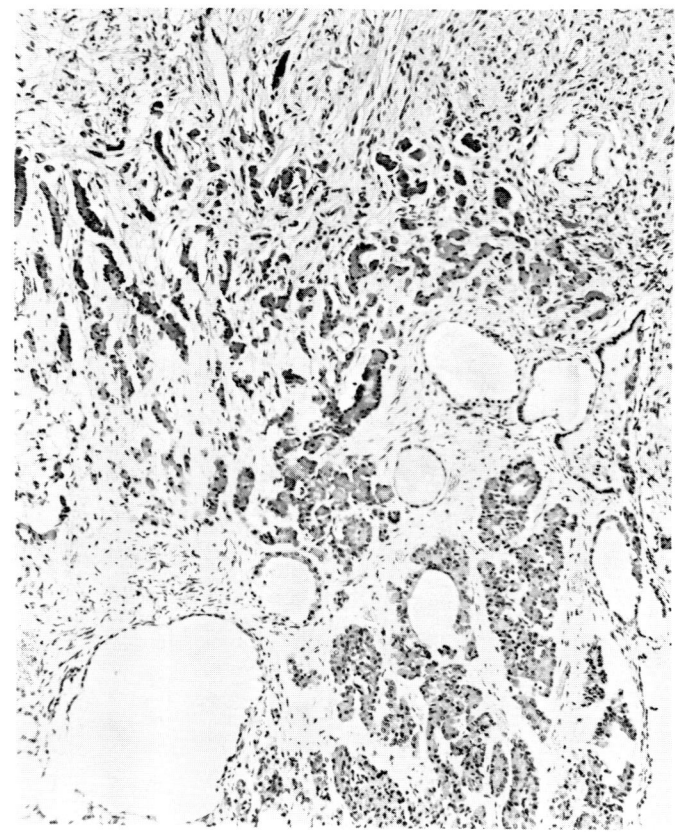

Figure 339. This field is taken from the junction between the two parts, the upper margin of the figure showing neural tissue and the bottom epithelium. This is the so-called pars intermedia. Note that there is no sharp delineation between epithelial and neural elements. The epithelial cells are large, and most are of a single kind with basophilic cytoplasm in H & E stains and with PAS positive cytoplasm in PAS-orange G stains. There are also small lakes of colloid material, which are normal for this area. *Pars intermedia* (× 80)

EPITHELIAL SOLIDS

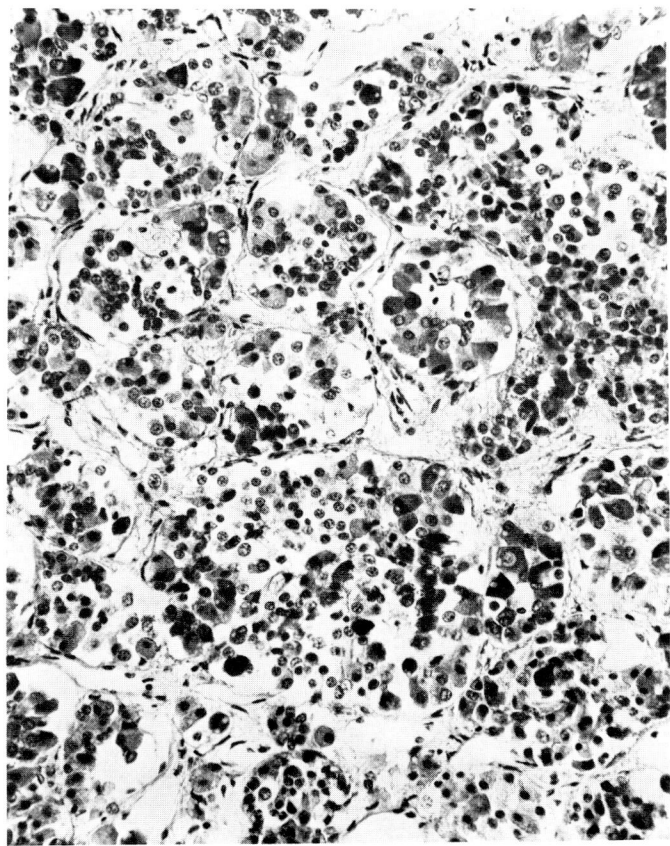

Figure 340. In the pars anterior, there is a tendency for cells to form islands or solid alveolar groups in a highly vascular, although scanty, stroma. H & E stains show a unique combination of eosinophilic, basophilic, and unstained (chromophobe) cells, with no particular or consistent localization. Staining by the PAS-orange G method (as here) produces a dark blue or purple color in cells that contain glycoprotein (PAS positive). This implies a content of FSH, LH, or TSH. ACTH is not a glycoprotein, except in its large precursor forms, but the cells producing ACTH are, by immunocytochemical identification, also basophils. The existence of large molecules, which give rise to both ACTH and lipotropins and to their hormone subunits and active metabolites, including MSH and endorphins, suggests that the presence of a variety of breakdown products may be responsible for difficulties in assigning specific functions to specific cells. Single cells may contain more than one active polypeptide, and ACTH and FSH have been reported in the same granules, as well as the same cell. In a PAS-orange G preparation, cells with all shades of staining intermediate between basophilic and orangeophilic can be identified. The orangeophilic cells in this photograph have a gray cytoplasm; they are related to growth hormone and prolactin, each apparently from different cells. The chromophobes are best seen just below the center of the plate as small round nuclei with minimal or no visible cytoplasm. *Anterior pituitary* (× 250)

EPITHELIAL SOLIDS – PITUITARY

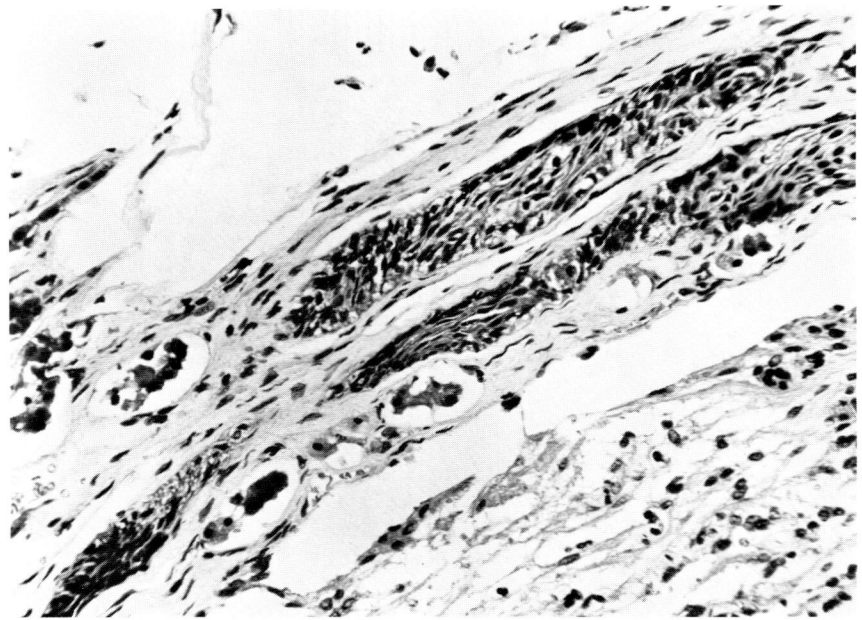

Figure 341. An epithelial extension of the pituitary gland runs up the stalk to constitute the pars tuberalis, (above). Here there are often islands of squamous cells with prickles or intercellular bridges. This type of tissue is believed to be related to the origin of the epithelial part of the pituitary from Rathke's pouch. *Pituitary stalk* (× 200)

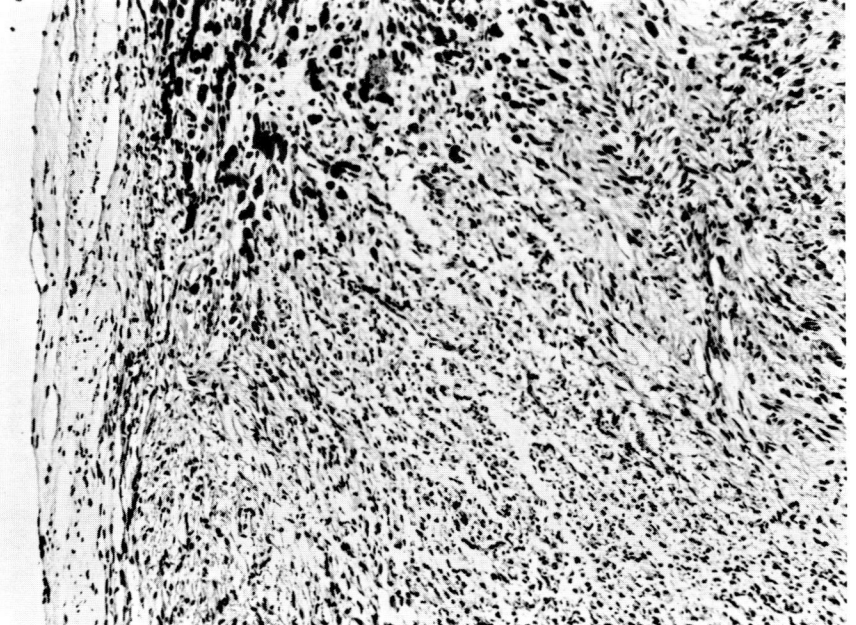

Figure 342. This is a finely fibrillary tissue containing glial fibers rather than collagen and thus belongs to the central nervous system. In the upper left corner, numerous epithelial cells merge insensibly with the neural component without intervening basement membrane. Some cells may contain pigment. *Posterior pituitary* (× 80)

NEURAL SOLIDS

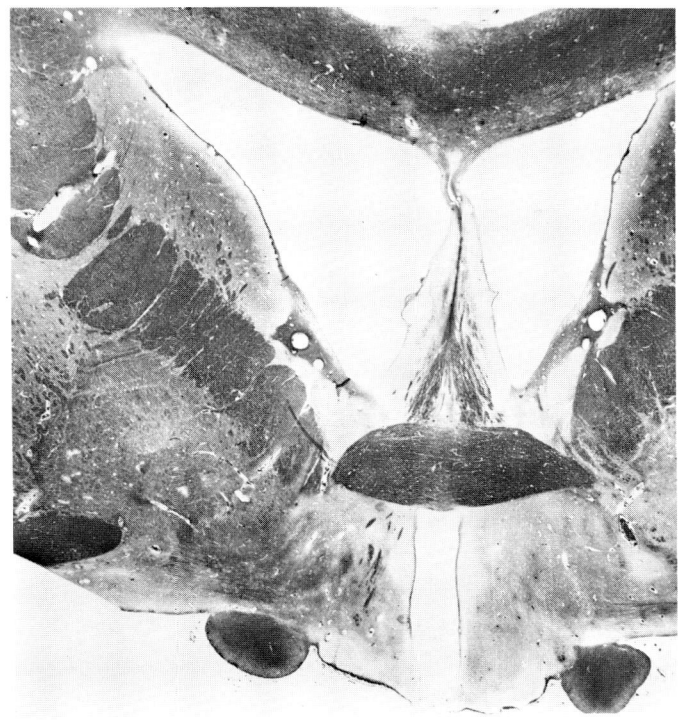

Figure 343. A myelin stain of brain at the level of the anterior commissure. (× 3)

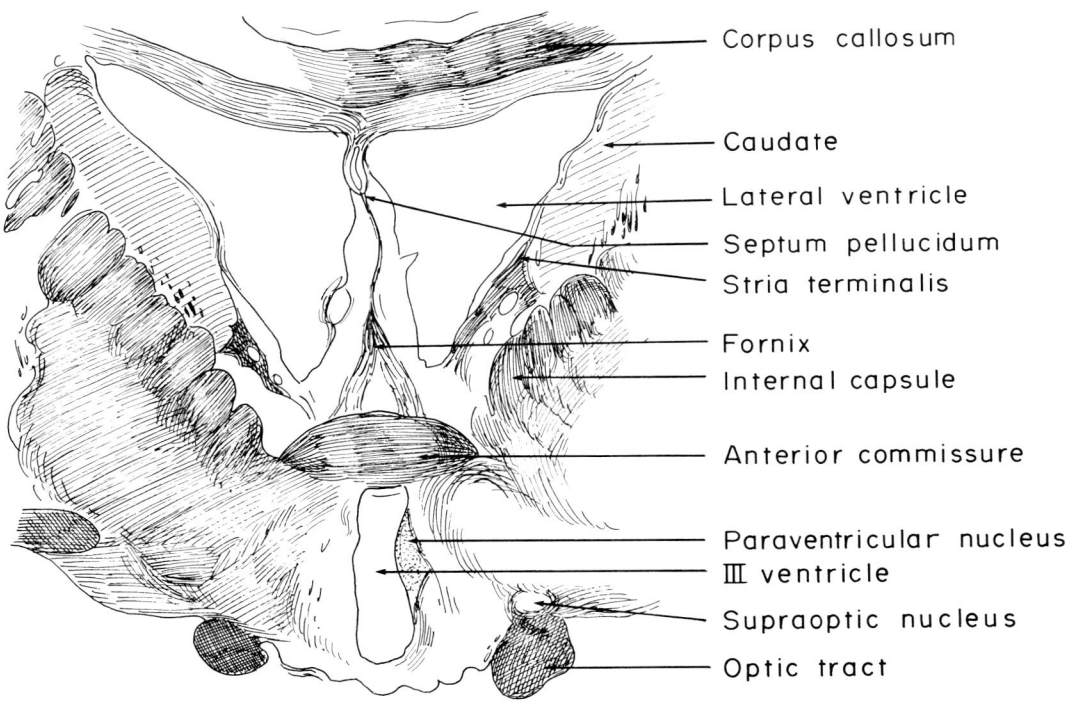

Figure 344. Identification of parts in Figure 343.

NEURAL SOLIDS

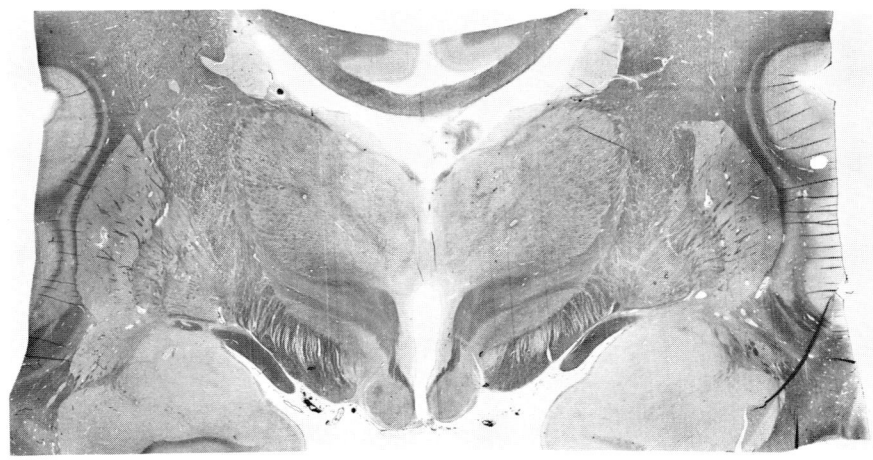

Figure 345. A more posterior view of the brain, at the level of the mammillary bodies. H & E (×1.7)

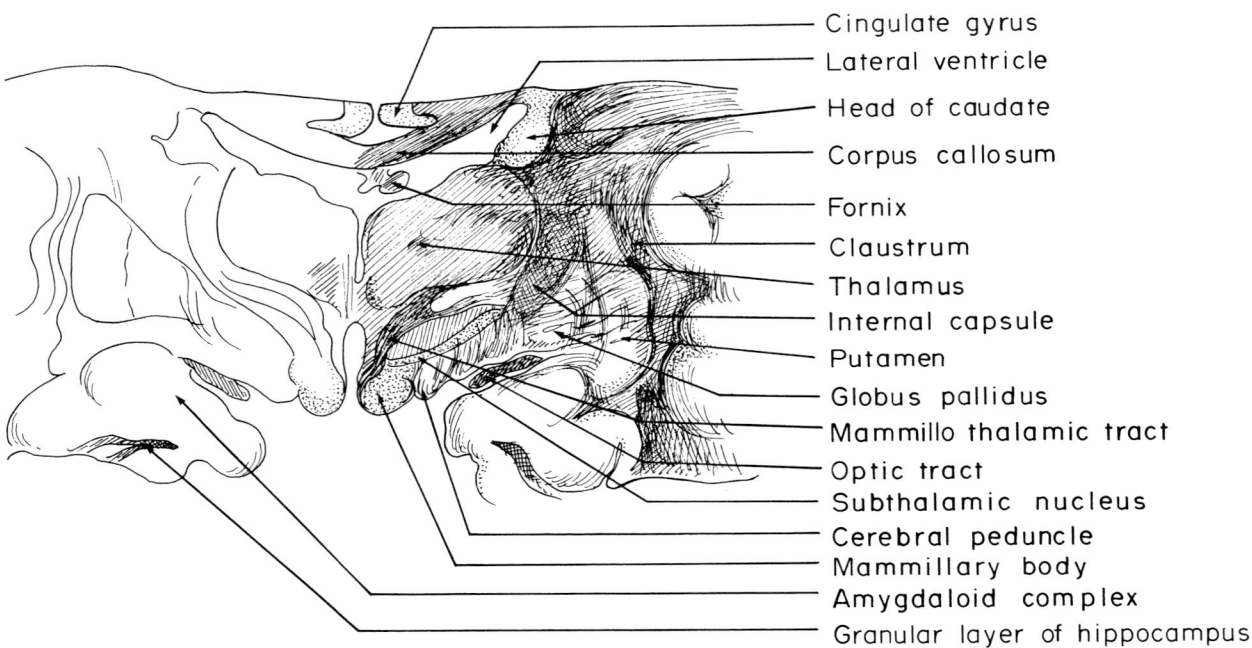

Figure 346. Identification of parts in Figure 345.

NEURAL SOLIDS

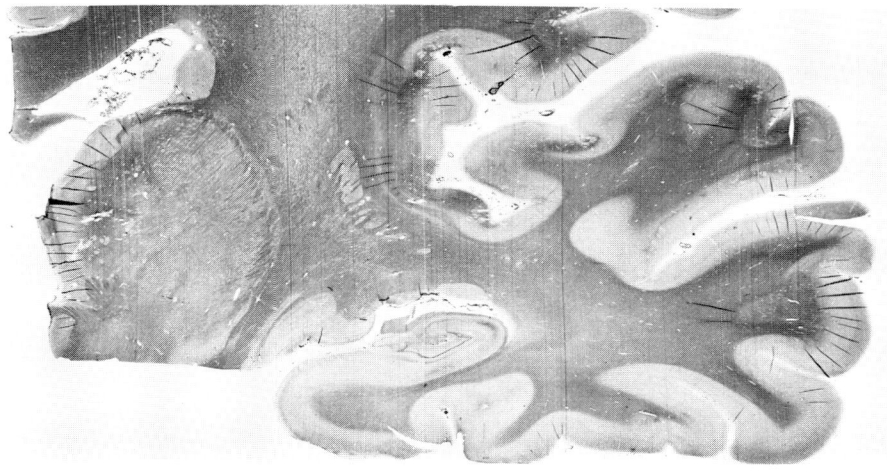

Figure 347. Insula, with lateral geniculate body and hippocampus. H & E (× 2.5)

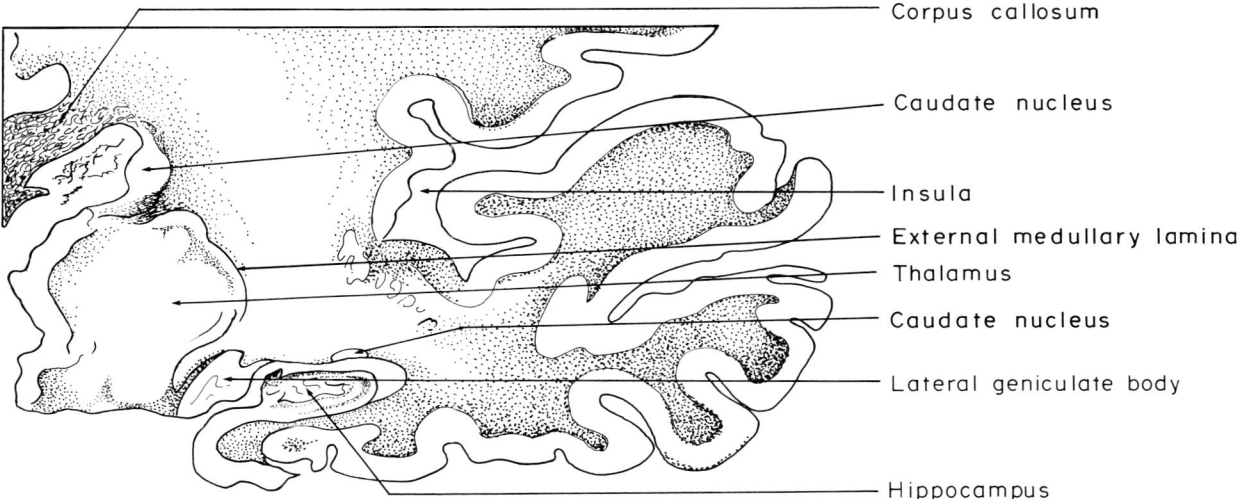

Figure 348. Identification of parts in Figure 347.

NEURAL SOLIDS

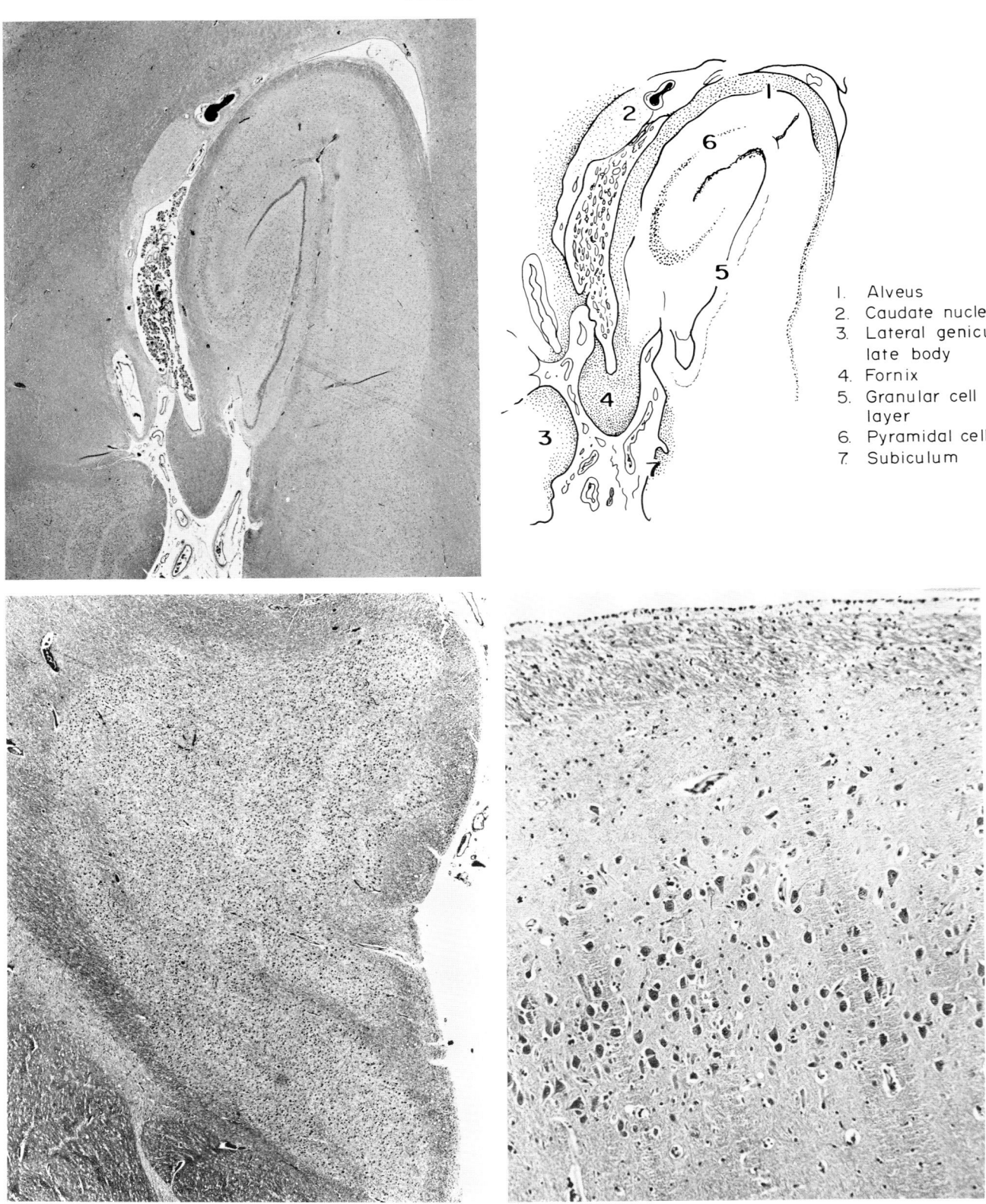

Figure 349. The three micrographs are from the region of the hippocampus. a. Low power shows the hippocampus (on the right), fornix (lower center), and the tricorne of the lateral geniculate body (lower left corner). (×6.5) b. Identification of parts in a. c. The tricorne of the lateral geniculate body shown at high power, illustrating its stratified nature. (×16) d. Shows a unique type of cortex, diagnostic of hippocampus because a fibrillary layer of white matter runs immediately beneath the surface ependyma (where the tissue projects into the ventricle) and superficial to the gray matter. (×80)

NEURAL SOLIDS

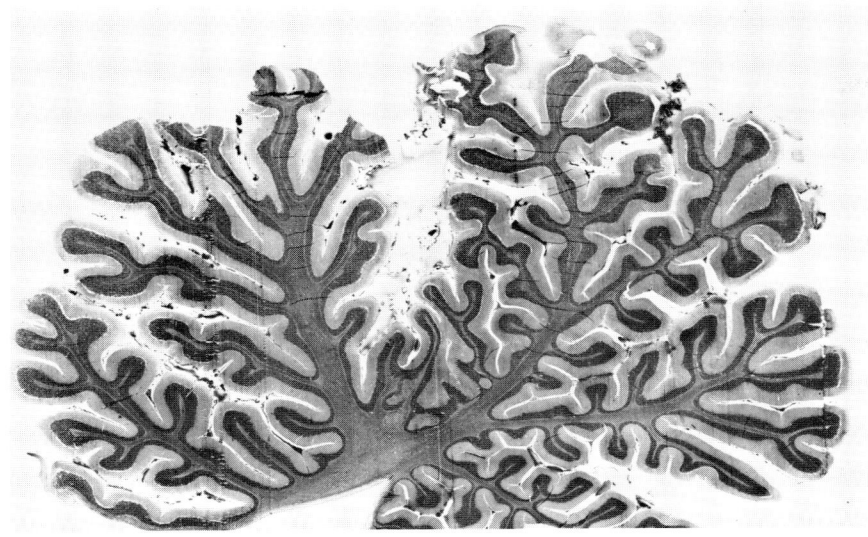

Figure 350. This distinctive pattern of multiple closely packed leaves of gray matter on a branching darker core of white matter is unique for the cerebellum, and the fan-shaped radiating appearance indicates the *vermis*. (× 3.5)

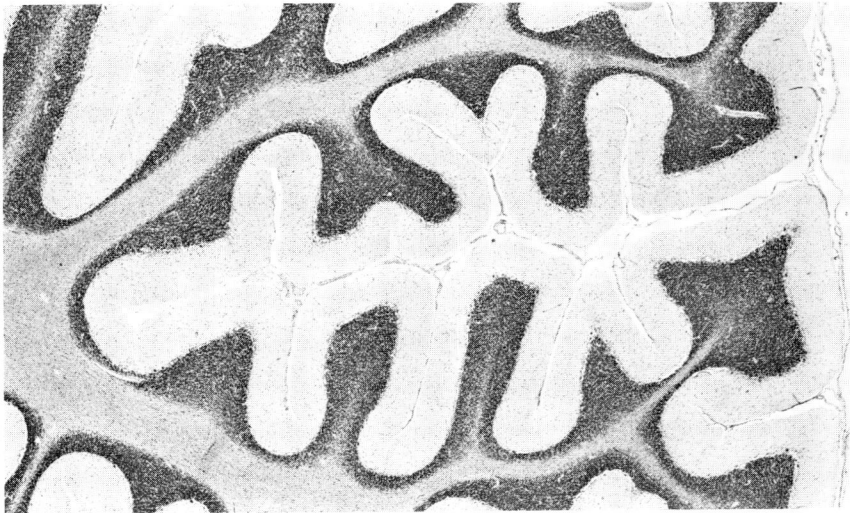

Figure 351. At higher power the fine delicate meninges are seen on the right. The relation of gray matter, external granular layer of small neurones, and branching white matter is demonstrated. (× 10)

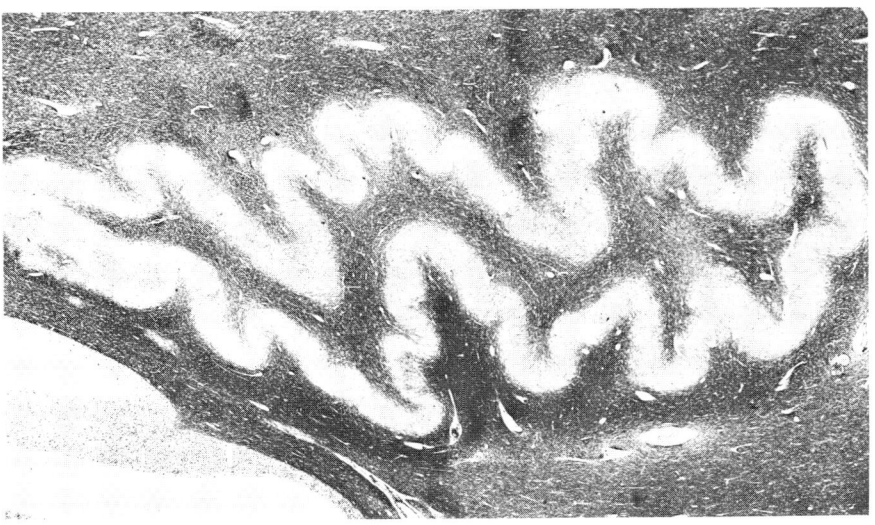

Figure 352. A large nucleus seen here in myelin stain as an undulating white band is the dentate (toothlike) nucleus of the cerebellum. (A smaller, rather more delicate, version is the inferior olive of the medulla.) *Dentate nucleus cerebellum*, myelin stain (× 9.5)

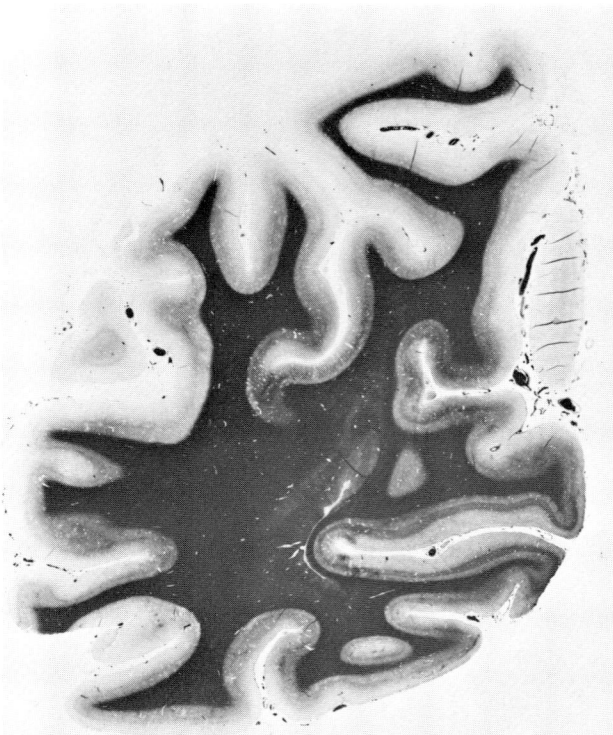

Figure 353. This is clearly a section of brain cortex with the relatively straight side on the right being the medial surface of one hemisphere. The inferior margin is convex, which identifies the occipital pole (the anterior pole is concave inferiorly). In the right lower quadrant, the gray matter contains a dark line which is the stria of Gennari and identifies the visual cortex. The deep sulcus running horizontally outward at the junction of the inferior and medial surfaces is the calcarine sulcus. *Visual cortex* (× 1.8)

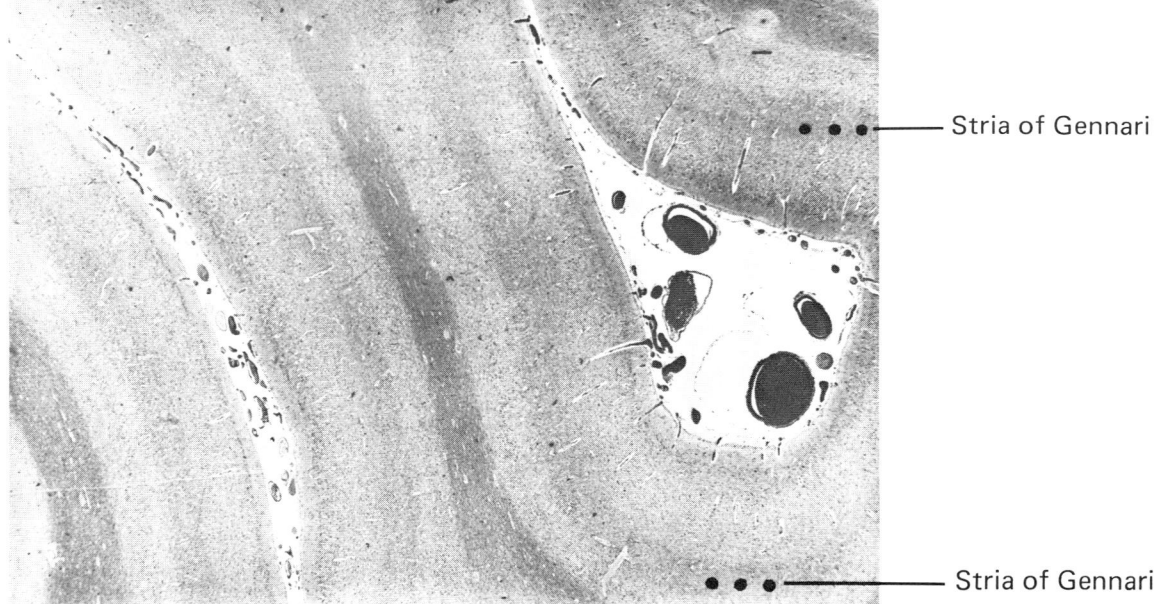

Figure 354. This is a higher power of the visual cortex showing open meningeal surfaces with blood vessels, convoluted gray matter, and dark bands of white matter (one in the left lower corner and the other running slightly obliquely down the center of the plate). The gray cortical matter is unique because it includes a dark band (not so dense as the white matter) caused by myelination of fibers. This is the stria of Gennari. *Visual cortex* (× 10)

NEURAL SOLIDS – NEURONE SHEETS

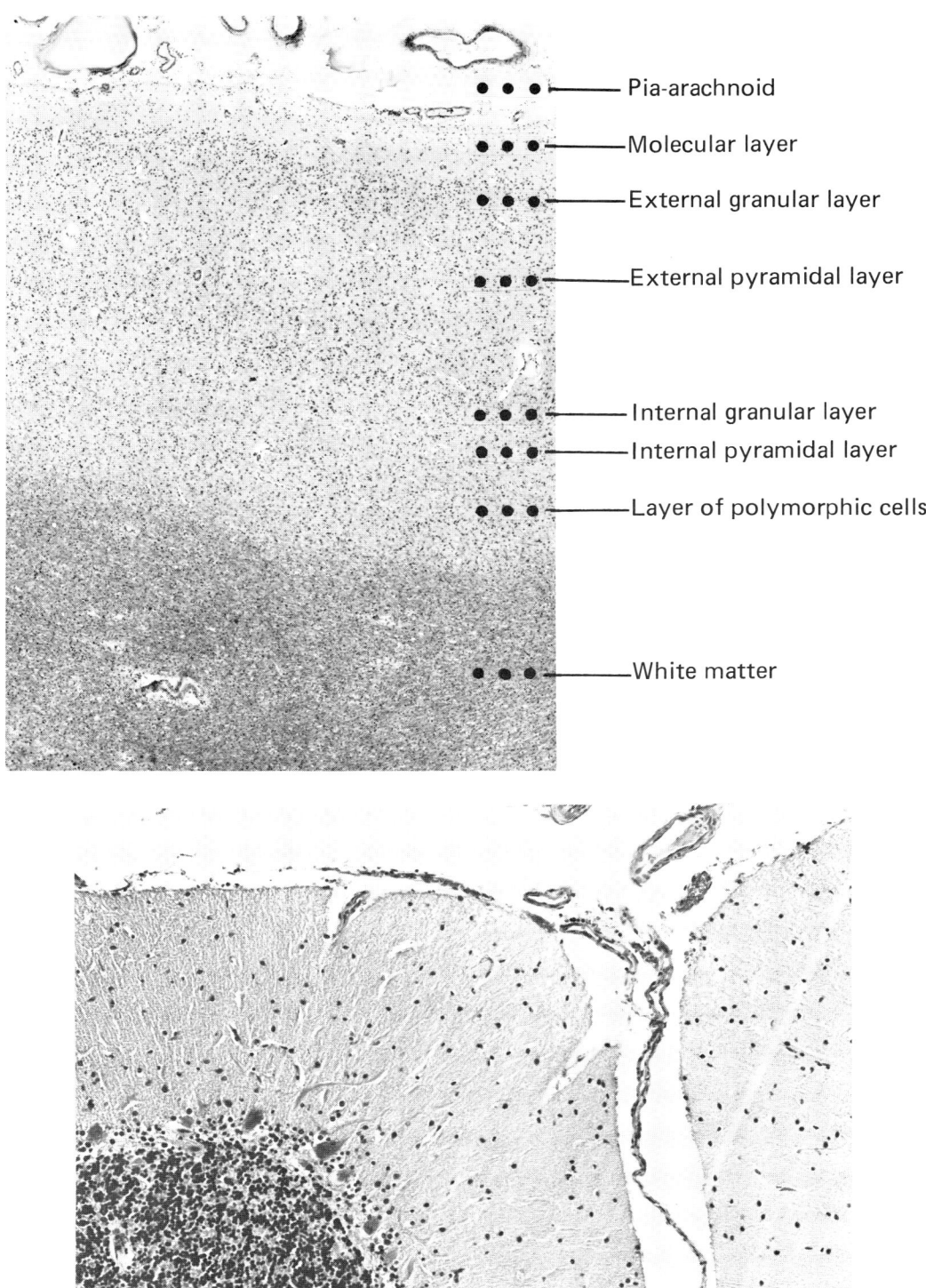

Figure 355. Two types of cortex. Both have overlying pia-arachnoid. a. The gray matter that lies directly over the darker staining fibrillary white matter is divided into six rather indistinct layers, as indicated. *Brain cortex*, H & E (× 27) b. A rind of gray matter overlying a granular layer of small neurones and at the junction showing large, typical Purkinje cells. *Cerebellar cortex* (× 100)

NEURAL SOLIDS

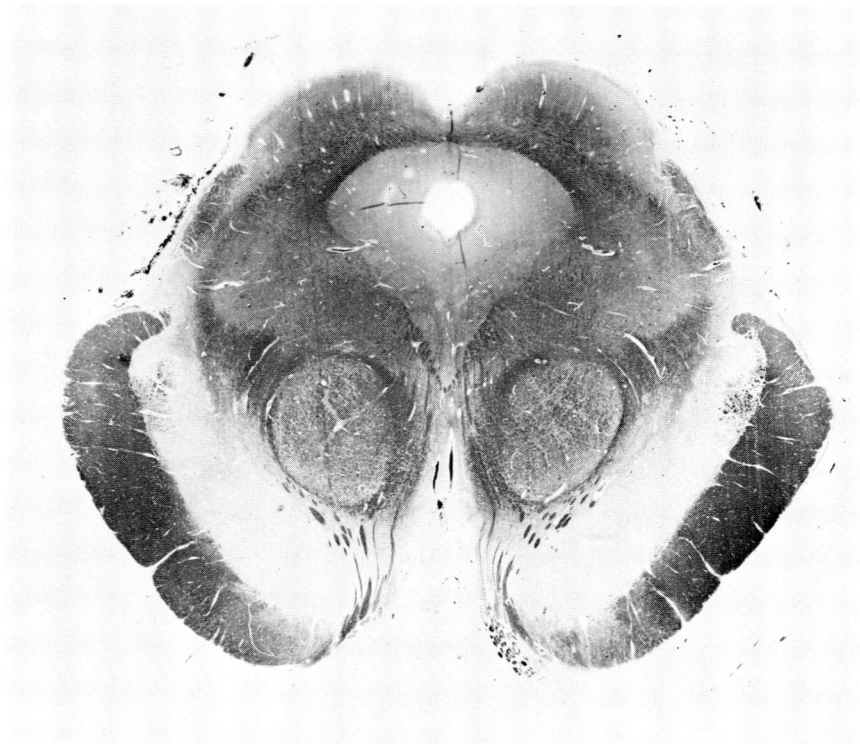

Figure 356. Midbrain at the level of the superior colliculus showing the aqueduct, red nuclei, and cerebral peduncles. Myelin stain (× 5)

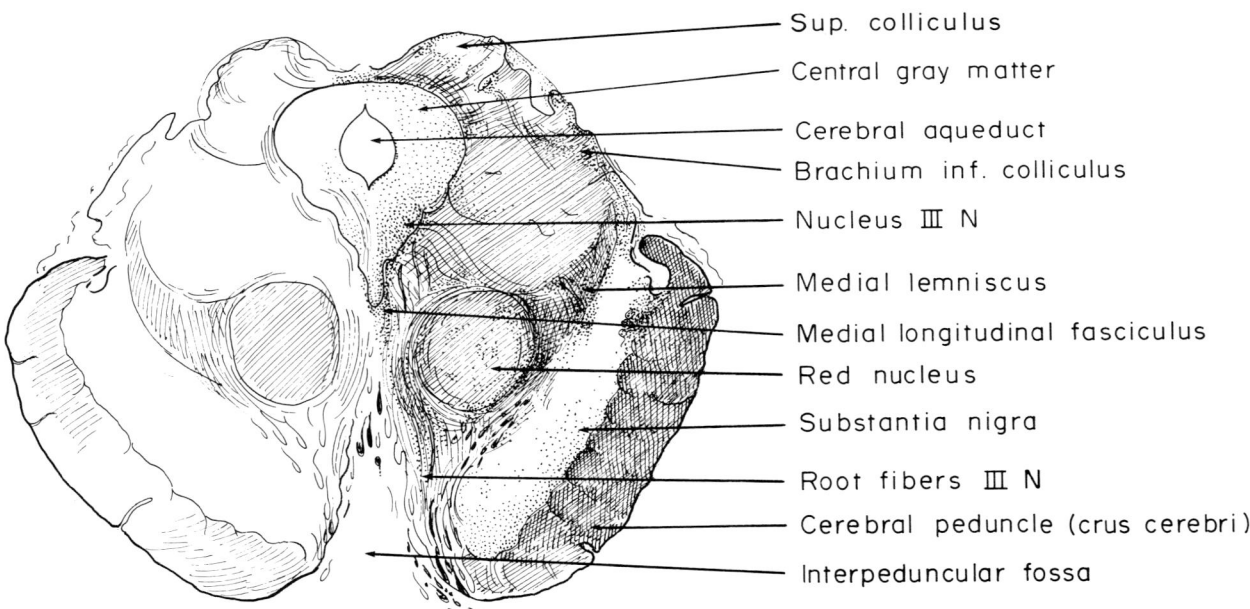

Figure 357. Identification of parts in Figure 356.

NEURAL SOLIDS

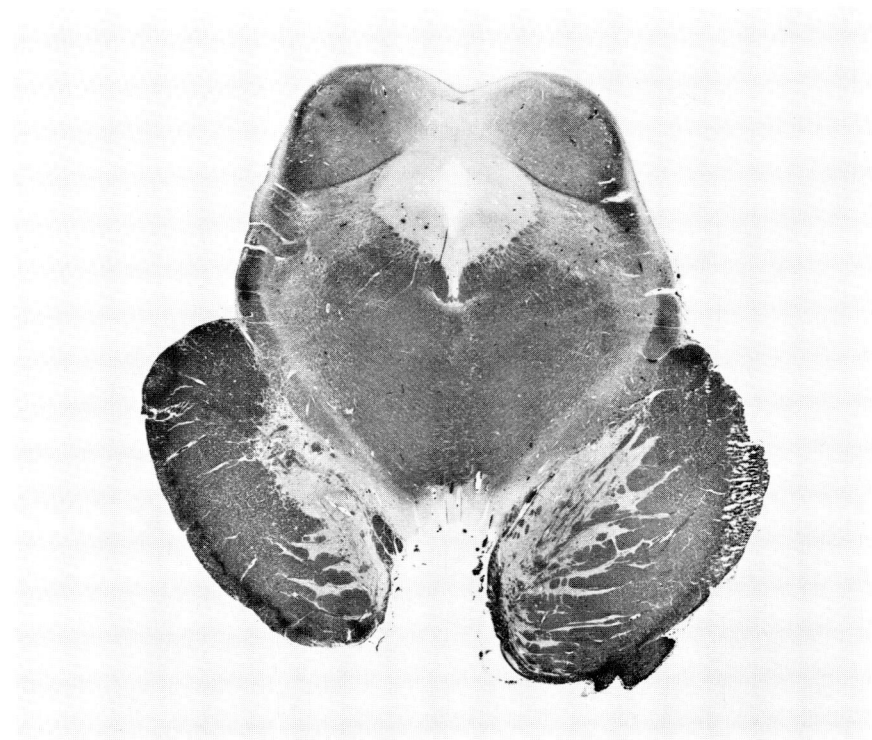

Figure 358. Midbrain at the level of the inferior colliculus. (× 3.8)

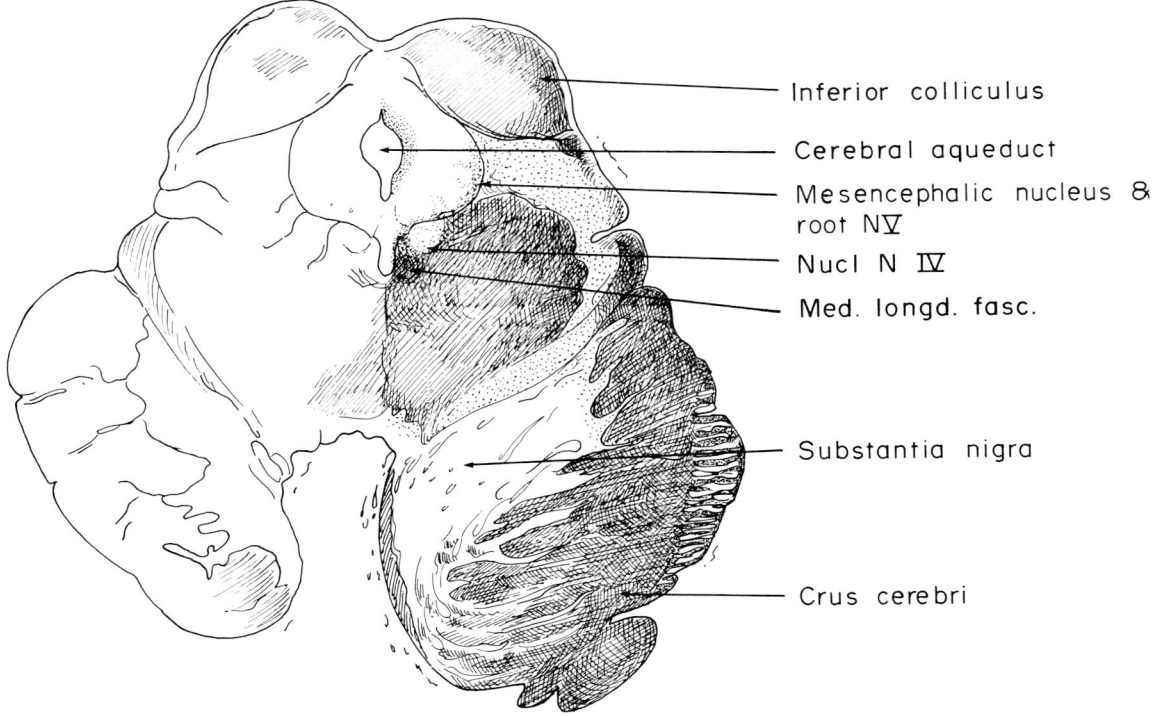

Figure 359. Identification of parts in Figure 358.

NEURAL SOLIDS

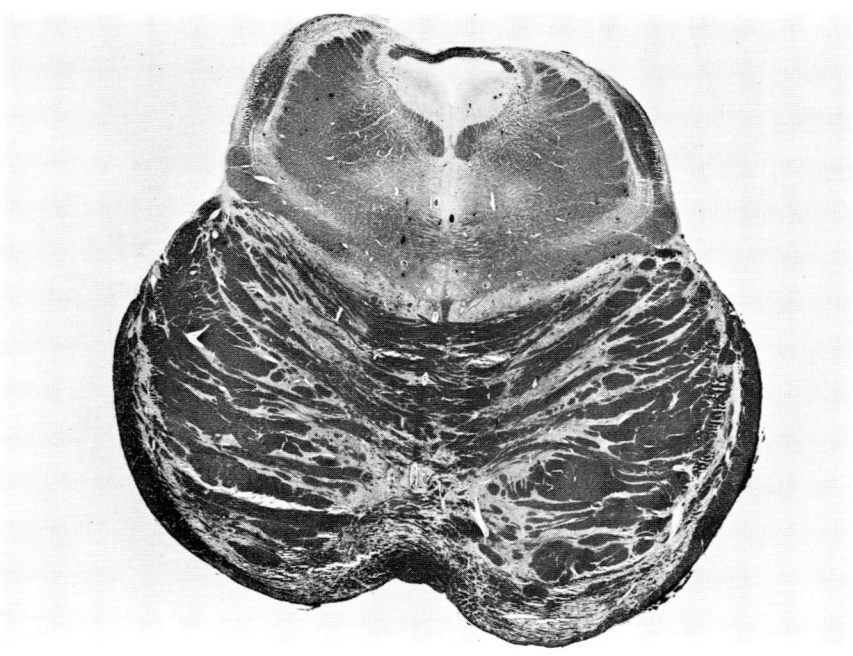

Figure 360. Section through the isthmus between midbrain and upper pons. (× 4)

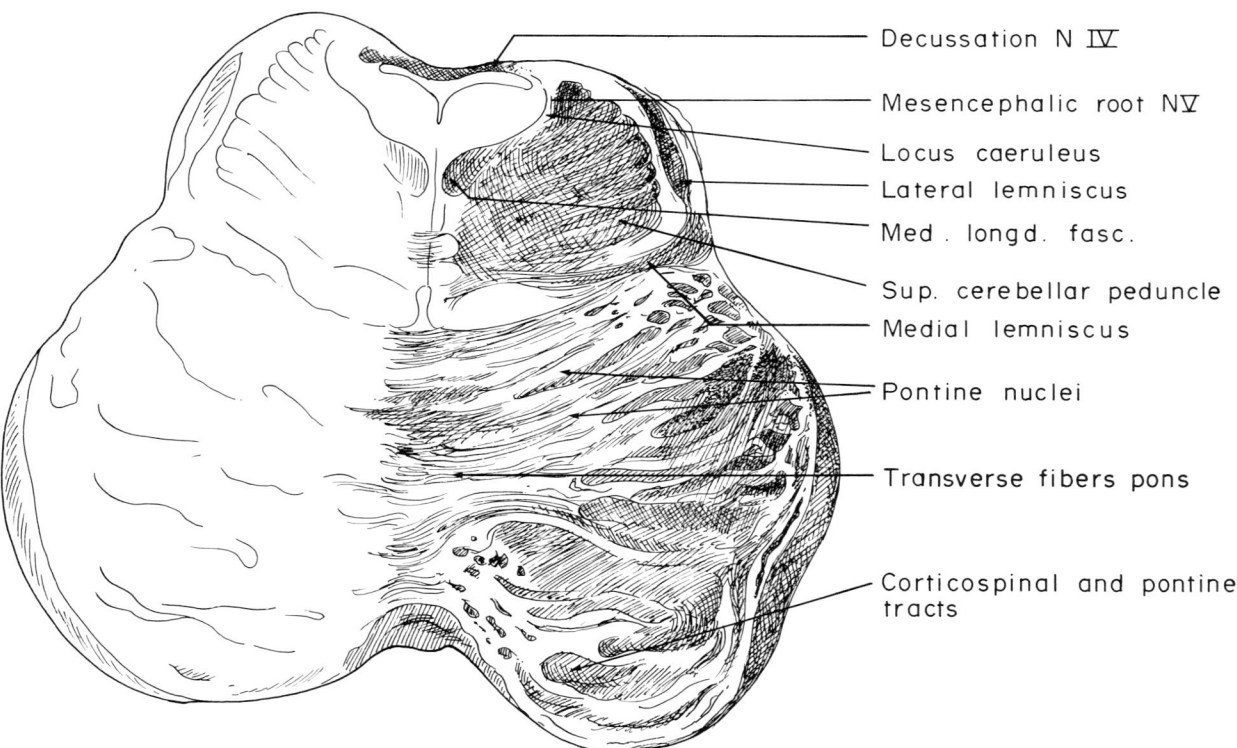

Figure 361. Identification of parts in Figure 360.

NEURAL SOLIDS

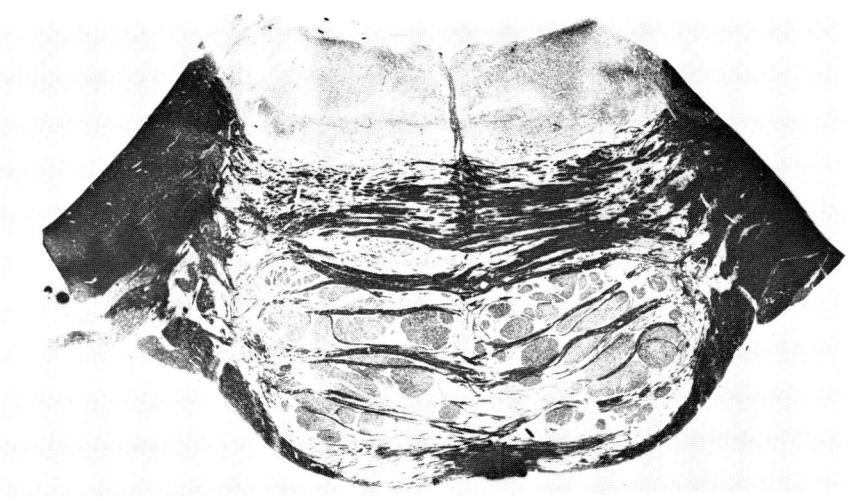

Figure 362. Section through pons at the emergence of the fifth nerve. (× 4)

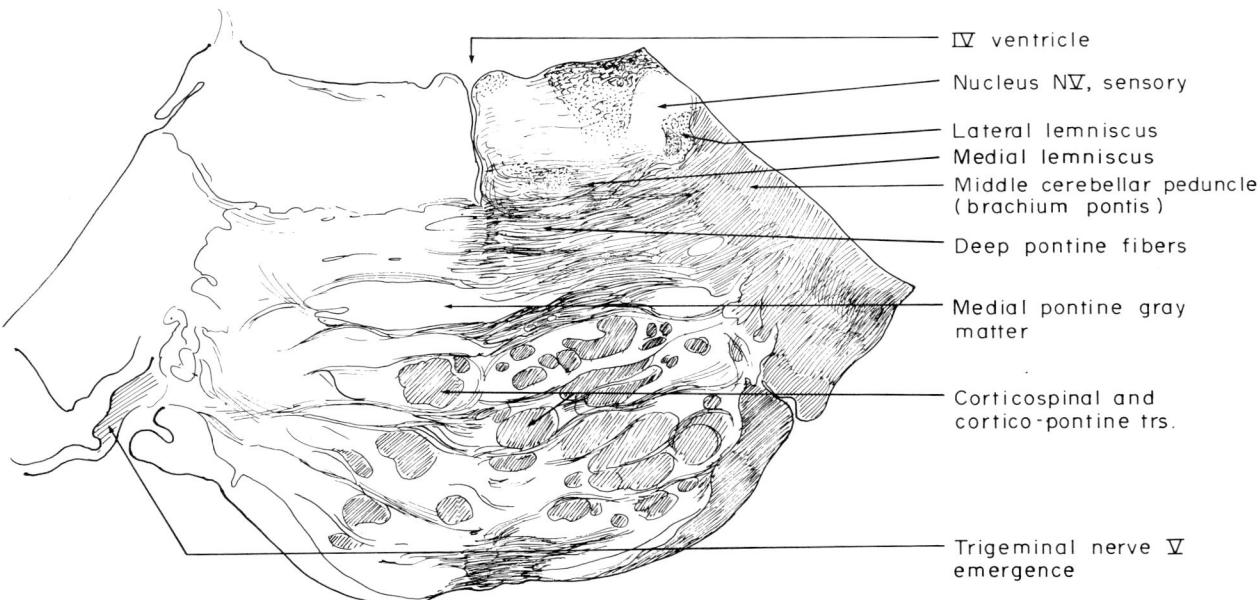

Figure 363. Identification of parts in Figure 362.

NEURAL SOLIDS

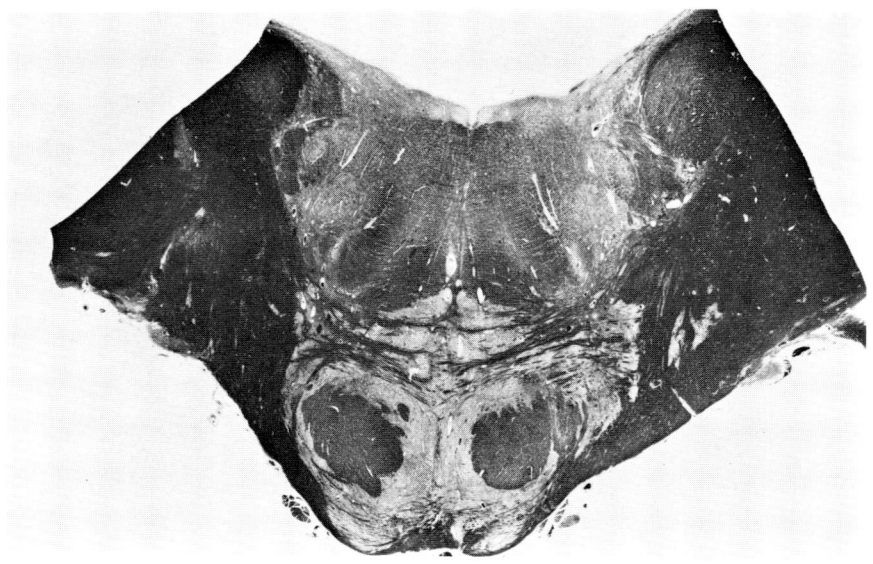

Figure 364. Section through pons at the emergence of the seventh nerve. (× 6)

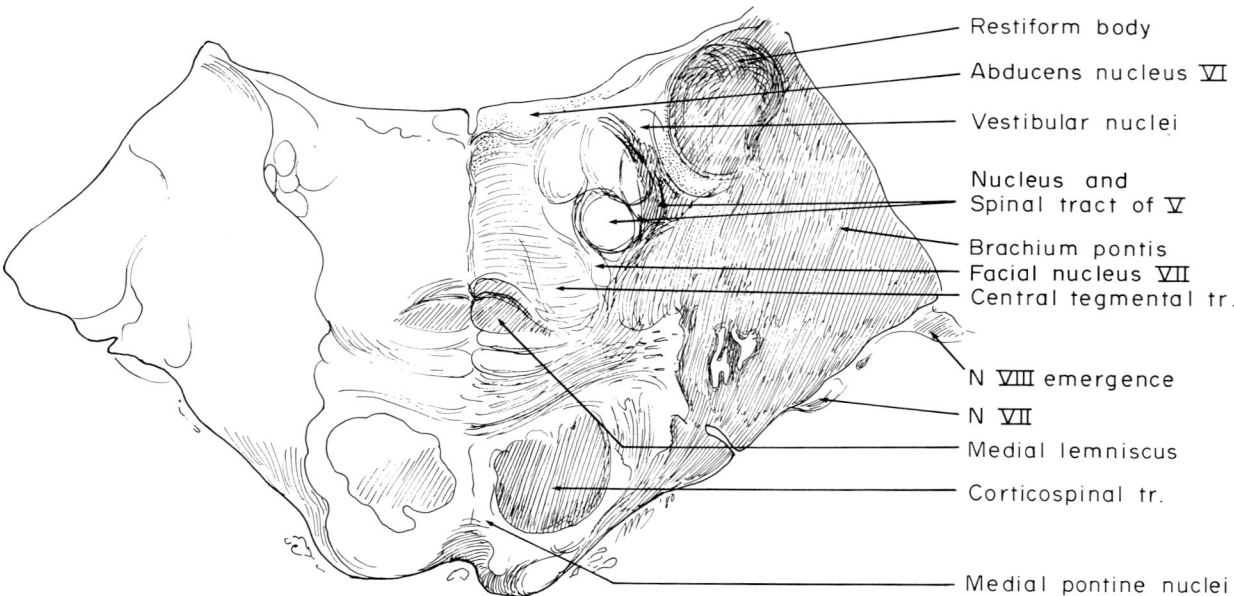

Figure 365. Identification of parts in Figure 364.

NEURAL SOLIDS

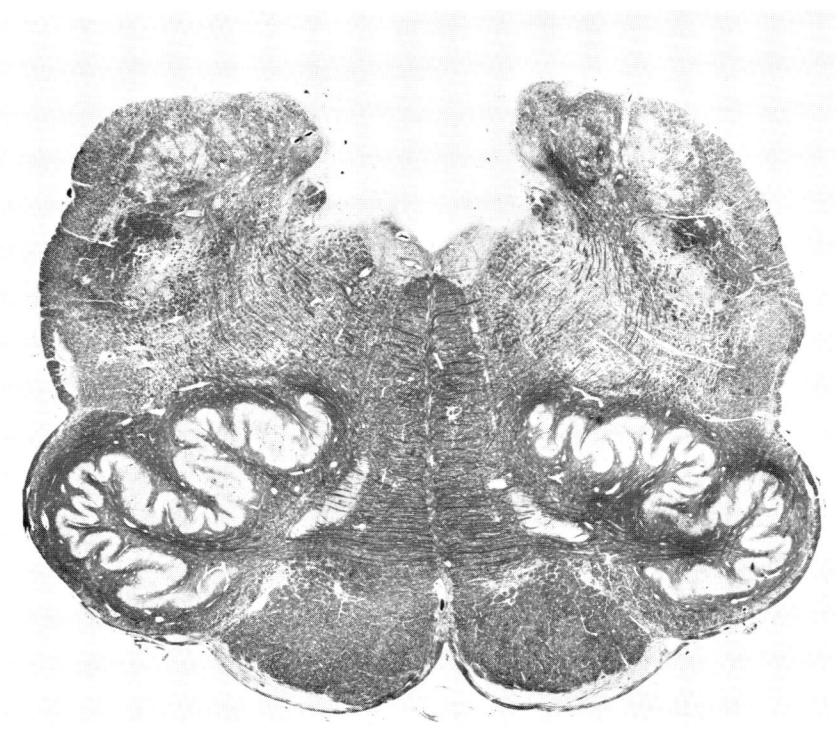

Figure 366. Section through the medulla at the level of the olives. (× 7)

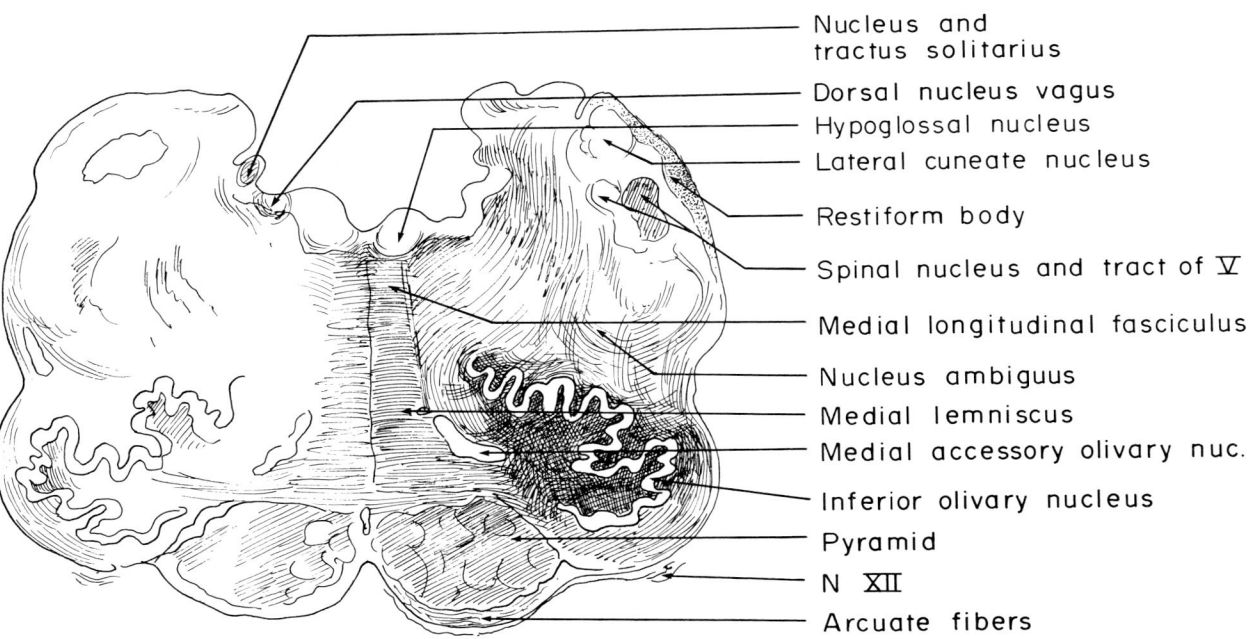

Figure 367. Identification of parts in Figure 366.

NEURAL SOLIDS

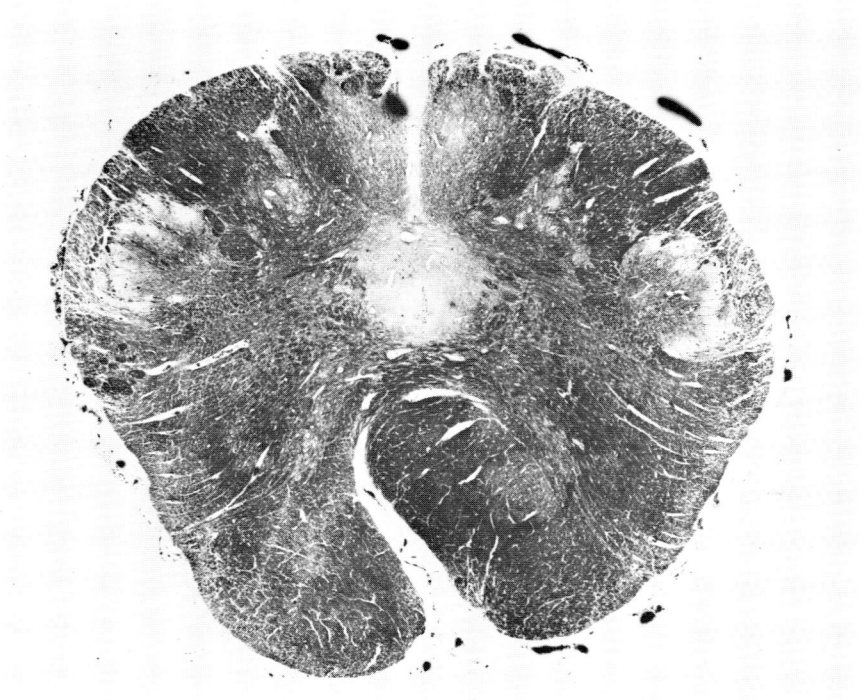

Figure 368. Section of the medulla at the decussation of the pyramid. (×9)

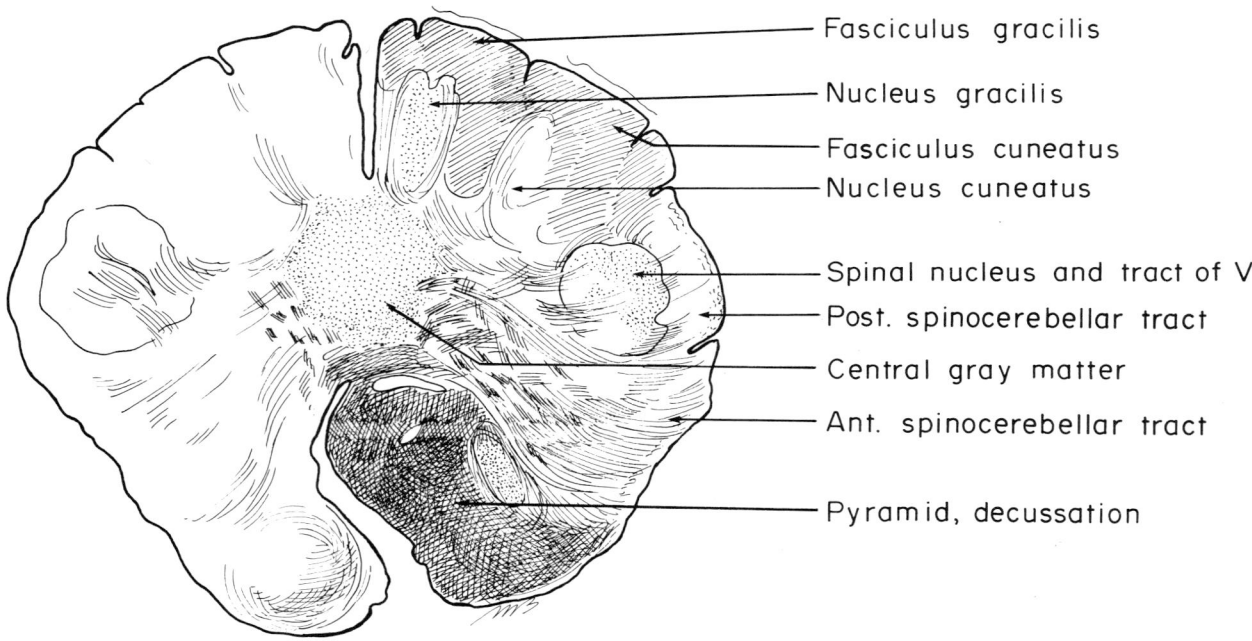

Figure 369. Identification of parts in Figure 368.

NEURAL SOLIDS

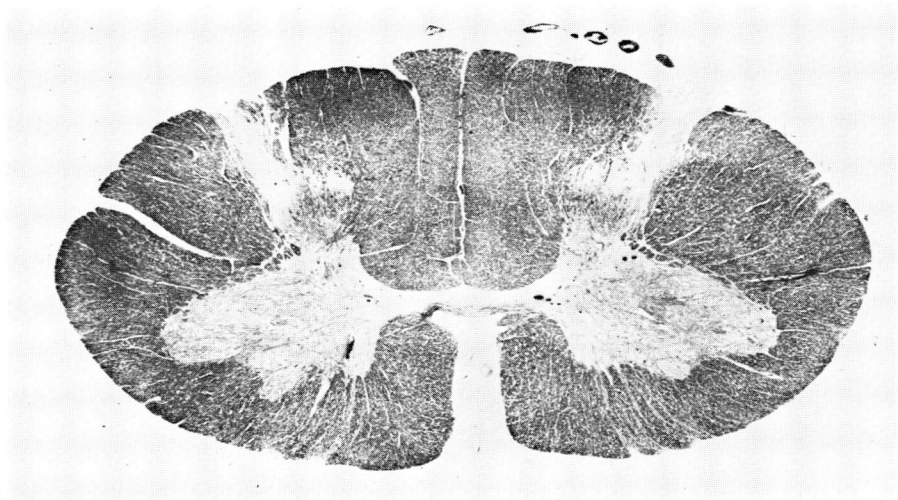

Figure 370. Spinal cord, cervical region. (×10)

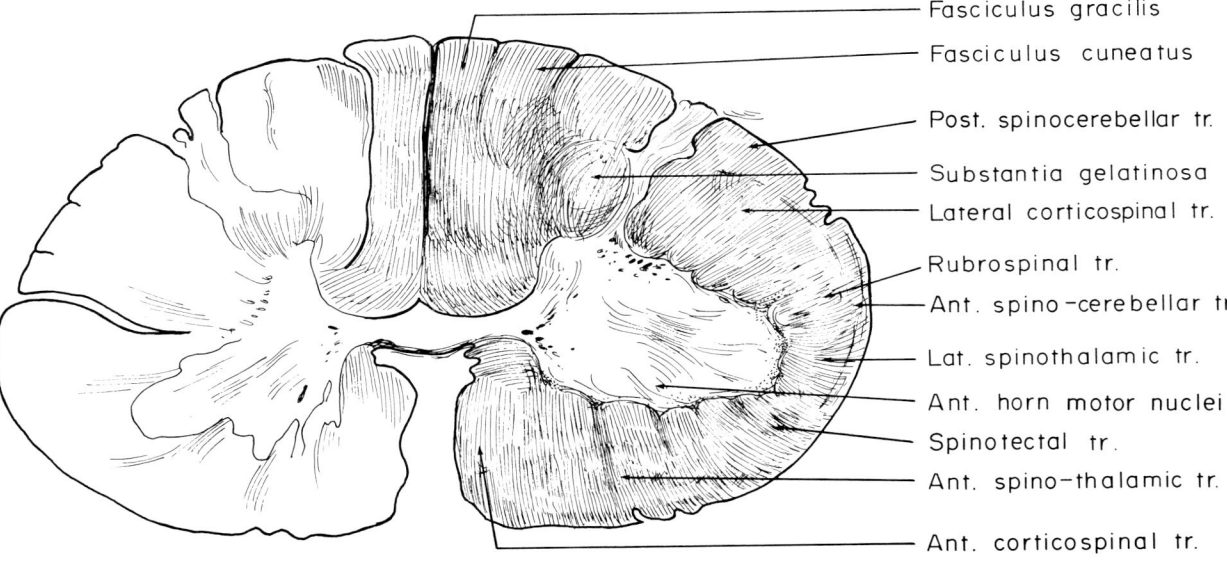

Figure 371. Identification of parts in Figure 370.

NEURAL SOLIDS

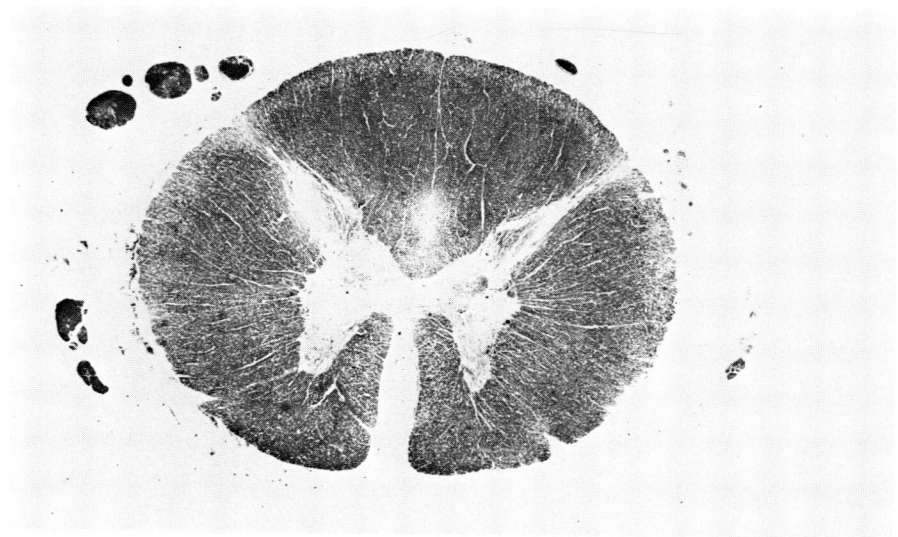

Figure 372. Spinal cord, thoracic region. (× 10)

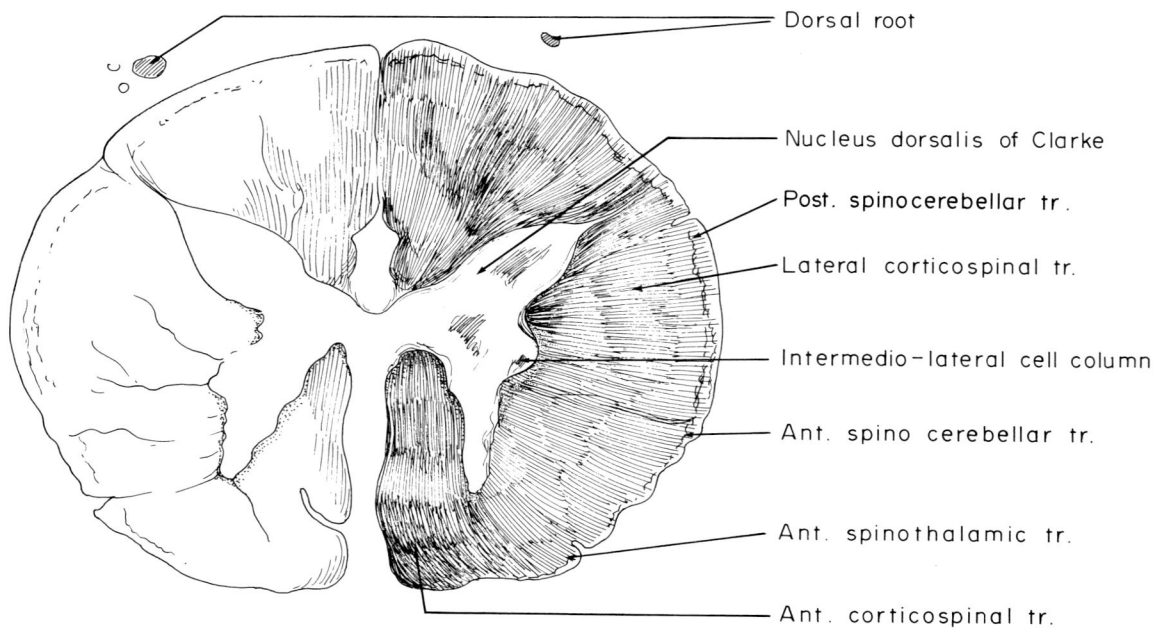

Figure 373. Identification of parts in Figure 372.

NEURAL SOLIDS

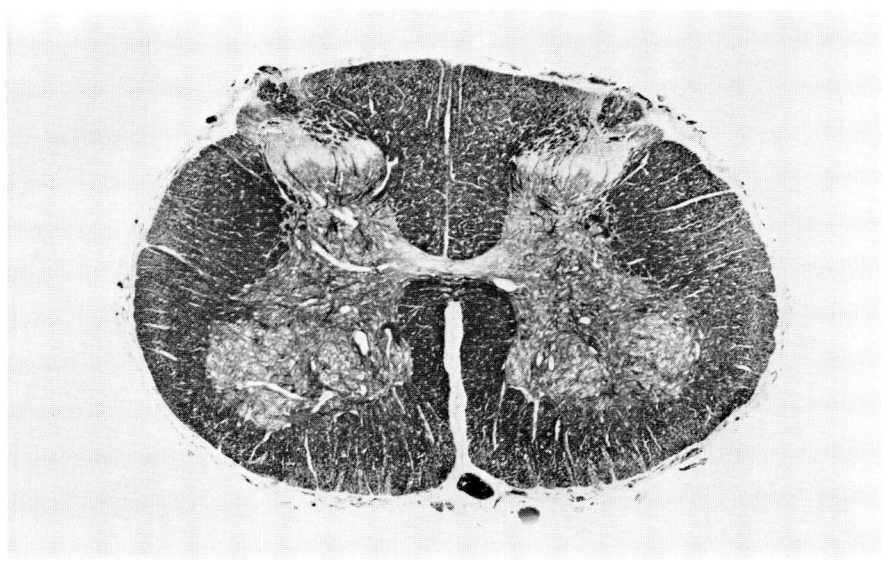

Figure 374. Spinal cord, lumbar region. (×10)

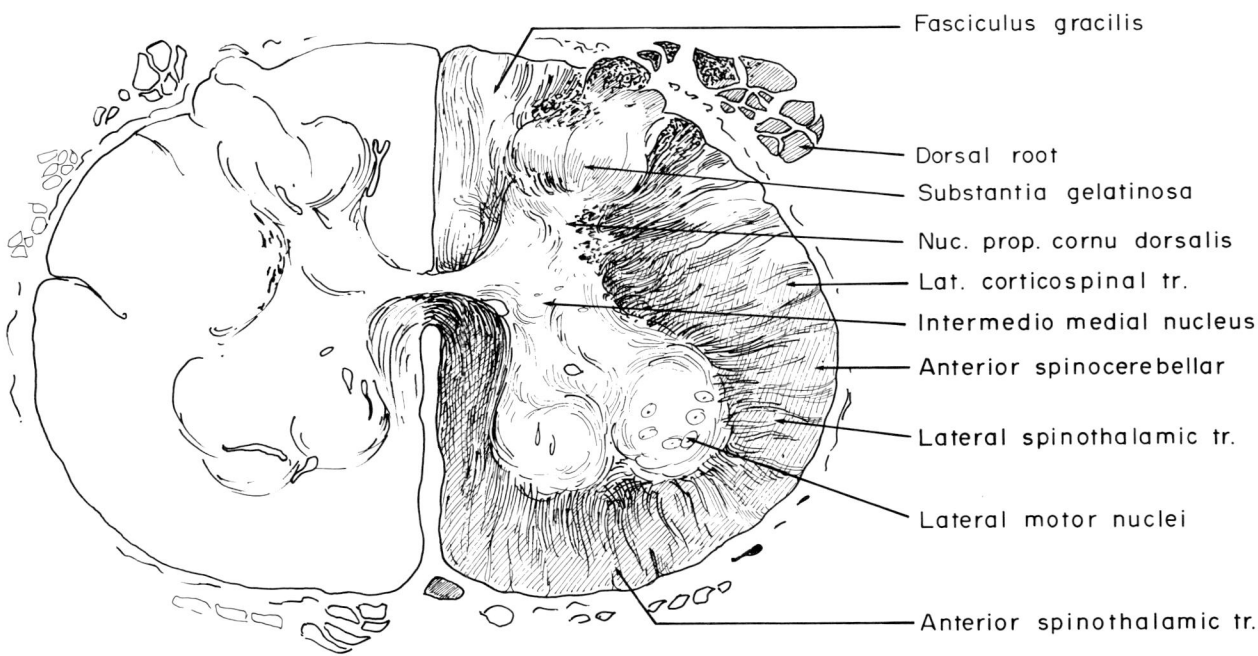

Figure 375. Identification of parts in Figure 374.

NEURAL SOLIDS

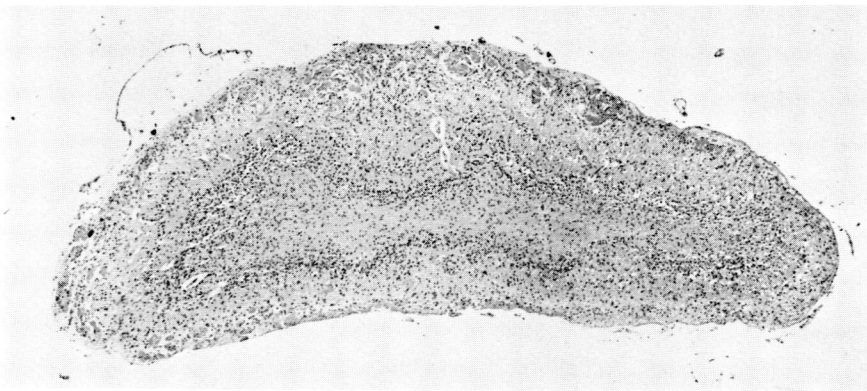

Figure 376. This is an insular structure of finely fibrillary nature with a strong suggestion of zonation. In the outer zone, whorls and fibers are known as glomeruli. Larger neurones are mitral cells. The adjacent small dark cells are part of the outer granular layer of small neurones. An inner undulating nuclear band in the central part of the structure is the inner granular layer. *Olfactory bulb* ($\times$ 27)

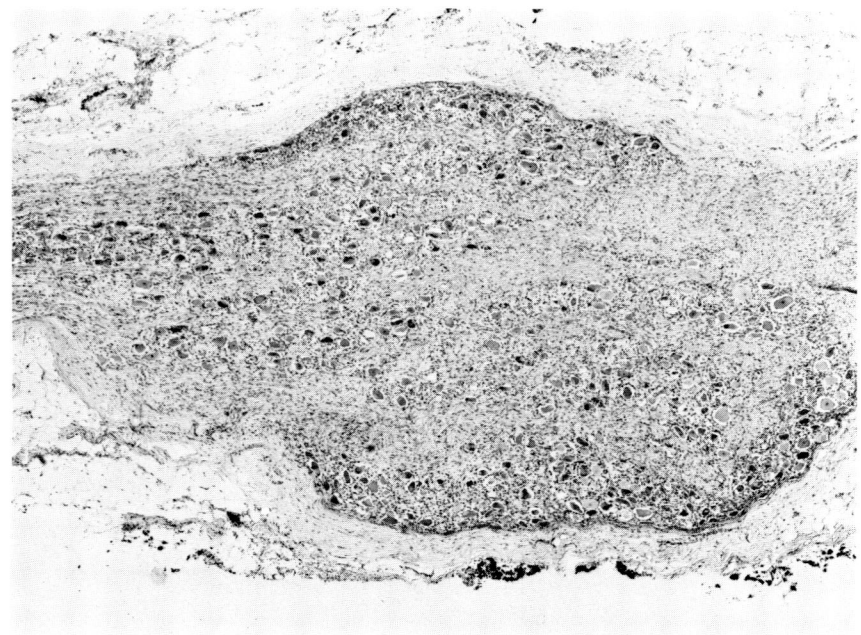

Figure 377. This is an ovoid solid with nerve fibers entering from the spinal cord (on the right) and fibers exiting on the left to join with the ventral root and form a peripheral nerve. This combination of neurones and peripheral nerve fibers is characteristic of a ganglion. *Dorsal root ganglion* ($\times$ 31)

NEURAL SOLIDS

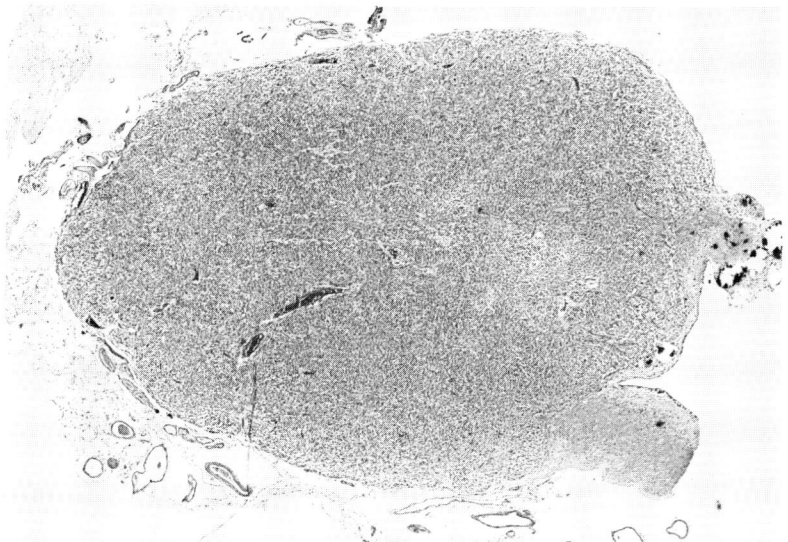

Figure 378. This is an insular solid without capsule but embedded in loose connective tissue (meningeal). On the right is part of the wall of the third ventricle with ependymal lining cells. The small black granules are calcified bodies. *Pineal*, eight-year-old boy (× 16)

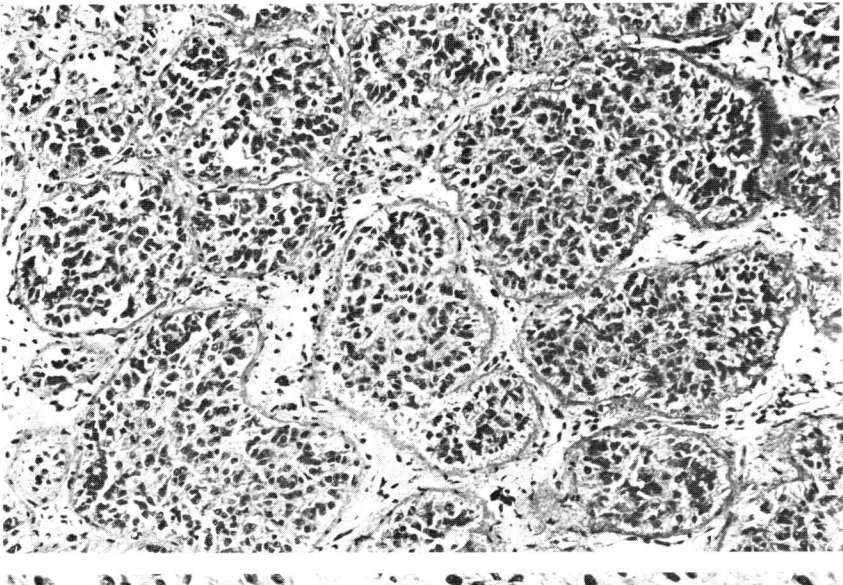

Figure 379. At higher magnification the cells are epithelioid in a glial matrix but delineated by fiber bundles, which prove to be collagenous. This combination is unique for the *pineal*. (× 120)

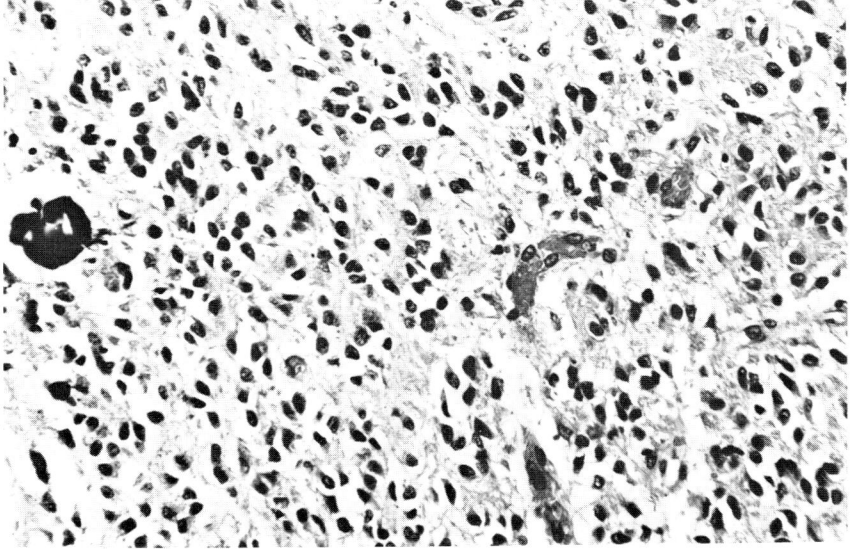

Figure 380. Another common arrangement shows pinealocytes or parenchymal cells in small clusters or in cords with a tendency to separate and simulate glands. Sand granules or corpora arenacea are typical. Some of the cells are astrocytes related to the glial matrix; others contain melanin granules. *Pineal* (× 250)

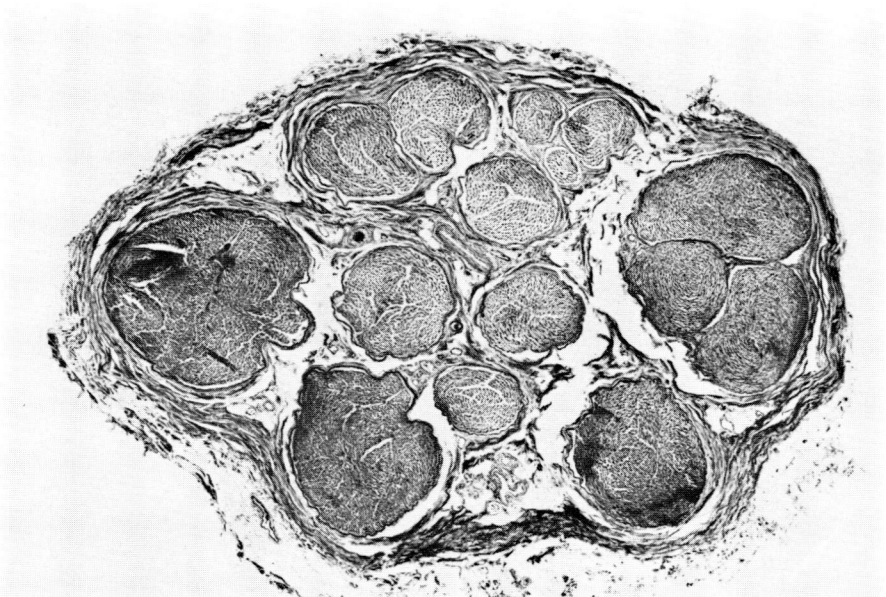

Figure 381. In transverse section, a peripheral ring of fibrous tissue is seen with some extensions inwards; this is the epineurium. Around each of the smaller nerve bundles is a narrow rim of perineural fibrous tissue. The tiny black dots within the fascicles represent axons cut transversely as seen after Bodian stain. Fibrocytes (not visible here) within each nerve bundle constitute the endoneurium. *Peripheral nerve*, cross section, Bodian ($\times 31$)

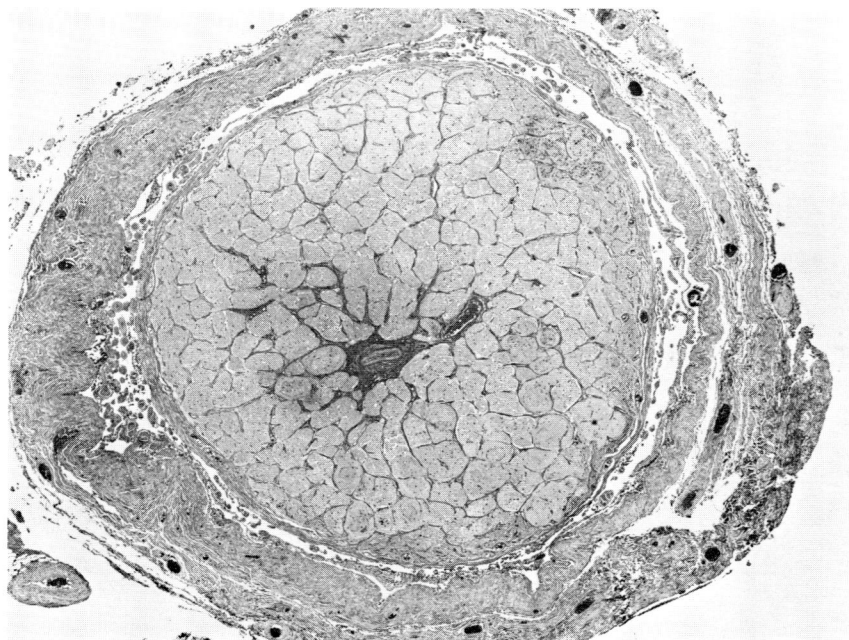

Figure 382. This is another insular solid embedded in a thick capsule of collagenous fibrous tissue from which it is separated by a small clear space with numerous small processes (arachnoid villi). The main structure in the center is divided by fine connective tissue septae and has a central artery. The bundles on higher power prove to be white matter. The whole is unique for the optic nerve with central (retinal) artery. *Optic nerve* ($\times 20$)

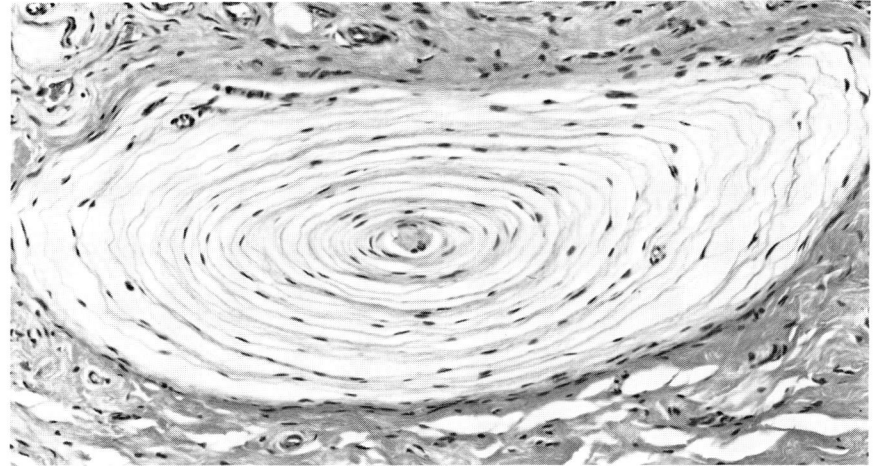

Figure 383. This section is from a fingertip and shows a unique lamellated body with layers of collagen around a central core in which there is an axon (not visible in this H & E preparation). *Pacinian corpuscle* (×110)

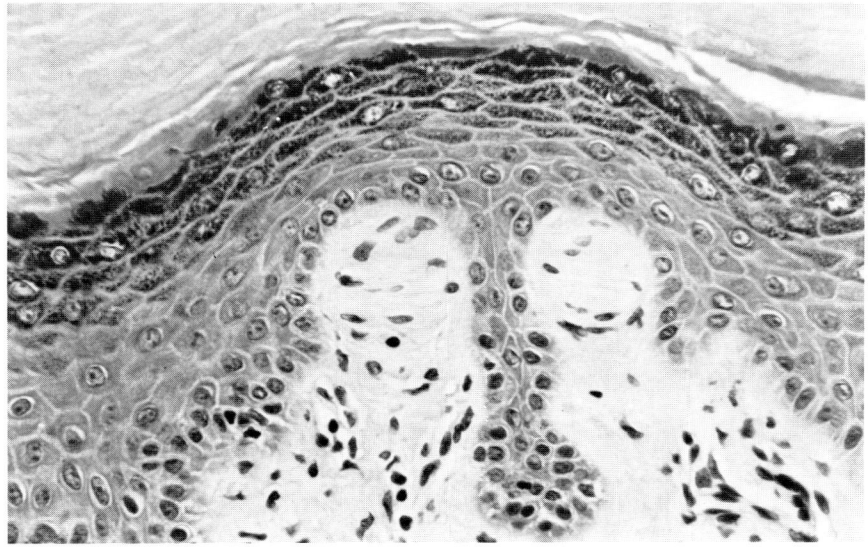

Figure 384. Here there is a portion of skin with two pale, rather zigzag structures immediately beneath the basal layer and in the apices of two dermal ridges. These are Meissner's corpuscles. *Fingertip, Meissner's corpuscles* (×320)

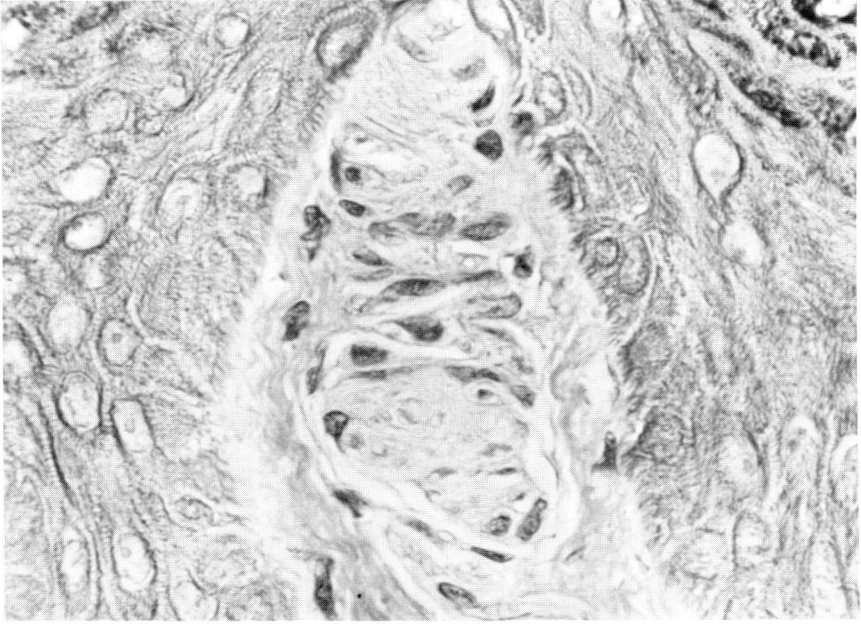

Figure 385. This is a high power of Meissner's corpuscle again from the finger showing the zigzag of collagen and demonstrating the intercellular prickles of the adjacent squamous cells. *Meissner's corpuscle*, Masson trichrome (×630)

MUSCLE SOLIDS

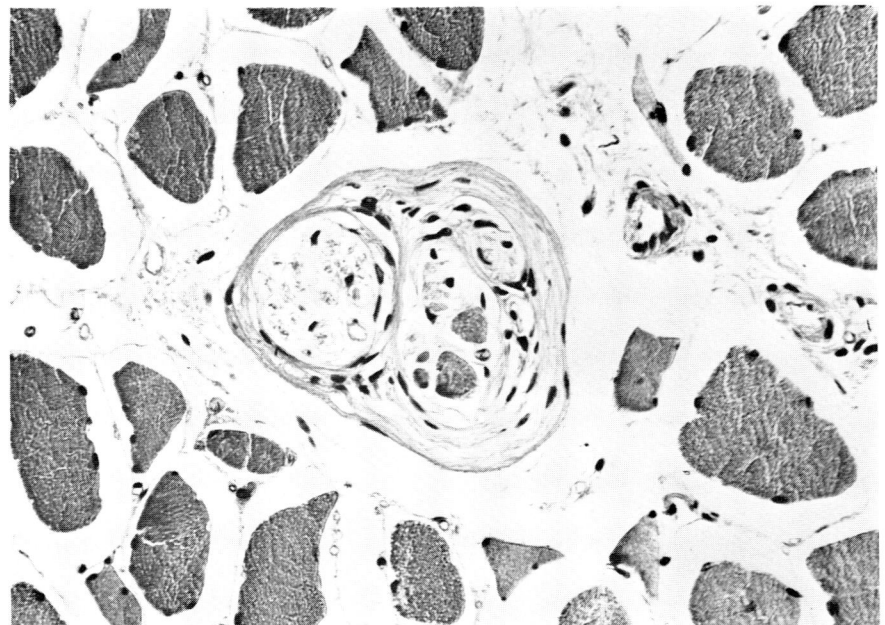

Figure 386. Within skeletal muscles there are specialized nerve endings (stretch receptors) having the three-dimensional form of a spindle. These are closely related to small nerves, as seen in this example, where the central, rather triangular spindle has a small nerve at its apex (left). The oval fibrous capsule encloses several darkly staining muscle fibers, even the largest being much smaller than the surrounding skeletal fibers. *Muscle spindle*, transverse (×300)

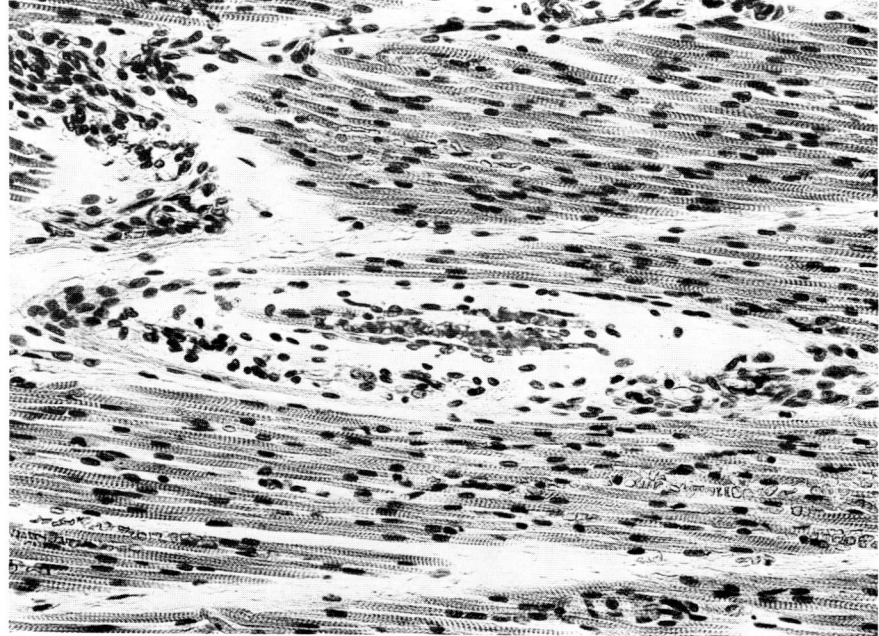

Figure 387. In longitudinal section the spindle shape is more apparent. The nuclei of the muscle cells in the center are aggregated to form what is known as a nuclear bag. The muscle fibers are extremely small, and their striations are very evident. This comes from an infant. *Muscle spindle*, longitudinal (×200)

MUSCLE SOLIDS

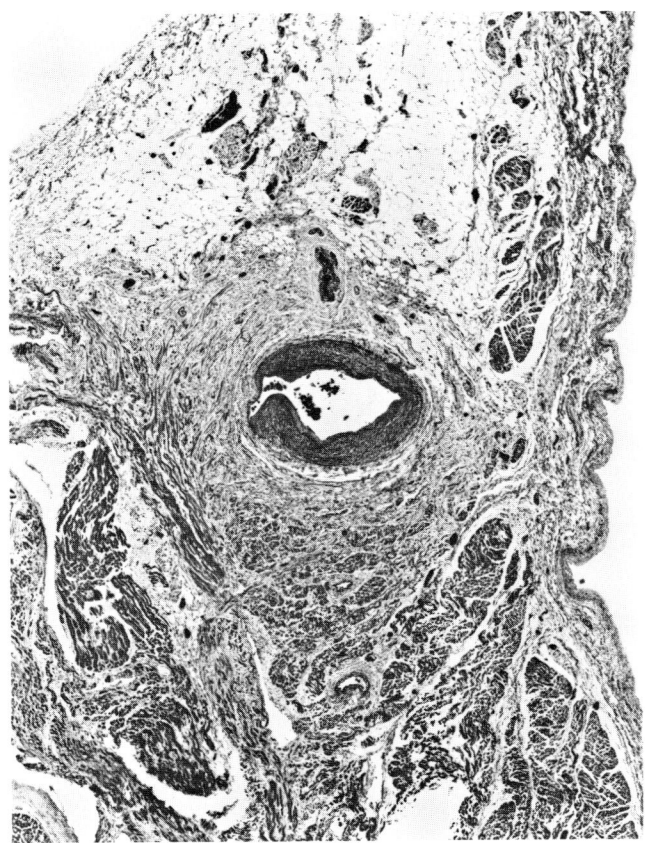

Figure 388. This section was taken from the junction of the right atrial appendage (below) with the superior vena cava (above). The epicardial surface is on the right margin with cardiac fibers extending in small groups beneath the intima of the vena cava. In the middle of the plate is a large artery (the central artery) with concentric fibrous tissue. Below this fibrous tissue is a triangular wedge of small cardiac muscle fibers, seen between two oblique bands of atrial muscle, and having a small artery at the apex. This is the *sinuatrial node*. (× 24)

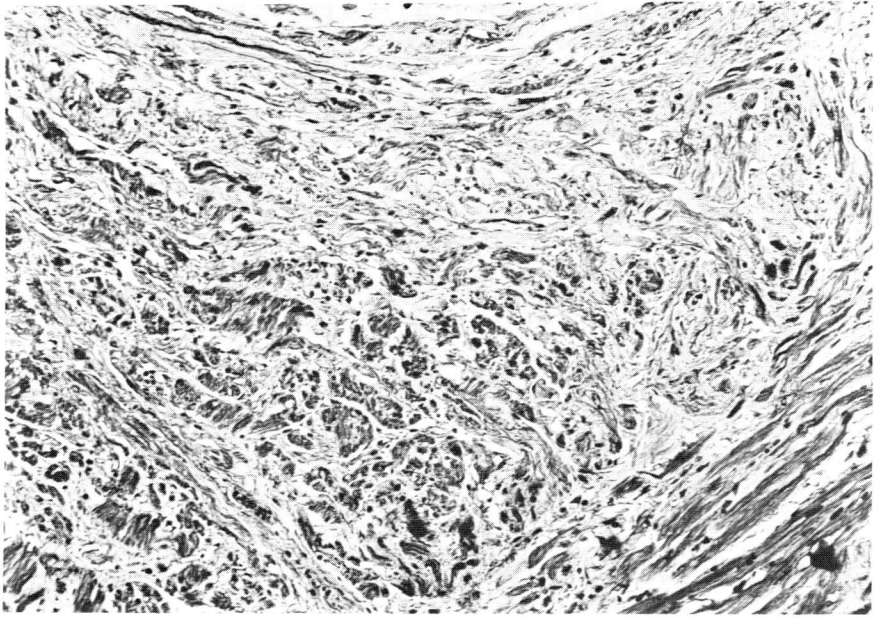

Figure 389. Higher power shows the relation between the small muscle fibers (dark) running in various directions and the fibrous tissue (gray) that separates and envelopes them. *S.A. node* (× 120)

CONDUCTING SYSTEM OF THE HEART

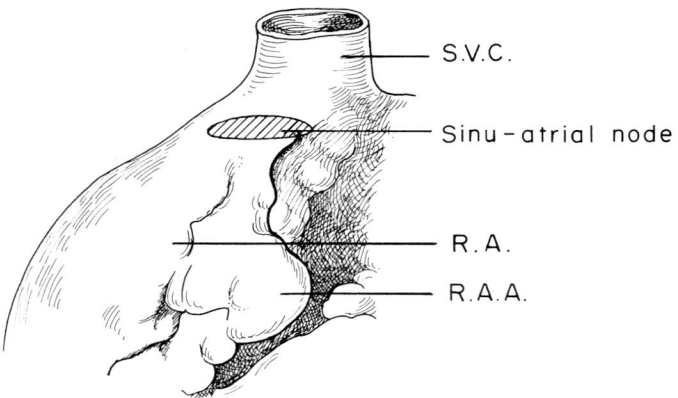

Figure 390. The nodes and bundles of the conducting system of the heart must be looked for in deliberately selected blocks, although the fibers themselves are distinctive when located. The sinuatrial (SA) node lies usually in the epicardial fat just to the right of the crest of the right atrial appendage, immediately below its junction with the superior vena cava. The fibers are small, tangled, and admixed with collagen and elastin. They are closely related to the small arterial ring that runs around the base of the vena cava, which forms a useful landmark. Adapted from Hudson, 1967.

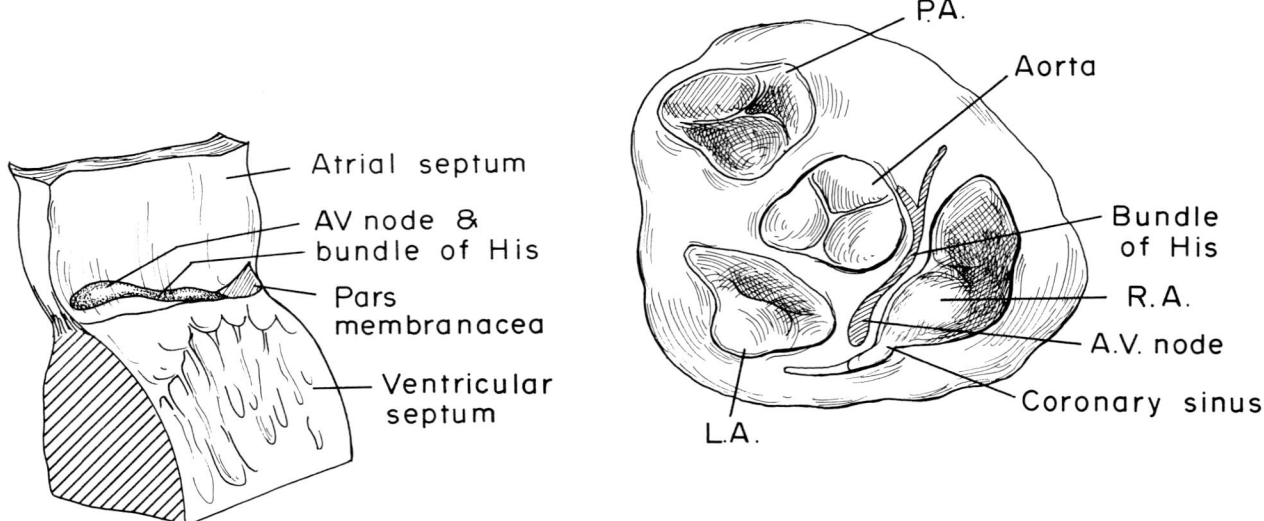

Figure 391. The artrioventricular node (AV) lies under the endocardium of the right atrium, against the central fibrous body, and just above the opening of the coronary sinus (in front, if the apex of the ventricle is pointed downwards during the dissection). His's bundle runs upwards along the crest of the interventricular septum, usually on the left and along the lower edge of the pars membranacea septi. A block of tissue approximately one inch square, including the crest of the interventricular septum from the coronary sinus to the pars membranacea, is taken and cut into serial blocks, vertical to the crest. The fibers of the node and bundle are cardiac in type but smaller and less regularly arranged than the ventricular fibers and again associated with elastin, collagen, nerves, and the nodal artery.

MUSCLE SOLIDS

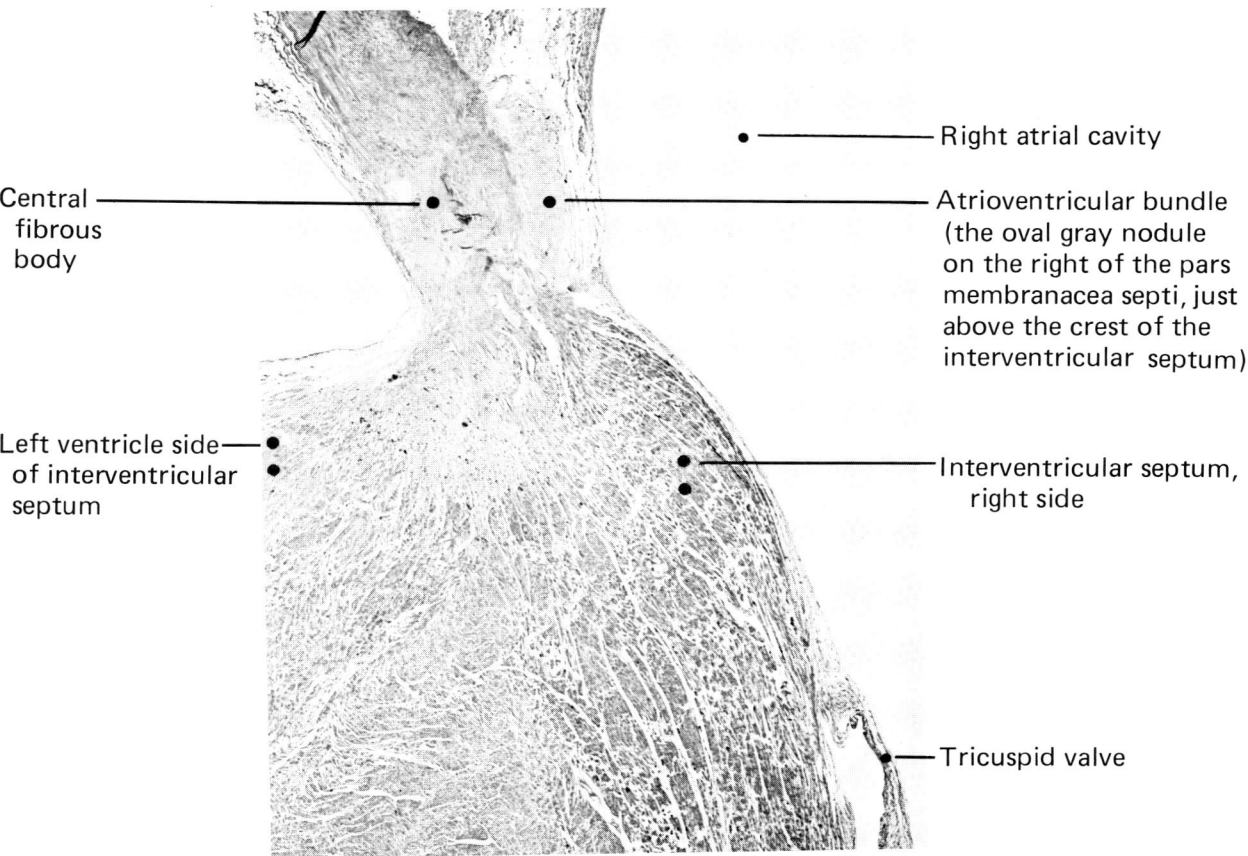

Figure 392. This section was deliberately selected to include the interventricular septum just in front of the opening of the coronary sinus. In the left upper part of the figure is a band of dense fibrous tissue with small oval cells, which suggests fibrocartilage. This is the central fibrous body. The oval, gray nodule on the right side of this, just above the crest of the interventricular septum, is the beginning of the atrioventricular bundle. Serial blocks would show this running upwards and forwards, finally forking over the septum to give right and left branches, which supply the ventricles. *His's atrioventricular bundle* (× 7.5)

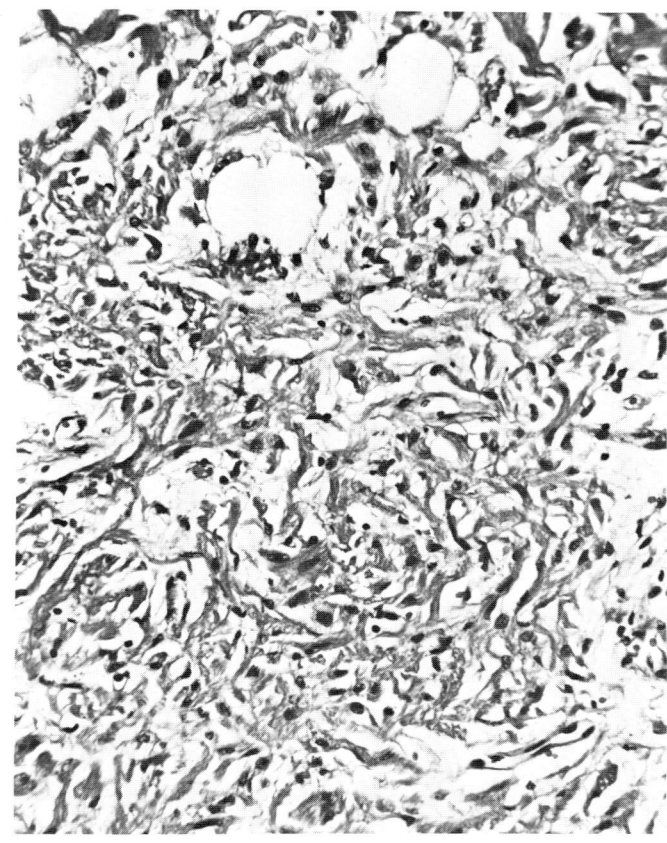

Figure 393. Bundle tissue is characterized by small, irregularly arranged, rather pale staining cardiac muscle fibers in a fibrous background, which contains much elastica and which is closely associated with nerves. *Conducting system* (× 200)

CONNECTIVE TISSUE SOLIDS

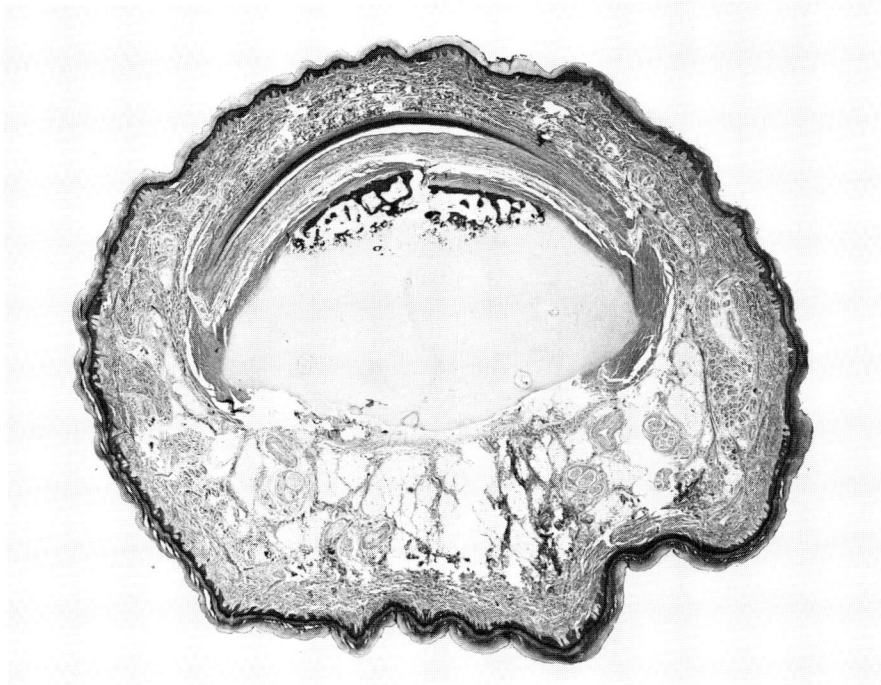

Figure 394. This is a solid island, dominated by different types of connective tissue and covered by stratified squamous epidermis. The central core is largely hyaline cartilage with a small amount of trabecular bone forming along its upper margin. In both lower quadrants there are pale areas of adipose tissue with nerves and blood vessels. Between the bone and the upper surface is a crescentic gray structure with stratified epithelium on both surfaces; this is unique for the nail bed and indicates a digit which has been cut through the terminal phalanx. *Finger, infant* (× 11)

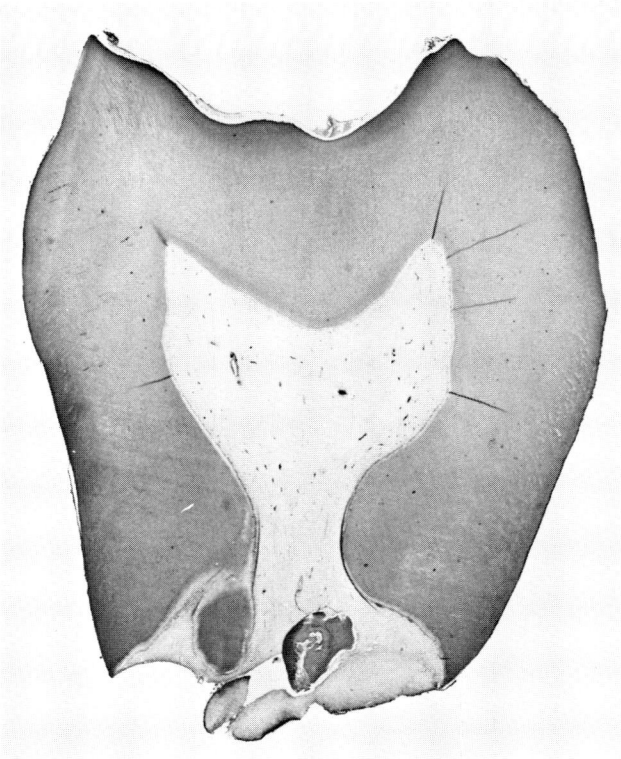

Figure 395. This section is from a decalcified, unerupted bicuspid tooth from an eight-year-old child. Only a few fragments of the protein residue of the enamel are seen along the upper concave margin. The broad dark band that constitutes most of the structure is dentine. The central white area is pulp, here with a goblet shape. This is a loose myxoid vascular connective tissue. At this age, the root of the tooth is not formed, and there is a relatively wide opening at the lower margin. *Tooth* (× 12)

CONNECTIVE TISSUE SOLIDS

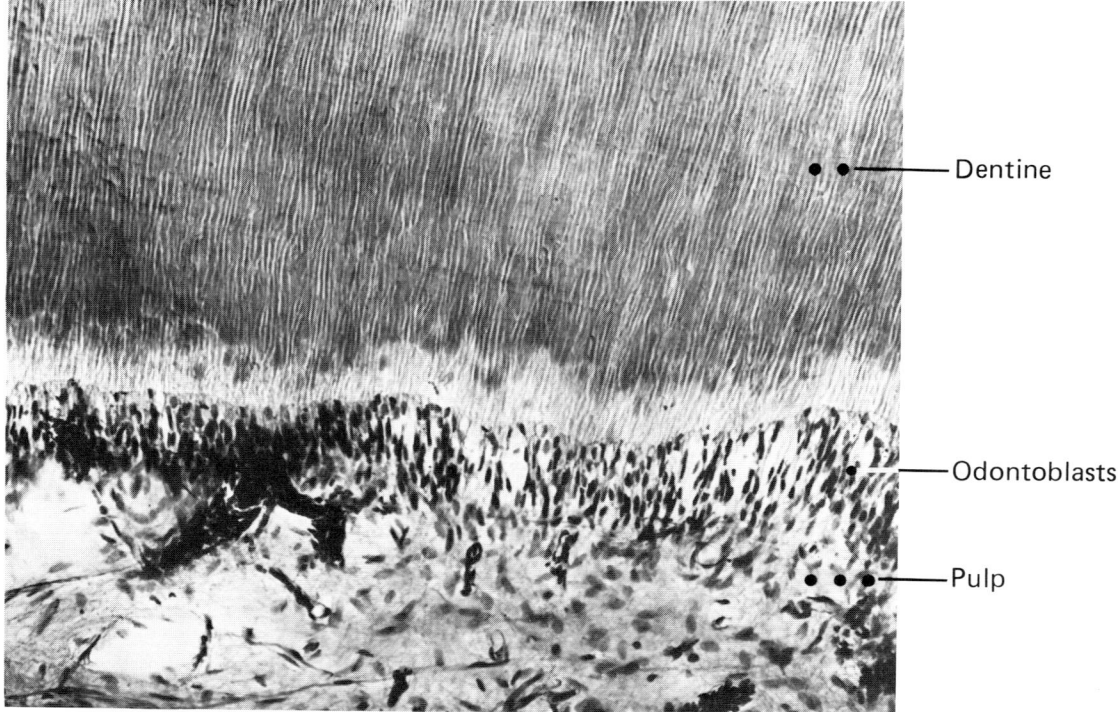

Figure 396. In this figure the upper half has a finely striated appearance and is dentine with its tubules. Below this the broad cellular zone contains the odontoblasts, whose cytoplasmic processes extend into the dentine tubules as Tomes' fibers. Below the odontoblast is the myxoid tissue of the pulp. *Tooth, inner aspect* (× 166)

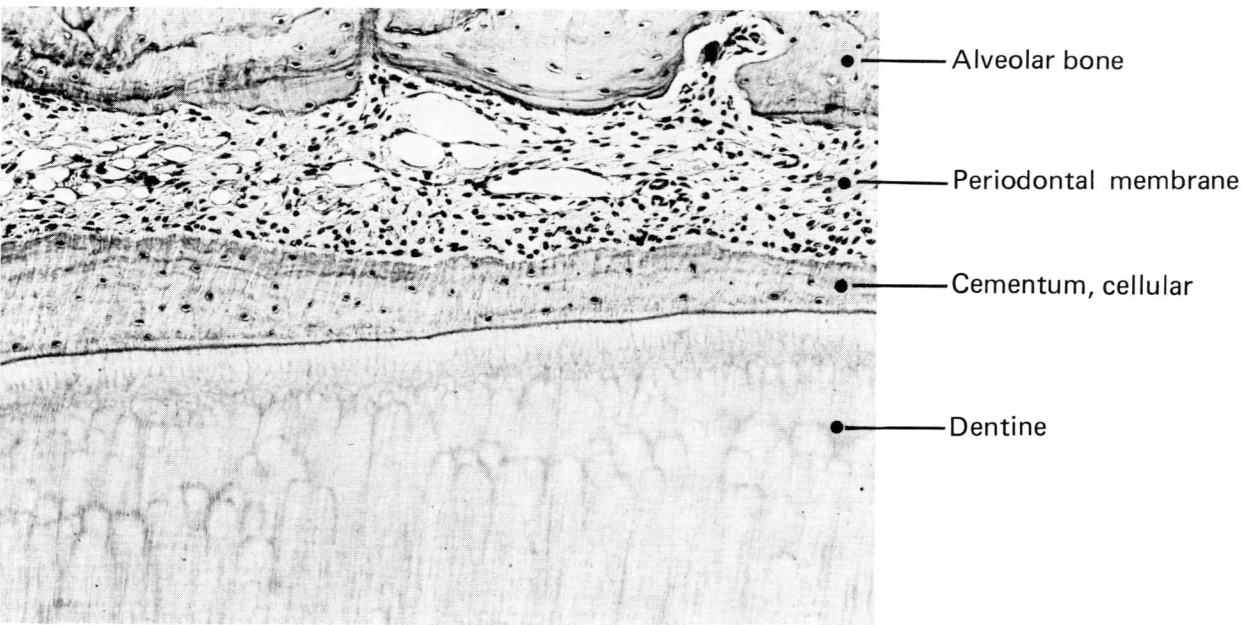

Figure 397. Here the lower part of the figure shows dentine tubules with a broad band of woven bone termed the cementum just above center. This is traversed by noncalcified collagen fibers of Sharpey. Cementum may be cellular (as shown here), but towards the crown of the tooth, it becomes acellular. The upper margin of the figure shows the ordinary alveolar bone of the jaw, and between this and the cementum is the fibrous periodontal membrane. *Tooth, root, outer aspect* (× 120)

CONNECTIVE TISSUE SOLIDS

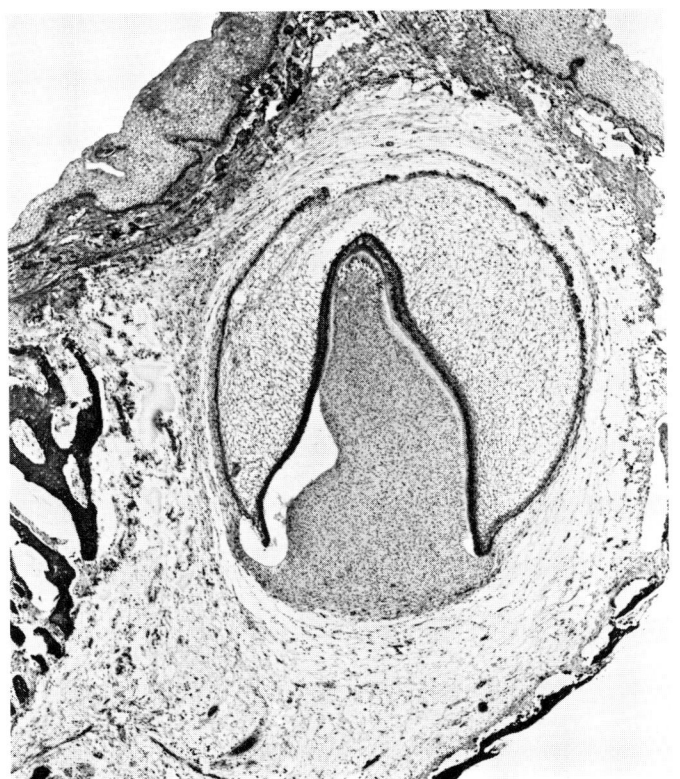

Figure 398. This is from the jaw of a fetus. The stratified squamous mucosa of the mouth is seen above on each side, and on the left margin there is some of the alveolar bone. The dark central pyramid is the developing tooth pulp. Enveloping this is a clawlike structure, the enamel organ, largely formed by stellate reticulum, whose outer margin is demarcated by a three-quarter circle of epithelial cells and whose inner aspect is delineated by a darker (inverted V) line of enamel epithelium. The whole structure can be compared to an epithelial funnel growing down into the mesenchyme as a sheath to the pulp and is known as the epithelial sheath of Hertwig. *Tooth bud* (×27)

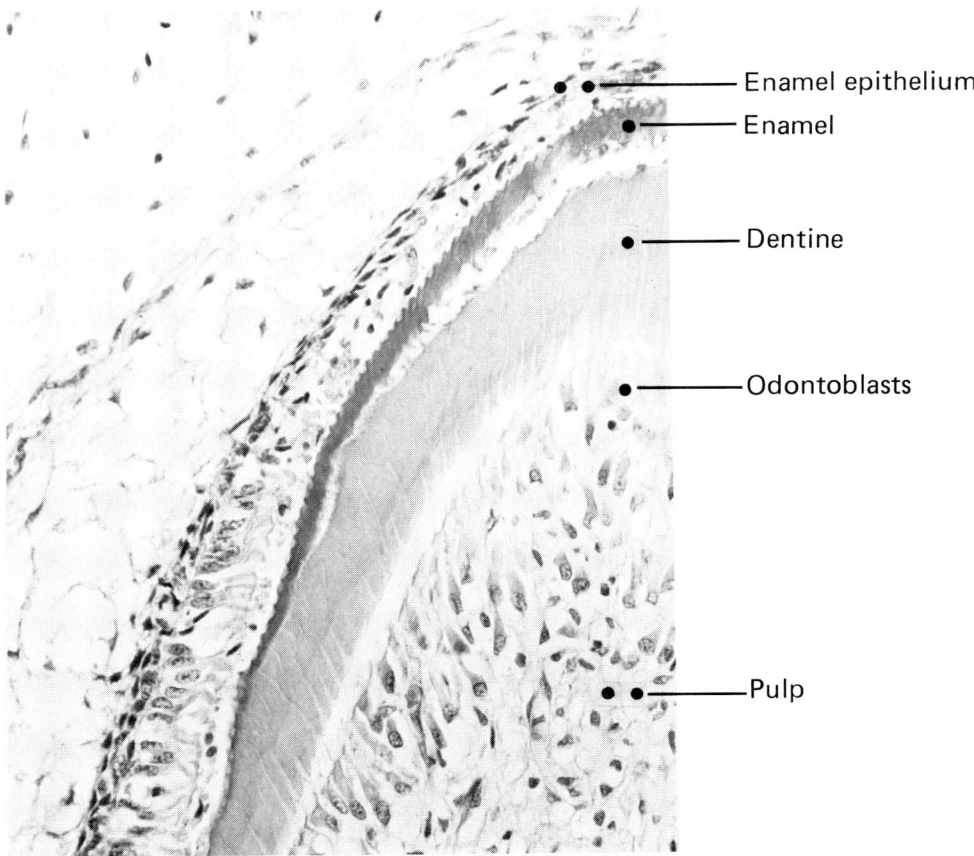

Figure 399. At the left lower margin, the inner part of the stellate reticulum is shown at higher power, separated from the dark enamel cap by a row of columnar ameloblasts. *Tooth bud* (×320)

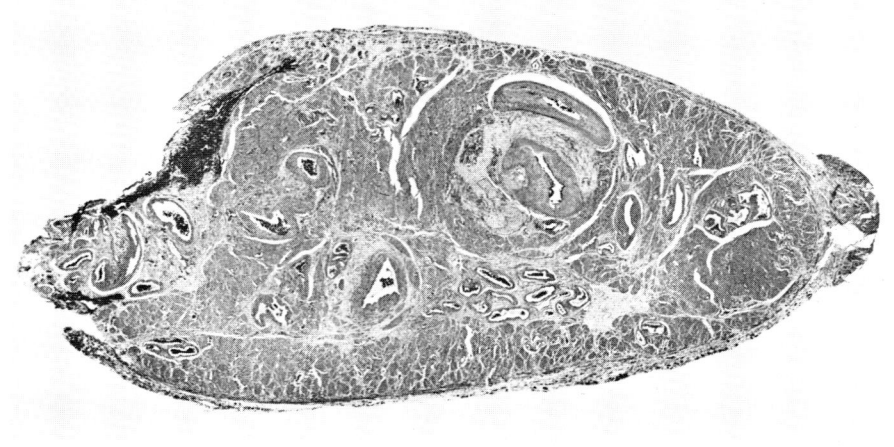

Figure 400. An ovoid island of nonuniform construction, including nonstriated muscle, conspicuous fibrous tissue, and large vessels, is the *round ligament* of the uterus. (× 9.5)

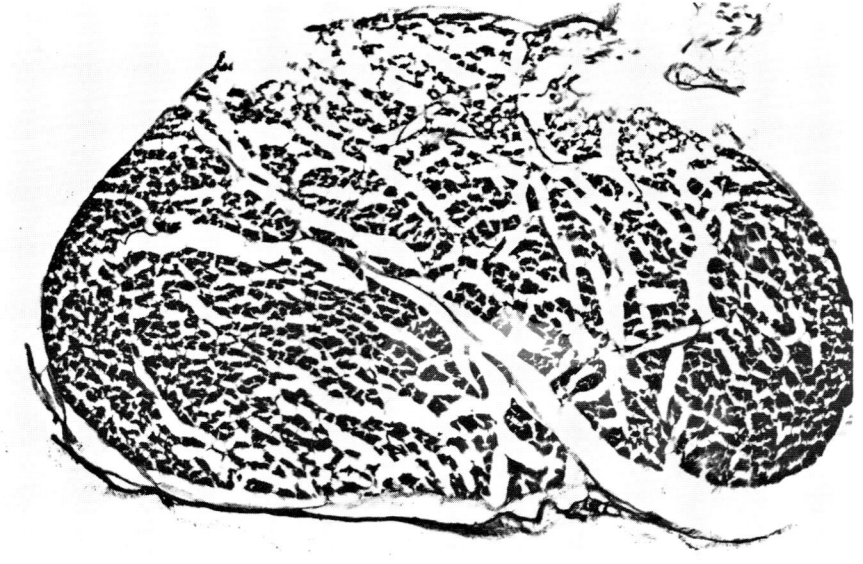

Figure 401. A round or oval island of relatively acellular, dense eosinophilic collagen bundles is a tendon. This is extremely difficult to cut in paraffin sections, and the specimen here is a frozen section. *Tendon* (× 12.5)

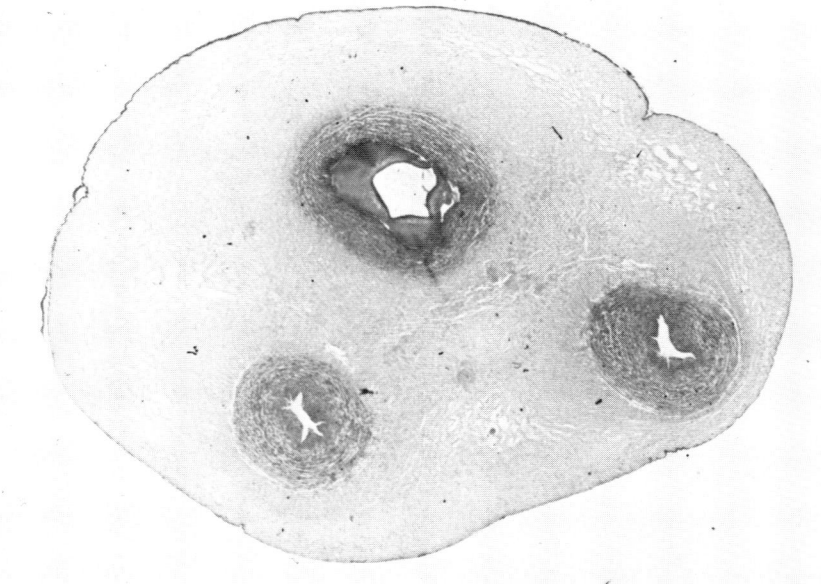

Figure 402. An island of myxoid tissue (Wharton's jelly) covered by a layer of cuboidal epithelium and containing two arteries and a single vein is the *umbilical cord*. The umbilical arteries are the only arteries without an internal elastica, except for those in glomera. (× 12)

CONNECTIVE TISSUE SOLIDS

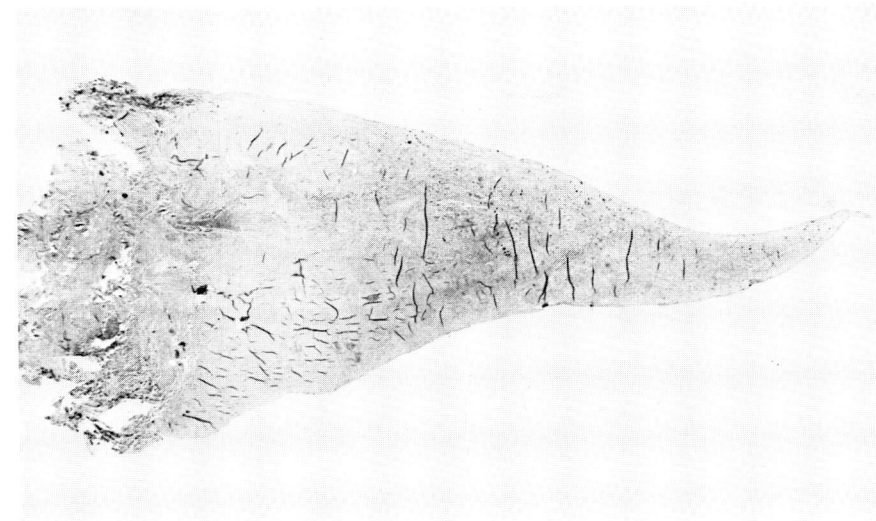

Figure 403. This is a small triangular or wedge-shaped solid, with an extremely sharp apex and a ragged base, where the structure has been dissected from neighboring tissues. The basic tissue is acellular fibrocartilage. The combination of size, shape, and substructure identifies this as one of the semilunar cartilages, or menisci, from a knee joint. *Meniscus*, knee joint ($\times 9.5$)

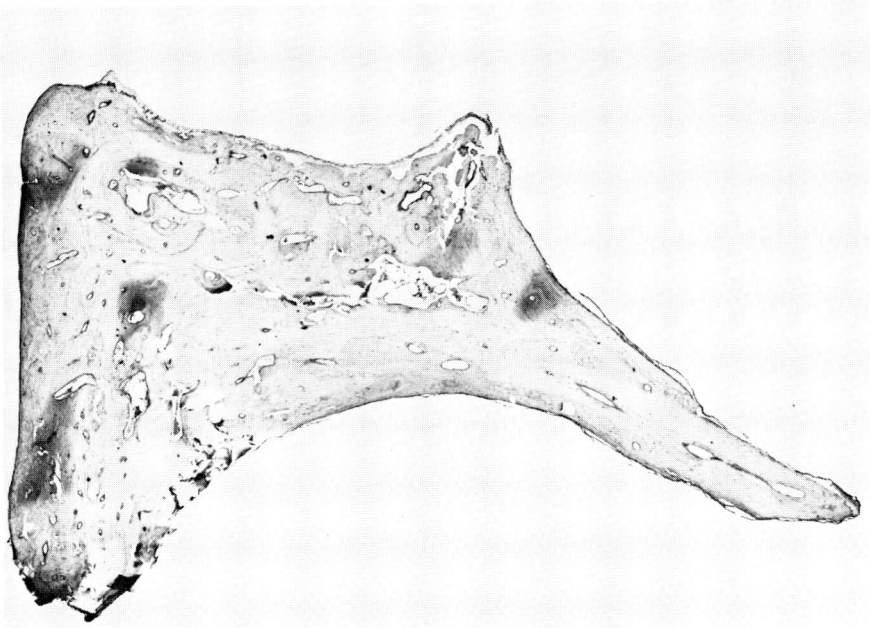

Figure 404. Some bones are small enough and have a contour that is sufficiently distinctive to enable them to be recognized in sections. This is a very small bone whose shape suggests that it is the incus, or anvil. Furthermore, it is woven rather than ordinary lamellar bone; there is no marrow, but there are a few spaces with connective tissue. Coarsely fibrillary or woven bone is normally found in the cortical bone of infants but in adults is restricted to the ossicles, the temporal bone, and the cementum of tooth. The ossicles have a narrow periphery of connective tissue with a flat epithelium. *Incus* ($\times 16$)

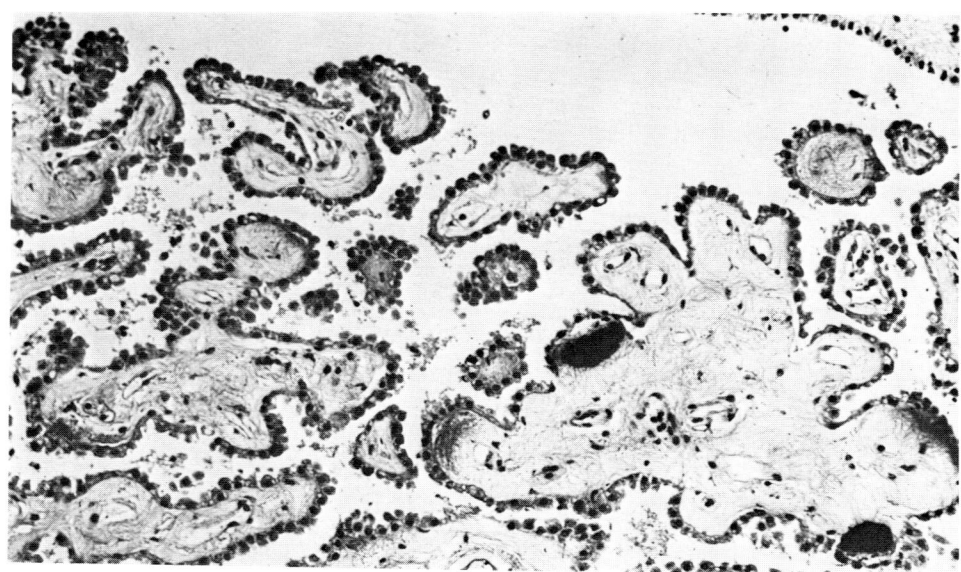

Figure 405. Multiple small islands of myxofibrous tissue, clothed with a cuboidal epithelium and possibly showing small spicules of calcium identify the *choroid plexus*. (×166)

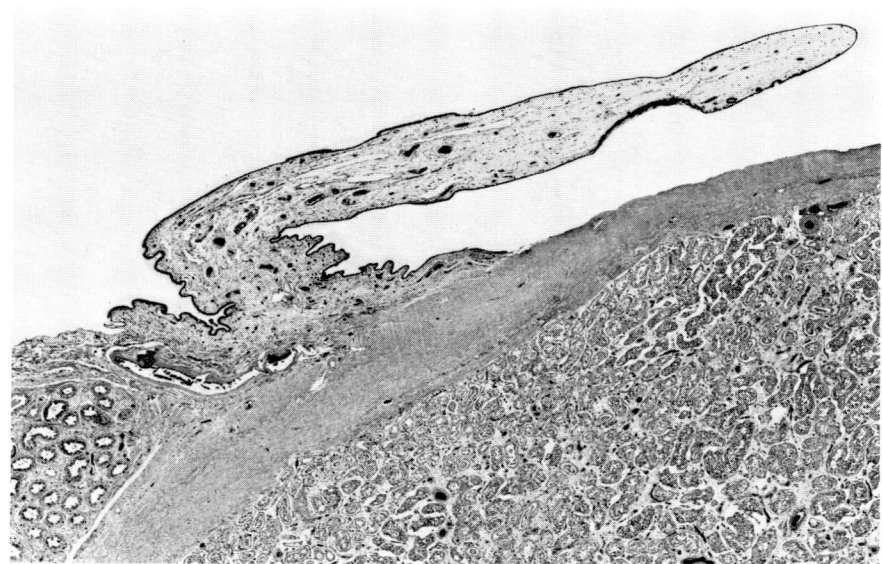

Figure 406. In 80 percent of males, a very small papillary excrescence is found in the groove between the epididymis and the body of the testis. Microscopically this appears as a fibrous peninsula, sometimes branching and sometimes with internal spaces. The core consists of connective tissue covered by low columnar epithelium. This is a Mullerian remnant known as the *appendix testis* (×250)

CONNECTIVE TISSUE SOLIDS

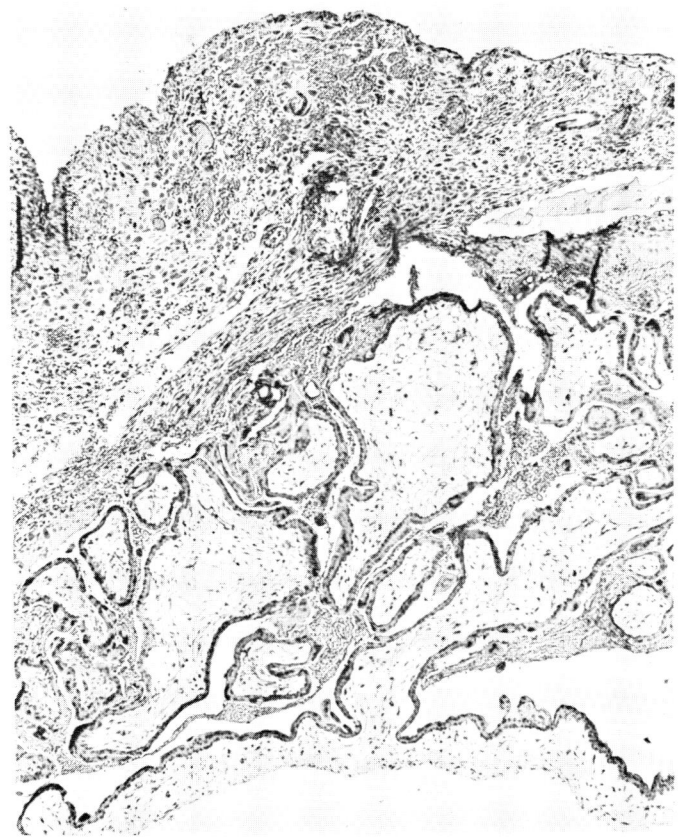

Figure 407. The small islands of pale tissue seen in the center of this figure, which have a reticulate pattern and are composed of myxoid tissue covered by an epithelium that includes multinucleated (syncytial) giant cells, are the chorionic villi. In early pregnancy, as here, the epithelium has two rows of cells — an outer syncytial layer in which giant cells appear as "knots" by clumping of nuclei, and an inner conventional cellular layer (Langhans) of cytotrophoblasts. The inner layer is lost at about sixteen weeks of gestation. The broad band of epithelioid cells running across the upper part of this figure is the endometrial decidua. The thinner lower band is the chorion, from which the amnion has been artefactually detached. The villi are seen as long extensions from this chorionic plate, and they project into maternal blood sinusoids. Vessels should be present in all villi by eight to ten weeks and may be seen here in the long fingerlike villus in the lower right field. *Placenta, immature* ($\times 50$)

CONNECTIVE TISSUE SOLIDS

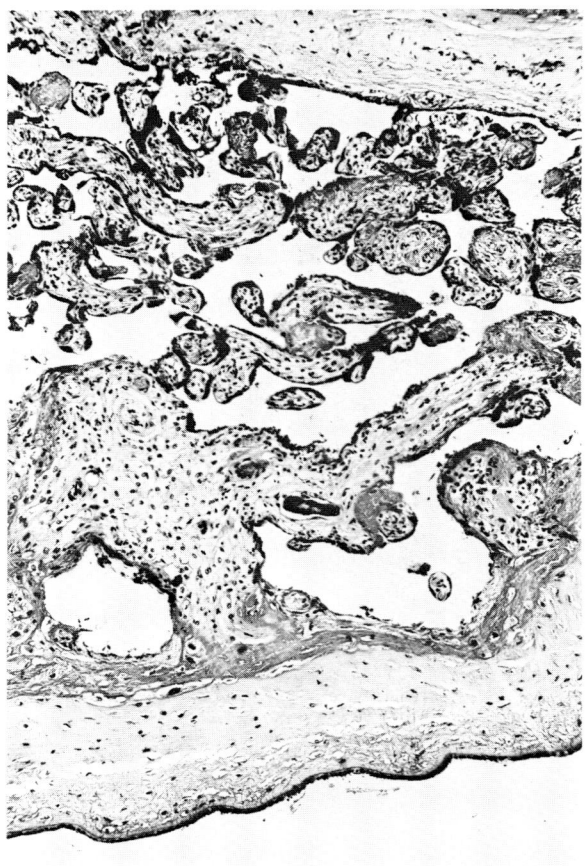

Figure 408. In the mature placenta, the fetal surface or roof plate is largely formed by the amnion, which has its own connective tissue and a covering of cuboidal amniotic epithelium (shown here below). This overlies the chorionic plate. The stroma of the villi has become more spindle celled and fibrous; the cells are known as Hoffbauer cells. Syncytial knots are prominent, and there is amorphous eosinophilic fibrinoid material not only between the villi but also forming a layer (Langhans layer) along the chorionic plate. *Roof plate*, placenta (×80)

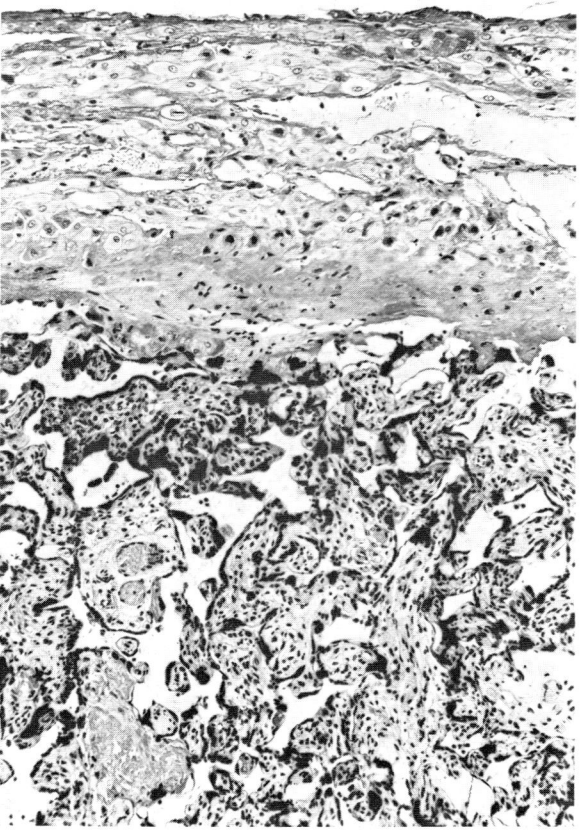

Figure 409. The uterine aspect of the placenta (floor plate) shows attached maternal decidua (above) containing large blood sinusoids. The horizontal amorphous layer of fibrinoid is known as Nitabuch's layer. The maternal and intervillous blood sinusoids are in communication, although not seen in this particular picture. *Floor plate*, placenta (×80)

CONNECTIVE TISSUE SOLIDS

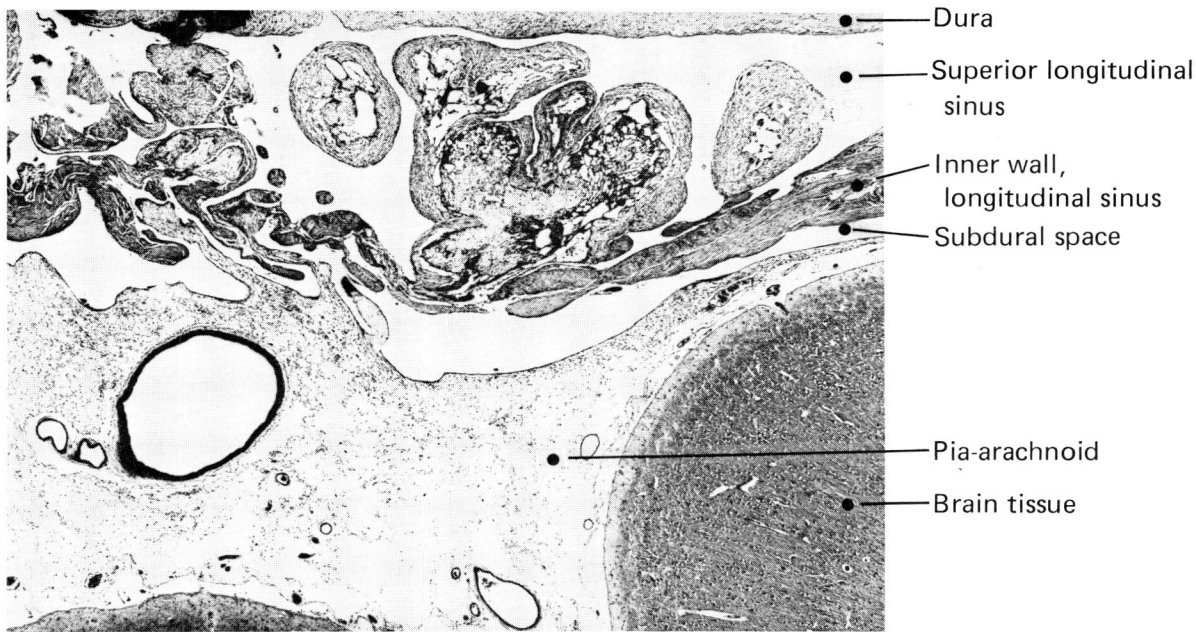

Figure 410. This is again a distinctive combination of small solids and spaces. In the bottom right is brain tissue. Adjacent to this, seen particularly in the left lower half, is loose tissue, which actually is a meshwork of spaces containing the cerebrospinal fluid. Along the upper margin is more dense fibrous tissue of the dura mater. The space beneath the dura mater is the superior longitudinal sinus, whose deeper wall adjoining the meninges is penetrated by irregular extensions of pia-arachnoid. These expand within the sinus to bulbous masses, many appearing as islands that are wrapped in fibrous tissue and then covered by endothelium. *Arachnoid villi*, Movat (× 20)

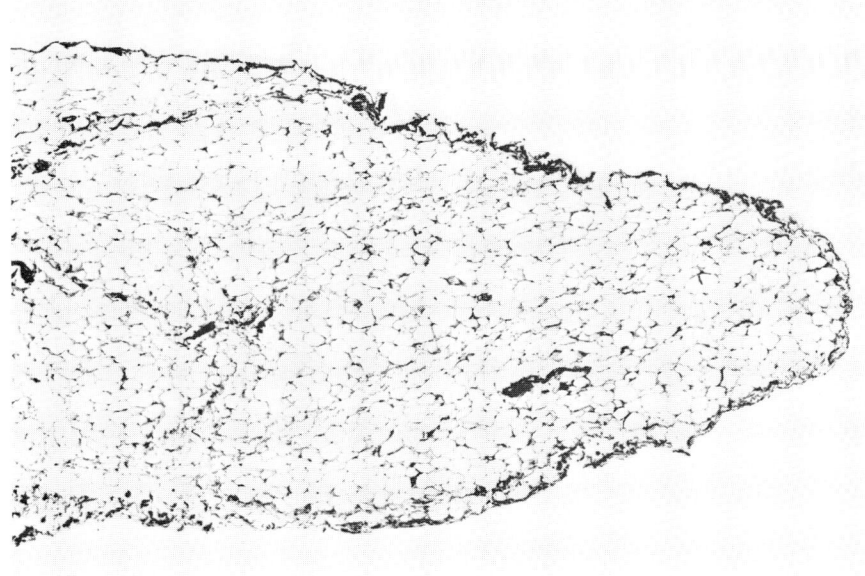

Figure 411. This specimen is dominated by adipose tissue, identified by the reticulate pattern. It is well demarcated and covered by a mesothelial surface (not distinguishable clearly). While adipose tissue forms a great deal of the supporting material of the body, it occasionally forms recognizable parts, as in the omentum, and in the appendices epiploicae, which are polypoid projections from the serosal coat of the large intestine. Part of an appendix is shown here. *Appendix epiploica* (× 32)

CONNECTIVE TISSUE SOLIDS

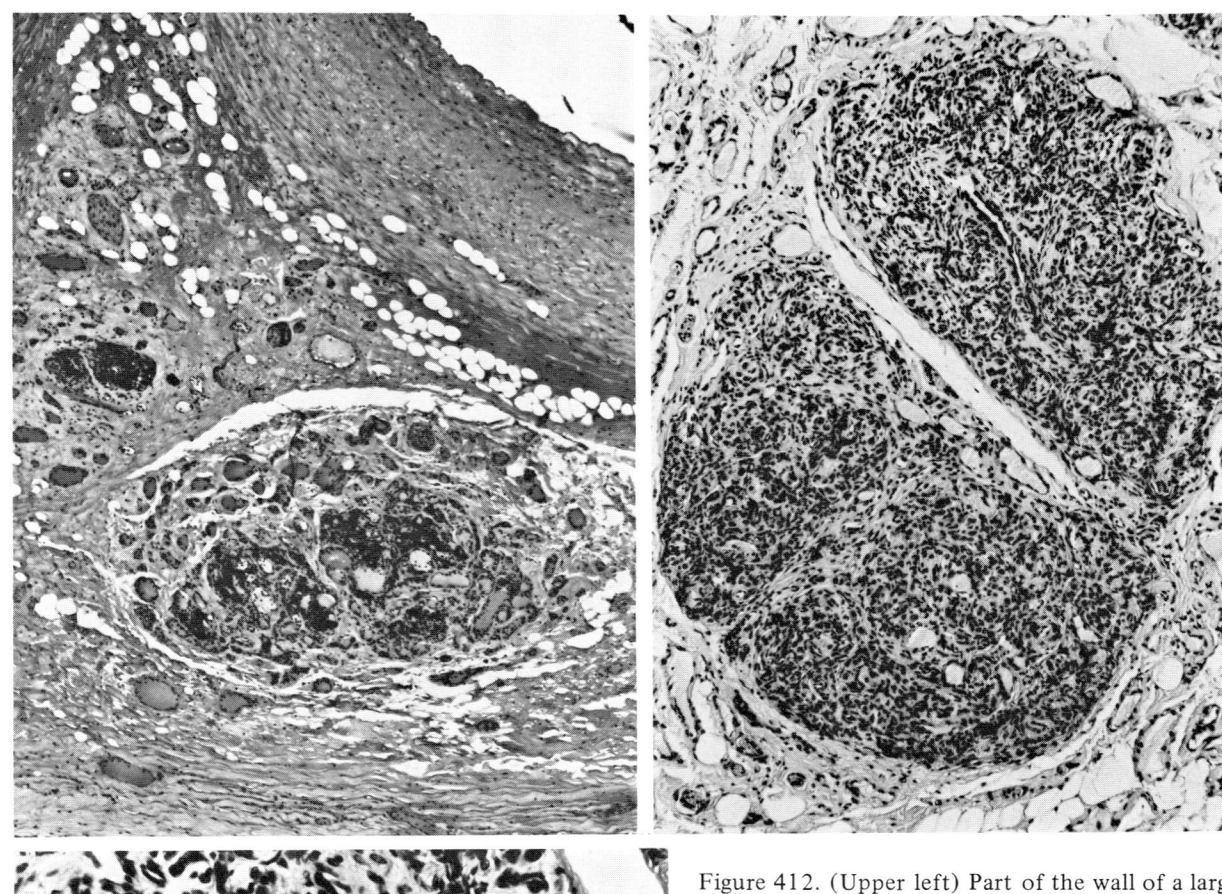

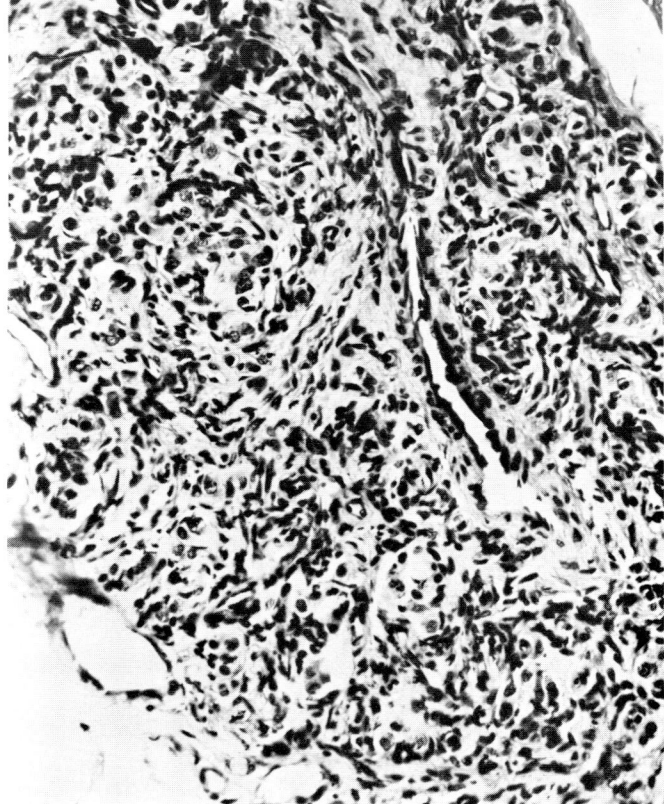

Figure 412. (Upper left) Part of the wall of a large artery (the carotid) runs across the upper right quadrant of this figure. In the lower center of the field is a cellular enclave, associated with numerous small vessels. *Carotid body* (× 40)

Figure 413. (Upper right) At slightly higher power, two cellular groups (from another specimen) are illustrated. (× 80)

Figure 414. (Lower left) The cells now appear as closely packed spindle and polyhedral cells, with the format of a segregated mesenchymal tissue and little suggestion of grouping. Two types of cells are seen in the carotid: type I — chief or glomus cells, and type II — sustentacular cells. The chief cells can be stained with lead hematoxylin. *Carotid body* (× 200)

CONNECTIVE TISSUE SOLIDS

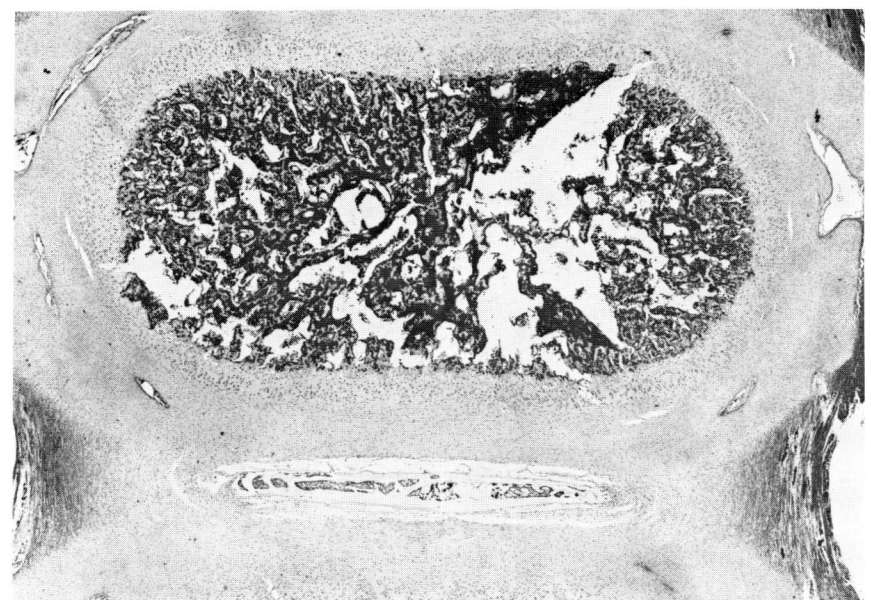

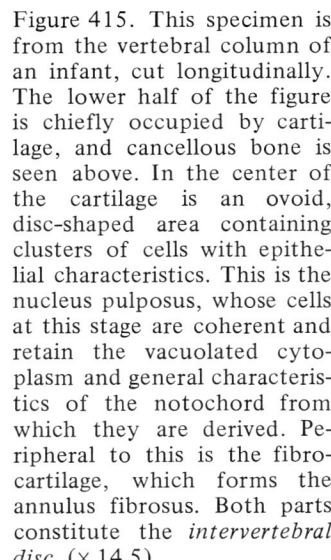

Figure 415. This specimen is from the vertebral column of an infant, cut longitudinally. The lower half of the figure is chiefly occupied by cartilage, and cancellous bone is seen above. In the center of the cartilage is an ovoid, disc-shaped area containing clusters of cells with epithelial characteristics. This is the nucleus pulposus, whose cells at this stage are coherent and retain the vacuolated cytoplasm and general characteristics of the notochord from which they are derived. Peripheral to this is the fibrocartilage, which forms the annulus fibrosus. Both parts constitute the *intervertebral disc*. (× 14.5)

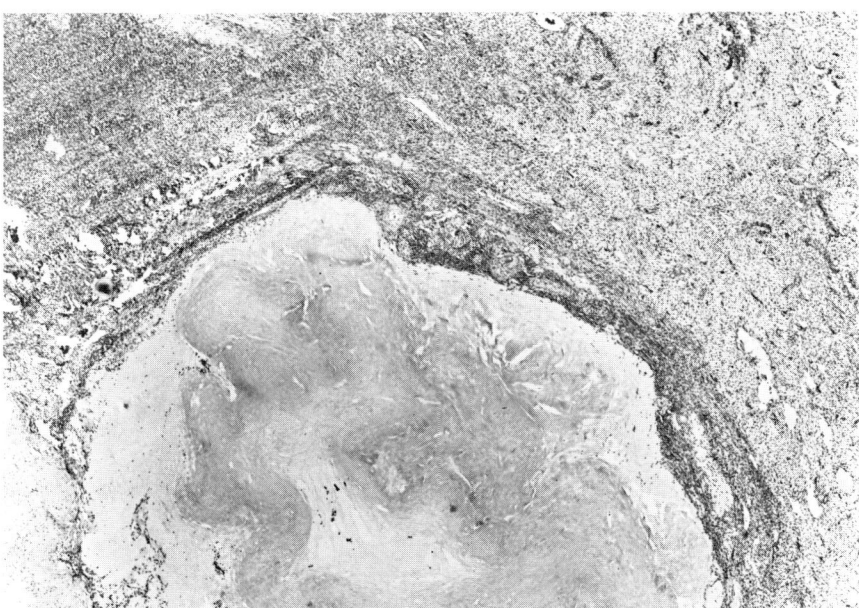

Figure 416. An island of hyalinized acellular collagenous tissue is seen lying within a more cellular fibrous tissue; this is typical of the corpus albicans of the ovary, which is the involuted terminal form of the corpus luteum, whose convoluted outline can still be seen. Corpora albicantia persist into old age and allow the identification of ovarian tissue even when other elements are atrophic and have disappeared. *Corpus albicans* (× 27)

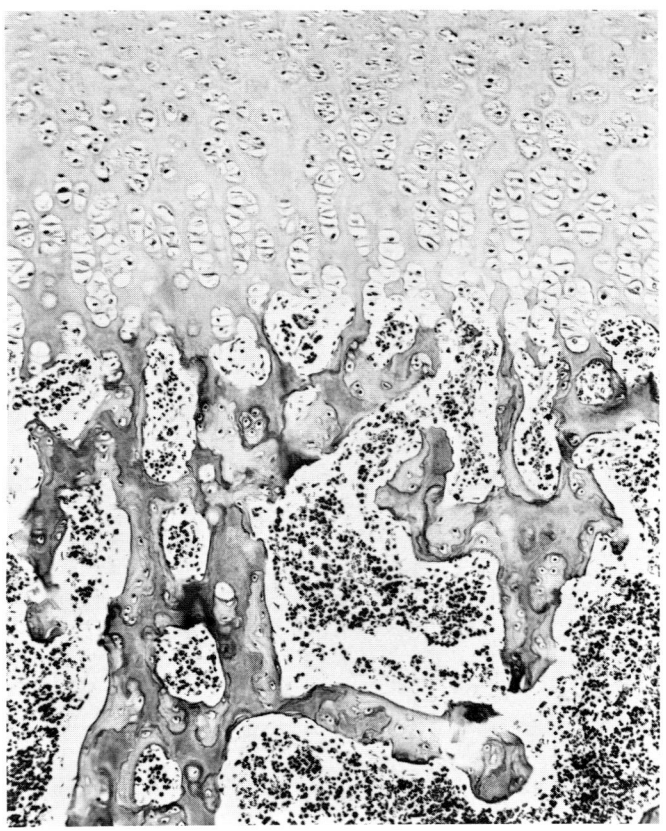

Figure 417. The upper part of this figure shows hyaline cartilage, with the cells as they are followed downwards becoming larger and lining up in rows. The matrix between the cells constitutes cartilage bars; these acquire calcium and consequently stain somewhat more darkly (just above the center line). The punctate tissue in the lower half of the figure is primitive bone marrow, lying among irregular trabeculae, which are partially ossified and represent the remains of the cartilage bars as they are replaced by bone. *Epiphyseal cartilage*, infant bone ($\times 80$)

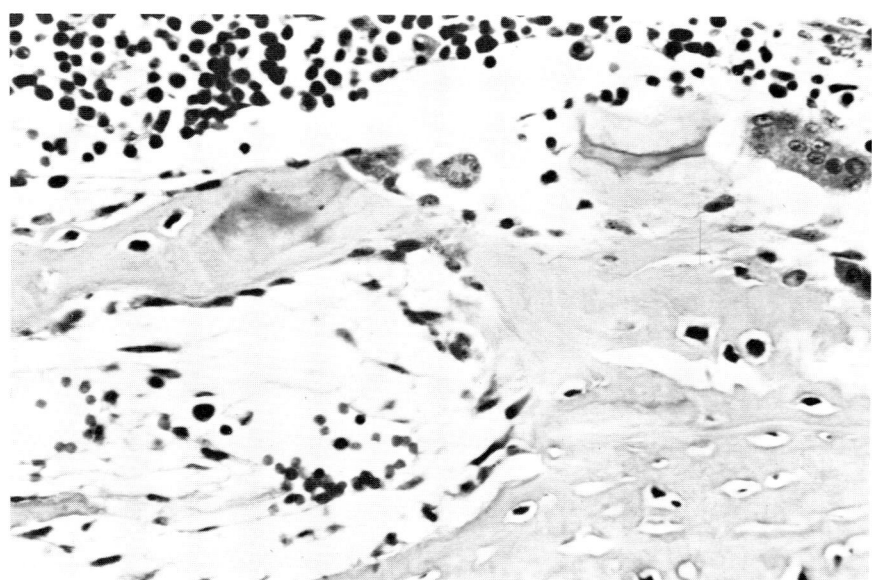

Figure 418. The area of bone adjacent to the epiphysis is known as the metaphysis and here active bone modelling takes place. This involves the removing of preexisting cartilage and bone by multinucleated osteoclasts, which can be seen in the upper right quadrant. The osteoblasts responsible for the formation of new bone can be seen forming rows of cells along each side of the trabecula in the left upper quadrant. The more mature cells enclosed within the trabeculae are the osteocytes. Between the bony plates is mesenchymal tissue with developing myeloid elements, but no fat has yet appeared, as expected in normal adult red marrow. *Metaphysis, fetus* ($\times 300$)

LYMPHATIC SOLIDS

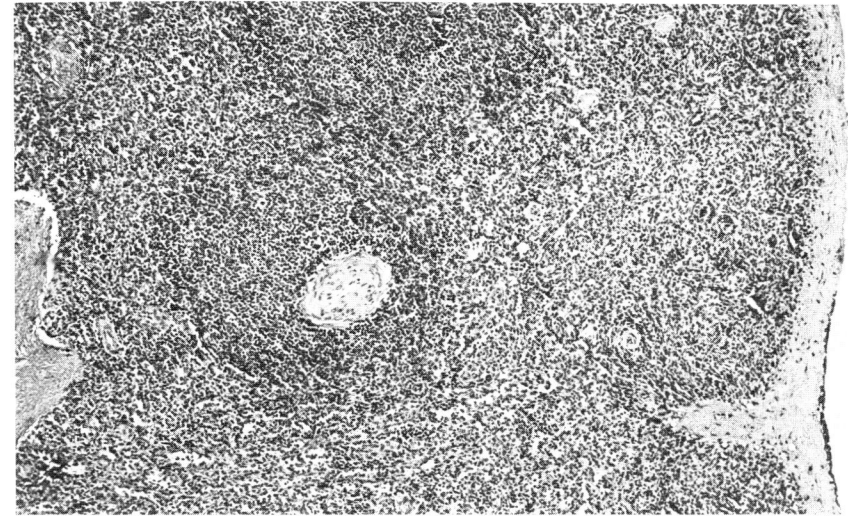

Figure 419. This shows a capsule of fibrous tissue with a surface of mesothelial cells along the right margin. Just above center is a fibromuscular band, representing part of the supporting framework, which extends in from the capsule on the right. *Spleen*, capsular surface (×80)

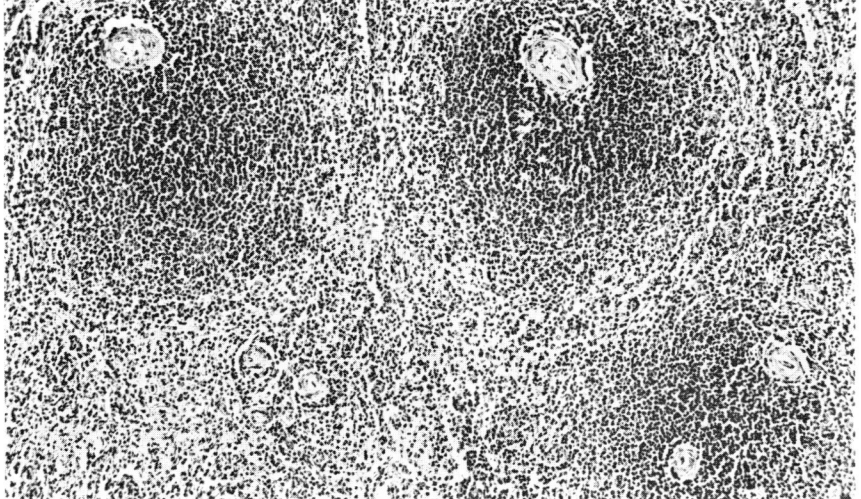

Figure 420. This shows nodular aggregates of lymphoid cells around the fibromuscular strands and around arteries; this perivascular arrangement is typical of spleen. The more dense lymphatic nodules constitute the white pulp, and the looser tissue between them is the red pulp, which is largely a collection of blood sinusoids, again unique to the spleen. *Spleen, lymphatic nodules* (Malpighian corpuscles) (×85)

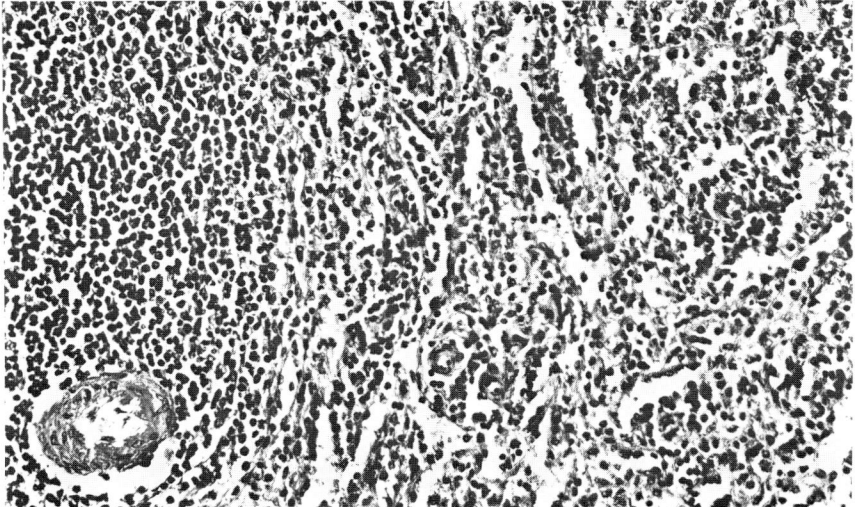

Figure 421. The splenic sinusoids are lined by plump phagocytic endothelial, or littoral, cells. All the sinusoids in this particular figure appear empty; others were stuffed with erythrocytes. (In other lymphatic tissues sinusoids contain lymph.) The more cellular areas between the sinusoids are known as Billroth's cords and contain not only lymphocytes and histiocytes but erythrocytes in an extravascular situation. *Spleen* (×200)

These three figures come from an apparent solid dominated by a punctate pattern, with lymphatic cells.

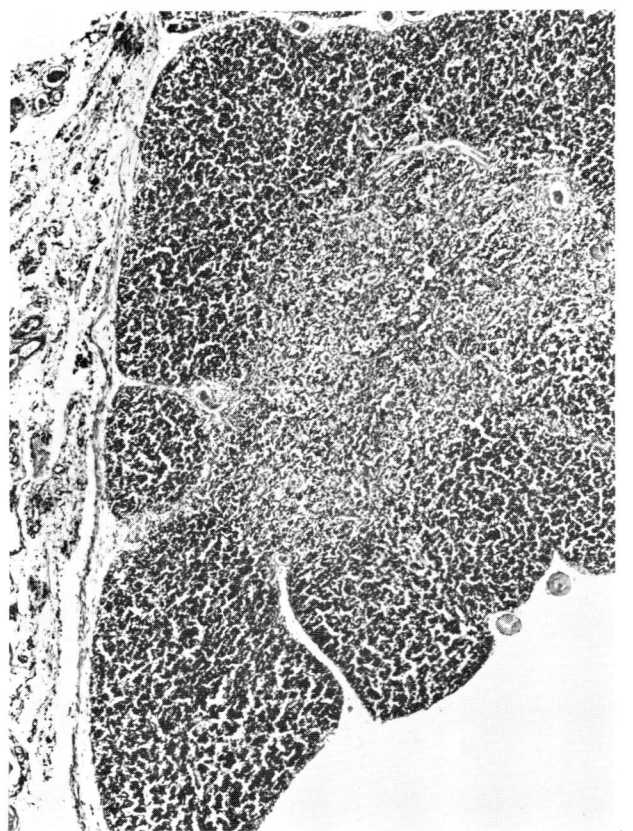
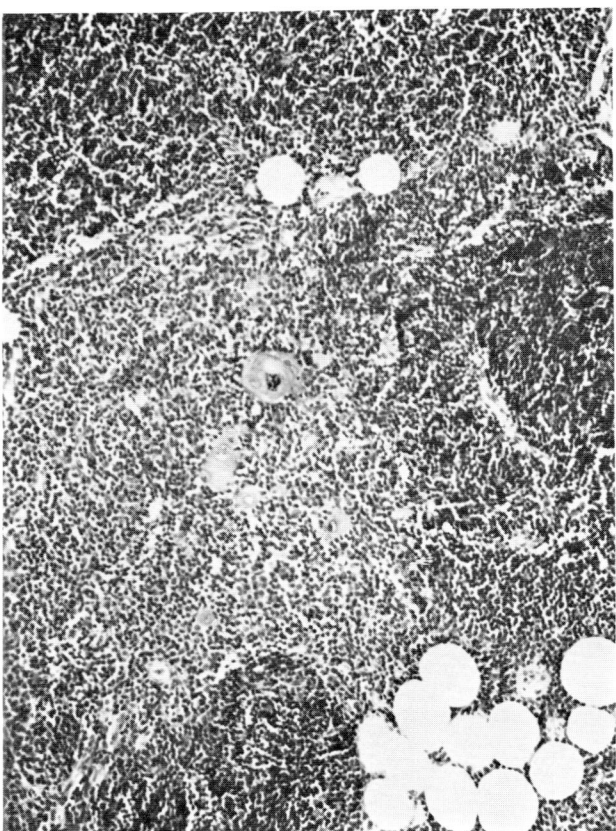
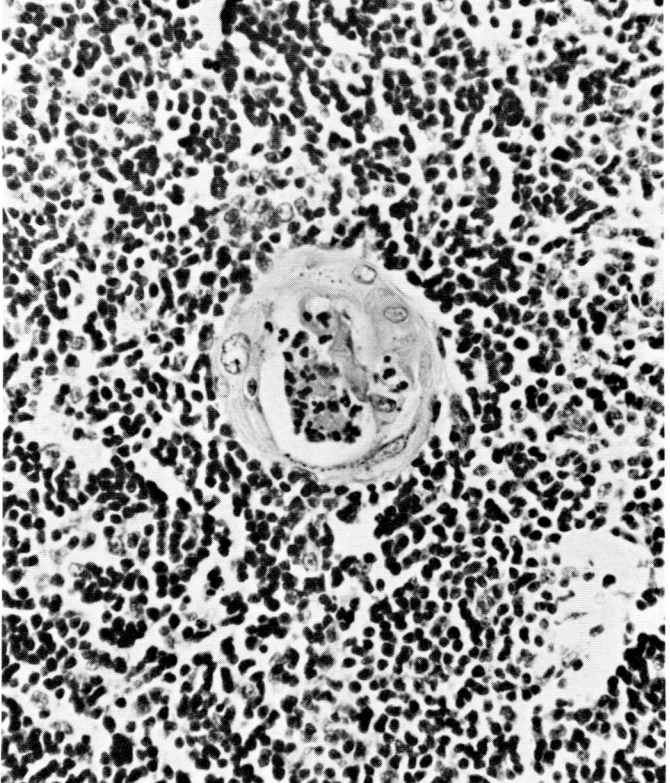

Figure 422. (Upper left) This is again a solid lymphatic structure with somewhat darker cortical zone and a paler medulla. It comes from the *fetal thymus*. (×40)

Figure 423. (Upper right) From puberty onwards, the thymus contains fat cells, seen here as empty spaces. In the center of the field is a small circular whorl of nonlymphoid nature (seen better in Figure 424.) *Thymus*. (×120)

Figure 424. (Lower left) At high magnification the whorl is formed of keratinizing cells enclosing a small amount of nuclear debris, which is often partly calcified. This is a Hassall's corpuscle. Among the smaller lymphocytes there are scattered, larger, pale-staining nuclei, which are also epithelial in nature and which are arranged in an open network, which gives rise to the term reticular cells. *Thymus* (×300)

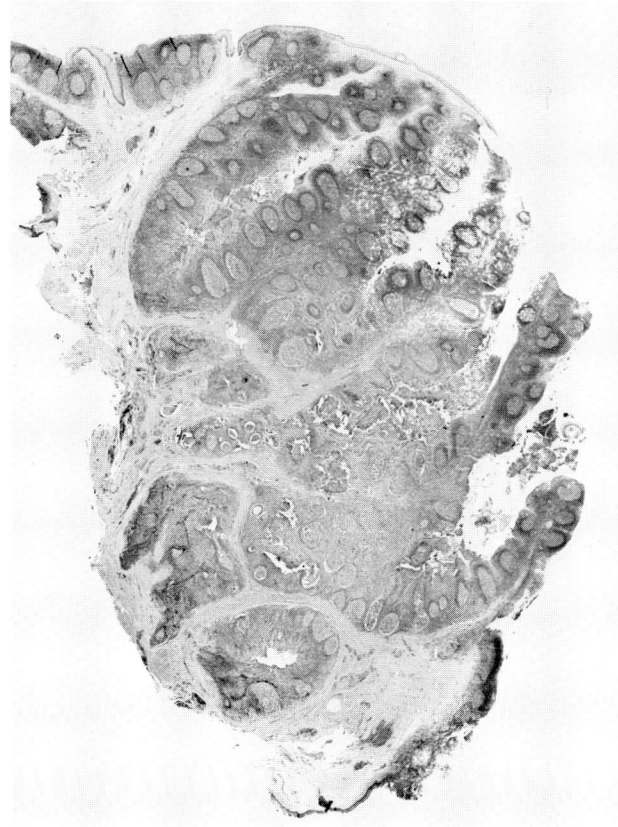

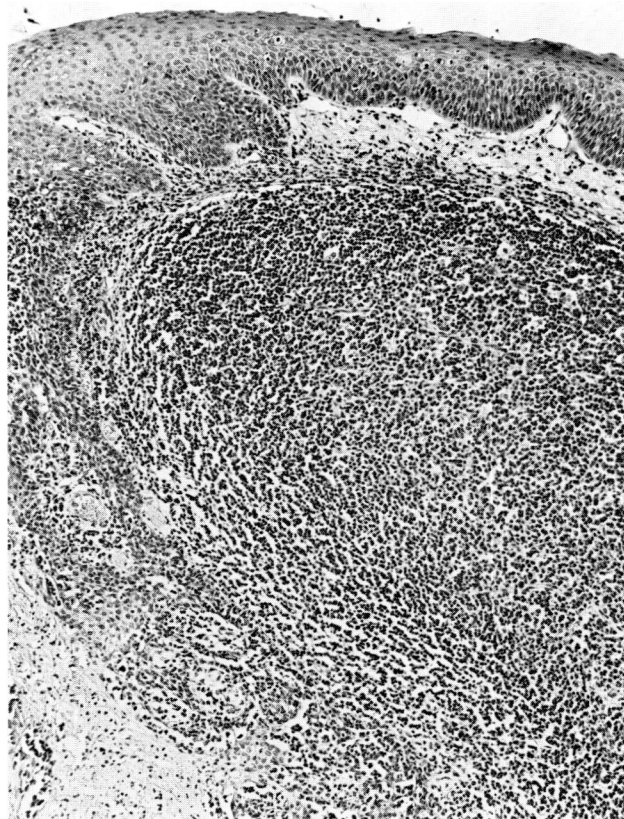

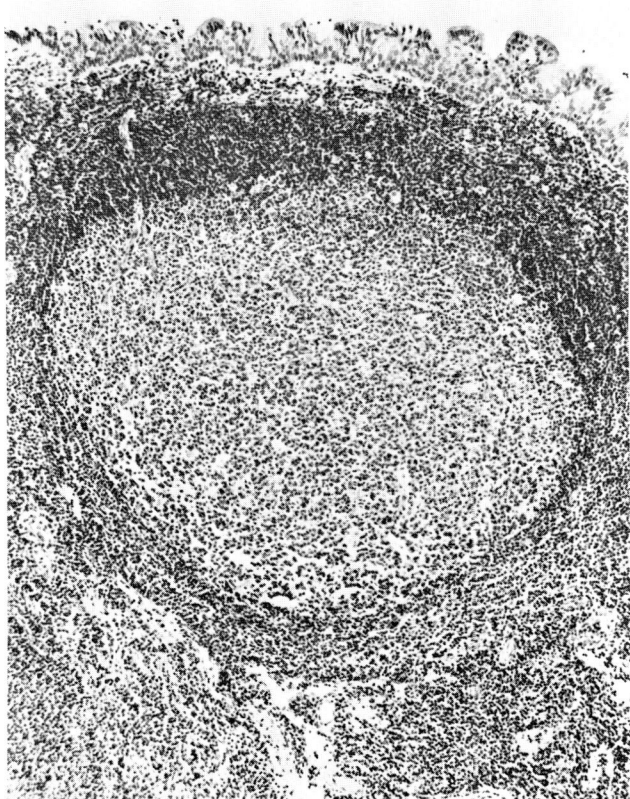

Figure 425. (Upper left) Set in a recess in a surface epithelium is a collection of lymphoid tissue, most obvious because of the nodules with germinal centers. From the surface there are deep branching crypts, structures that are unique to the adenoids or tonsils. The distinction between them depends on the nature of the surface and crypt epithelium. Where this is stratified ciliated and of respiratory type, it indicates origin from the nasopharynx, and the structure is an adenoid. Where the surface is a stratified squamous mucosa it comes from the oral pharynx, and the structure is the tonsil. *Tonsil* (× 6)

Figure 426. (Upper right) The epithelium here is clearly stratified squamous mucosa, and the structure is therefore tonsil. Part of the wall of a crypt runs obliquely down the left side to the lower center, and here there is a unique and intimate admixture of lymphocytes apparently passing through the epithelial cells. *Tonsil* (× 80)

Figure 427. (Lower left) The overlying epithelium here is respiratory; otherwise, the structure is similar to that of the tonsil. *Adenoid* (× 80)

LYMPHATIC SOLIDS

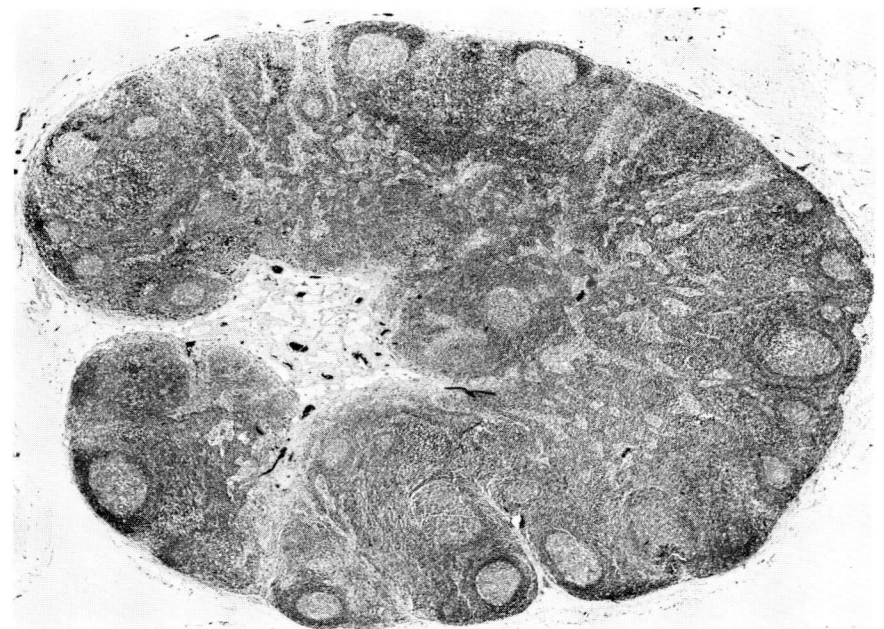

Figure 428. This is a well-demarcated island of punctate format, embedded in a loose connective tissue. The pale circular and oval areas at the periphery, each with a darker rim of cells, are lymphatic nodules with germinal centers. The pale slits that appear to meander through the substance of the structure are sinusoids which drain towards the hilus of the node that is seen on the left. The lymph that enters the gland passes around the cortical sinus seen immediately beneath the capsule and from here drains to the medulla and from the hilus to the general lymphatic system. *Lymph node* ($\times 14$)

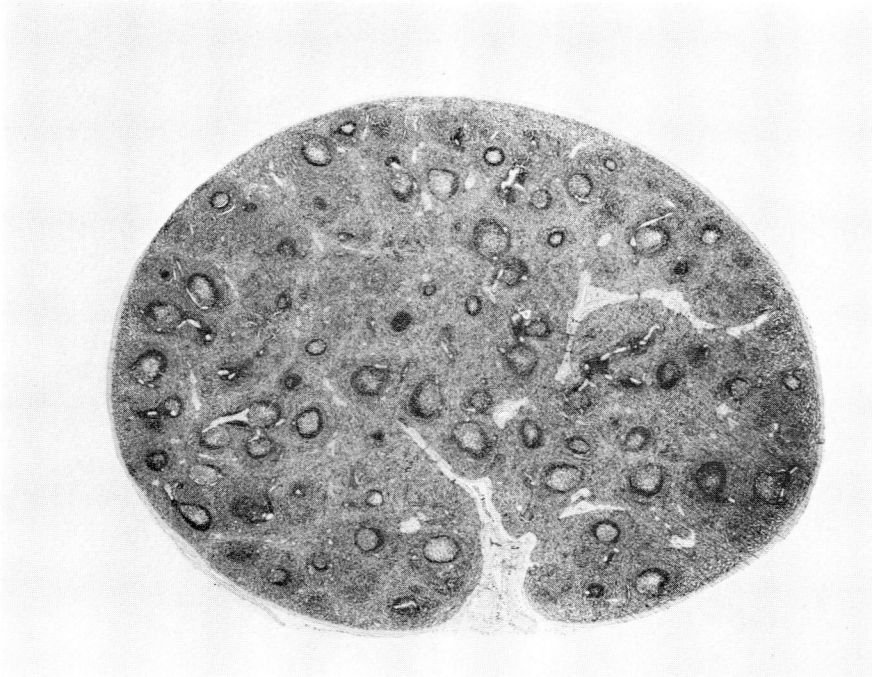

Figure 429. This is a somewhat similar ovoid encapsulated mass with a fibrous periphery, strongly suggestive of a lymph node. However, the external surface is a mesothelial covering indicating that it projects into some serous cavity, thus excluding lymph node. The presence of arteries within the lymphatic nodules and the erythrocytes within the sinusoids establish this as an *accessory spleen (spleniculus)*. ($\times 7$)

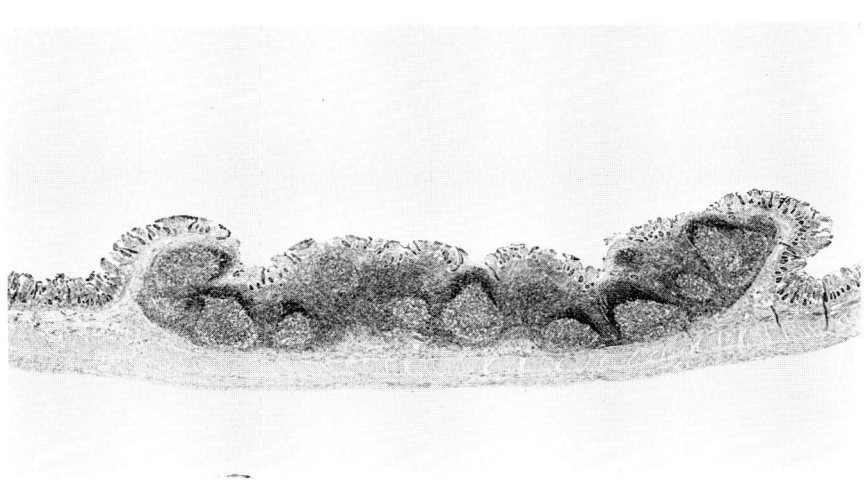

Figure 430. Small shallow craters can be seen by the naked eye in the mucosa of the terminal ileum; they are oval in configuration, with their long axes running longitudinally. Microscopically these areas have collections of lymphoid tissue in the submucosa, with partial loss of the muscularis mucosa, and they are known as Peyer's patches. In this case, the lymphoid nodules have large prominent germinal centers in which histiocytes appear as tiny clear spaces. The nodules are capped above by darkly staining masses of small lymphocytes. *Peyer's patch* (× 12)

III
SUMMARY

HISTOLOGIC identification begins by asking whether the section is lineate, annulate, multiperforate, or solid; whether it has any characteristic size and shape; is cut out from some large part; or is only a small tissue fragment.

1. If the section is *lineate*, with a flat open surface the first consideration is whether the surface is microscopically smooth or is ruffled, and the next consideration is the type of epithelium.

Examples of Structures with Smooth Surfaces

Stratified squamous epidermis	Skin
Stratified squamous mucosa	Openings into body cavities. Esophagus
Transitional epithelium	Bladder
Pseudostratified ciliated epithelium	Respiratory mucosa
Stratified columnar epithelium	Conjunctiva
Cuboidal epithelium	Amnion; lens
Simple squamous epithelium	Serous cavities and vessels
No epithelium	Synovium

Examples of Structures with Ruffled Surfaces

Single row columnar epithelium	Stomach
	Gallbladder
	Small and large intestine
	Uterus

2. If the section is *annulate*, the first consideration is whether the lining is smooth or ruffled, followed by consideration of the type of epithelium and the type of supporting tissues.

Examples of Structures with Smooth Linings

Stratified squamous epidermis	External auditory canal
Pseudostratified ciliated epithelium	Bronchus
Squamous epithelium	Vessel

Examples of Structures with Ruffled Linings

Transitional epithelium	Ureter
Stratified columnar epithelium	Vas deferens
Single columnar epithelium	Appendix
	Fallopian tube
	Bile duct

3. If the section is *multiperforate*, the first consideration is whether the spaces are large or small; the next questions concern the contour of the spaces, whether tubular or spheroidal and whether regular or irregular. The most important considerations are the type of epithelium lining the space, the contents, and the supporting tissues.

Examples of Structures with Large Spaces with Predominantly Tubular Profiles

Stratified polygonal epithelium, sperm	Testis
Ciliated/pseudociliated epithelium	Epididymis
Single/double flat epithelium, irregular contour	Rete testis
Squamous epithelium, irregular contour	Erectile tissue

Examples of Structures with Large Spaces with Predominantly Circular Profiles

Double layer epithelium, regular	Apocrine glands
Double layer epithelium, irregular	Prostate
Single layer, with colloid	Thyroid

Examples of Structures with Small Spaces with Predominantly Circular Profiles

(These are further identified by considering the numerical density of the spaces, the type of epithelial lining cells, the type of stroma, and sometimes the anatomic location.)

Eccrine sweat glands
Breast
Lacrimal glands
Salivary glands
Pancreas
Brunner's glands
Bartholin's glands
Cowper's glands

4. If the section is *solid*, the first consideration is the predominant tissue family. Sometimes size and shape are unique by themselves.

Examples of Structures Dominated by Epithelial Tissues –

with large cells	Liver
	Adrenal
	Corpus luteum
	Skin appendages
with small cells	Parathyroid
	Islets of pancreas
with mixed cells	Pituitary

Examples of Structures Dominated by Neural Tissues —

with glial supporting tissue	Brain
	Cerebellum
with neurilemmal and fibrous supporting tissue	Peripheral nerve
	Nerve endings
with glial and fibrous supporting tissue	Optic Nerve
	Pineal

Examples of Structures Dominated by Muscle Tissues —

with striated fibers	Skeletal muscles of limbs
	Heart
with nonstriated (visceral) fibers	Uterus

Examples of Structures Dominated by Connective Tissue —

with segregated matrix (further identification depends chiefly on the nature of the intercellular material, but sometimes on cell content)	Bones
	Cartilages
	Umbilical cord
	Fat
with free punctate format	Myeloid component of marrow
	Thymus, spleen, tonsils, adenoids, lymph nodes, and Peyer's patches

REFERENCES

1. Baker, J.R.: *Principles of Biological Microtechnique.* A study of fixation and dyeing. New York, John Wiley and Sons, Inc., 1958.
2. Drury, R.A.B. and Wallington, E.A.: *Carleton's Histological Techniques.* Oxford University Press, 4th ed., 1967.
3. Fernandez Pascual, J.S.: A New Method for Easy Demonstration of Argyrophil Cells. *Stain Technol., 51:*231-35, 1976.
4. Feyrter, F.: Über die Peripheren endokrinen (parakrinen) Drusen des Menschen; einführendes Referat. *Krebsarzt, 13:*169-180, 1958.
5. Gabe, M.: *Histological Techniques.* Masson, Springer-Verlag, 1976.
6. Hudson, R.E.B.: Surgical pathology of the conducting system of the heart. *Br Heart J, 29:*646-670, 1967.
7. Lillie, R.D. and Fullmer, H.M.: *Histopathologic Technic and Practical Histochemistry.* New York, McGraw-Hill Book Co., 4th ed., 1976.
8. Lillie, R.D.: *Conn's Biological Stains.* Baltimore, The Williams and Wilkins Co., 9th ed., 1977.
9. Luna, L.G.: Manual of Histologic Staining Methods of the Armed Forces Institute of Pathology. New York, McGraw-Hill Book Co., 3rd ed., 1968.
10. Pearse, A.G.E.: *Histochemistry: Theoretical and Applied,* 2 vols. Baltimore, The Williams and Wilkins Co., 3rd ed., 1972.
11. Pearse, A.G.E.: The diffuse neuroendocrine system and the apud concept: related "endocrine" peptides in brain, intestine, pituitary, placenta, and anuran cutaneous glands. *Med. Biol., 55:*115-125, 1977.
12. Taylor, C.R.: Immunoperoxidase Techniques. *Arch Pathol. Lab Med, 102:*113-21, 1978.
13. Thompson, S.W.: *Selected Histochemical and Histopathological Methods.* Springfield, Charles C Thomas, 1974.

INDEX

A
Adenoid, Fig. 427
Adipose tissue, Figs. 76, 129, 308, 411
Adrenal, Figs. 65, 66, 324-326
Alveoli, Figs. 302-305
Ameloblast, Fig. 399
Amnion, Figs. 61, 173, 174
Annulate sections, 49, Figs. 141, 216-250
Anterior commissure, Figs. 343, 344
Aorta, Figs. 181, 182
Apocrine sweat glands, Fig. 306
Appendix, Figs. 227, 228
Appendix epiploica, Fig. 411
Appendix testis, Fig. 406
Aqueduct, sylvian, Figs. 356-361
Arachnoid, Figs. 175, 382, 410
Areolar connective tissue, Fig. 127
Argentaffin cells, Fig. 201
Arrangement, modes of, 7
Arrector pili muscles, Fig. 150
Artery, Figs. 231-234
Astrocytes, Figs. 77, 79, 100-102
Atria, lung, Fig. 304
Atrioventricular node, Figs. 391-393
Atrium, Fig. 179
Auditory canal, Figs. 216, 217
Auerbach's myenteric plexus, Figs. 108, 196, 204
Axon, Fig. 78

B
Bands, Z, H, &, I, Fig. 114
Bartholin's gland, Figs. 54, 55, 323
Basal cells, Figs. 44, 45
Basement membrane, Figs. 264, 265
Basophils, pituitary, Figs. 70, 339, 340
Beta cells, pancreas, Figs. 335, 337
Betz cells, Figs. 30, 79
Bile duct, Figs. 229, 230
Billroth's cords, Fig. 420
Bipolar cells
    Olfactory mucosa, Fig. 170
    Retina, Figs. 246, 247
Bladder, urinary, Figs. 120, 167, 168
Body
    Amyloid, Fig. 14
    Calcific, Figs. 15-17, 289, 389, 405
    Carotid, Figs. 71, 412-414
    Ciliary, Figs. 240, 242, 244
    Geniculate, Figs. 347-349
    Mammillary, Figs. 345, 346
    Nissl, Fig. 79
    Nonnucleated, Figs. 14-17, 286, 287
    Tingible, Fig. 139
Bone
    Cortical, Figs. 88-90
    Fibrillary, Figs. 94-96, 404
    Marrow, Figs. 91, 133, 134
    Temporal, Fig. 96
    Trabecular, Figs. 91-93, 418
Bowman's capsule, Figs. 263, 265
Bowman's glands, Fig. 170
Bowman's membrane, Fig. 242
Brain
    Amygdaloid, Figs. 356, 357
    Anterior commissure, Figs. 343, 344
    Aqueduct, Figs. 356-361
    Basal ganglia, Figs. 345, 346
    Caudate nucleus, Figs. 345-349
    Cerebellum, Figs. 80, 131, 350-352, 355b
    Colliculus, Figs. 356-359
    Corpus callosum, Figs. 101, 343-348
    Cortex, Figs. 77-79, 353-355
    Dentate fascia, Figs. 132, 349
    Fornix, Figs. 343-346, 349
    Geniculate body, Figs. 347-349
    Gennari, stria, Figs. 353, 354
    Globus pallidus, Figs. 83, 345, 346
    Gray matter, Figs. 77, 78
    Hippocampus, Figs. 132, 347-349
    Insula, Figs. 347, 348
    Internal capsule, Figs. 100, 101, 343, 344
    Locus caeruleus, Figs. 360-362
    Mammillary bodies, Figs. 345, 346
    Medulla, Figs. 366-369
    Mesencephalon, Figs. 356-359
    Olfactory bulb, Fig. 376
    Olive, Figs. 366, 367
    Pons, Figs. 84, 360-365
    Posterior pole, Fig. 354
    Putamen, Figs. 82, 345, 346
    Pyramids, Figs. 366-369
    Red nucleus, Figs. 356, 357
    Subiculum, Fig. 349
    Substantia gelatinosa, Figs. 370, 371
    Substantia nigra, Figs. 81, 356-359
    Supraoptic nucleus, Figs. 343, 344
    Thalamus, Figs. 345, 346
    Tracts, Figs. 360-375
    Vermis, Fig. 350
    Visual cortex, Fig. 354
    White matter, Figs. 100, 101, 349c
Breast, Figs. 152, 239, 308-313, 331
    Atrophic, Fig. 312
    Lactating, Figs. 310, 311
    Male, Fig. 313
Bronchus, Figs. 220, 221
Bronchiole, Figs. 304, 305
Brown fat, Fig. 76

Bruch's membrane, Fig. 247
Brunner's glands, Figs. 194. 312
Brush border, Fig. 265
Bulb, olfactory, Fig. 376
Bulbourethral glands, Fig. 322

C

Calcific bodies, Figs. 15-17, 380, 405
Calyx, renal, Fig. 262
Canal
    Auditory, Figs. 216, 217
    Haversian, Figs. 88-90
    Schlemm, Figs. 244, 245
    Semicircular, Figs. 251, 252
    Volkmann, Fig. 88
Cardiac muscle, Figs. 117-119
Carotid artery, Figs. 231, 232
Carotid body, Figs. 71, 412-414
Cartilage, types, Figs. 85-87, 403, 417
Caudate nucleus, Figs. 345-349
Cells, identification, 15
    By cytoplasmic and nuclear characteristics, Figs. 32-43
    By eponyms or letters, 20 (Table 3)
    By shape and surface modifications, Figs. 22-31
    In other ways, 19 (Table 2)
    Types
        Acidophil, Figs. 69, 70, 340
        Alpha pancreas, Figs. 335, 337
        Ameloblasts, Fig. 399
        Argentaffin, Fig. 201
        Astrocytes, Figs. 77, 79, 100
        Basket, Fig. 309
        Basophil, Figs. 70, 340
        B cells, Figs. 138, 139
        Beta, Figs. 70, 335, 336
        Betz, Figs. 30, 79
        Bichromic, Fig. 319
        Bipolar olfactory, Fig. 170
        Bipolar, retina, Figs. 246, 247
        C cells, Figs. 295, 296
        Centroacinar, Fig. 319
        Chondrocytes, Figs. 85-87
        Chromophobe, Figs. 70, 340
        Ciliated, Figs. 24, 53, 59, 60, 220, 320
        Clara, Fig. 305
        Claudius, Fig. 258
        Columnar, Figs. 22, 23, 54-56, 186-215
        Cones, Fig. 247
        Cuboidal, Figs. 27, 61
        Decidua, Figs. 76, 174
        Enterochromaffin, Fig. 201
        Erythroblasts, Figs. 134-136
        Ganglion, Figs. 106-108, 130
        Goblet, Figs. 29, 47, 58, 197-205
        Granular, Figs. 263, 265, 266
        Granulosa, Figs. 51, 269-272
        Hair, Figs. 257, 258
        Hensen, Fig. 258
        Hepatocytes, Figs. 63, 64, 332
        Hilus, Fig. 73
        Histiocytes, Figs. 137-139
        Hofbauer, Figs. 136, 408
        Immunoblasts, Fig. 139
        Interstitial, Figs. 72, 73, 279
        Islet, Fig. 68
        Juxtaglomerular, Figs. 263-266
        Kulchitsky, Fig. 201
        Kupffer, Fig. 332
        Langhans, Fig. 407
        Leydig, Figs. 72, 279
        Lutein, Fig. 67
        Megakaryocyte, Fig. 134
        Melanocyte, Fig. 45
        Meningocyte, Fig. 175
        Mitral, Fig. 376
        Muscle, Figs. 109-122
        Myelocyte, Fig. 134
        Myoepithelial, Figs. 234, 239, 306, 307, 309
        Neurones, Figs. 77-81
        Odontoblast, Fig. 396
        Oligodendrocytes, Figs. 79, 100
        Osteoblasts, Figs. 93-96
        Osteocytes, Figs. 88-96
        Oxyphil, Figs. 34, 191, 192, 334
        Paneth, Fig. 200
        Paracrine, Figs. 201-203, 295, 296
        Parietal, Figs. 191, 192
        Peg, Fig. 226
        Pillar, Fig. 258
        Pinealocytes, Figs. 379, 380
        Prickle, Figs. 26, 44-48, 385
        Purkinje, Figs. 31, 80, 355b
        Pyramidal, Figs. 30, 79, 355a
        Rod, Fig. 247
        Satellite, Figs. 106, 107
        Schwann, Fig. 103
        Serous, Figs. 316, 317
        Sertoli, Figs. 280, 281
        Squamous, Figs. 28, 62, 175, 176
        Sustentacular, Figs. 170, 414
        T cells, Fig. 138
        Trophoblasts, Fig. 52
        Zymogenic, Figs. 191, 192, 319
Cementum, Fig. 397
Cerebellum, Figs. 80, 131, 350-352. 355b
Cerebral cortex, Figs. 77-79, 353-355a
Ceruminous glands, Fig. 217
Cervix uteri, Figs. 46, 214, 215
Chorion, Figs. 173, 174, 407
Chorionic villi, Figs. 52, 136, 407
Choroid, Figs. 246, 247
Choroid plexus, Figs. 15, 405
Chromophobes, Fig. 342
Cilia, Figs. 53, 59, 60, 220, 320
Ciliary body, Figs. 240, 242, 244
Circumvallate papillae, Fig. 159
Clara cells, Fig. 305
Clarke's column, Figs. 372, 373
Clitoris, Fig. 297
Cochlea, Figs. 251, 252, 254-256
Coeliac ganglion, Fig. 106
Collagen, Figs. 90, 123, 124, 127, 401
Colliculus, cerebral, Figs. 356-359
Colliculus seminalis, Fig. 286
Colloid, Figs. 293-295
Colon, Figs. 204, 205
Coloring procedures, 5 (Table 1)
Conducting system, Figs. 388-393

Cones, Fig. 247
Conjunctive, Fig. 47
Connective tissue, Figs. 123-129
Construction
    Levels, Fig. 1-4
    Modes, 7
Convoluted tubules, Figs. 263, 267
Cord
    Bilroth, Fig. 420
    Spinal, Figs. 370-375
    Umbilical, Figs. 128, 402
    Vocal, Fig. 171
Cornea, Figs. 48, 240, 242, 244
Corona radiata, Fig. 272
Corpora amylacea, Figs. 14, 17, 288, 289
Corpora arenacea, Figs. 16, 380
Corpora cavernosa, Figs. 238, 298
Corpus albicans, Figs. 99, 274, 416
Corpus callosum, Figs. 101, 345, 346
Corpus cavernosum, Figs. 238, 297, 298
Corpus luteum, Figs. 67, 273-275
Corpus spongiosum, Fig. 238
Corpuscles
    Hassall's, Figs. 423, 424
    Meissner's, Figs. 148, 384, 385
    Malphigian
        Kidney, Figs. 261, 263
        Spleen, Fig. 420
    Pacinian, Fig. 383
Cortex
    Adrenal, Figs. 65, 66, 324, 325
    Bone, Figs. 88-90
    Cerebellar, Figs. 80, 131, 355b
    Cerebral, Figs. 77, 78, 353-355
    Ovarian, Figs. 126, 267, 268
    Renal, Fig. 261
Corti, organ, Figs. 254, 257, 258
Cowper's gland, Fig. 322
Crypts
    Lieberkuhn, Figs. 200, 201
    Tonsil, Fig. 425
Crystals, Reinke, Fig. 72
Cytoplasm, 15

D
Decidua, Figs. 74, 174, 407
Demilunes, Fig. 316
Dentate gyrus, Fig. 132
Dentate nucleus, Fig. 352
Dentine, Figs. 395-397
Descemet's membrane, Figs. 242, 244, 245
Diaphragm, Fig. 177
Dichorionic membranes, Fig. 173
Disc
    Intervertebral, Fig. 415
    Optic, Fig. 243
Discus proligerus, Figs. 270-272
Disse, spaces, Fig. 332
Distal convoluted tubule, Figs. 263, 265
Ducts
    Alveolar, Fig. 304
    Bartholin, Fig. 54
    Bile, Figs. 229, 230
    Cochlear, Figs. 254-256
    Ejaculatory, Fig. 286
    Hepatic, Fig. 332
    Mammary, Figs. 239, 331
    Pancreatic, Fig. 318
    Salivary, Figs. 161, 315-317
    Sebaceous gland, Fig. 330
    Sweat, Fig. 307
    Thoracic, Fig. 237
Ductuli efferentes, Figs. 276, 277, 284, 285
Ductus deferens, Figs. 222, 223, 289
Ductus endolymphaticus, Fig. 251
Ductus epididymis, Figs. 276, 282, 283
Duodenum, Figs. 193, 194
Dura mater, Fig. 410
Dyeing, 3

E
Ear, Figs. 251, 252
    External canal, Figs. 216, 217, 251, 252
    Inner, Figs. 251, 252, 254-260
    Middle, Figs. 251-253, 404
    Petrous temporal bone, Fig. 96
    Pinna, Figs. 86, 145
Eccrine gland, Fig. 307
Elastic arteries, Figs. 181, 182, 231
Elastic cartilage, Figs. 86, 163, 171, 216
Elastic fibers, Figs. 125, 181, 182
Elastic ligaments, Fig. 125
Enamel organ, Figs. 398, 399
Endocervix, Figs. 214, 215
Endometrium, Figs. 60, 74, 75
    Phases, 91 (Table 4), Figs. 206-213
Ependyma, Figs. 15, 349c
Epidermis, Figs. 44, 45, 144-154, 216, 217
Epididymis, Figs. 276, 277, 282-285
Epiphysis, Fig. 417
Epiglottis, Fig. 163
Epineurium, Fig. 381
Epithelium
    Anuclear derivative, Figs. 18-21
    Columnar, Figs. 56-60
    Cuboidal, Figs. 61, 294
    Double row, Figs. 55, 239
    Germinal, Fig. 270
    Pseudostratified ciliated columnar, Figs. 53, 169, 170
    Simple squamous, Figs. 175-185
        Squamous, keratinizing, Figs. 44, 45
        Squamous, nonkeratinizing, Figs. 46-48
    Stratified columnar, Figs. 54, 222, 223, 238
    Transitional, Figs. 49, 167, 168, 218, 219
Erectile tissue
    Clitoris, Fig. 297
    Penis, Figs. 238, 298
Erythroblasts, Fig. 136
Esophagus, Figs. 165, 166
External auditory canal, Figs. 216, 217, 251, 252
Eye, Figs. 124, 240-250
Eyelid, Figs. 153, 330

F
Fallopian tube, Figs. 59, 224-226
Fasciculus
    Cuneate, Figs. 368-372
    Gracile, Figs. 368-372

Medial longitudinal, Figs. 356-361
Fat
  Adult, Figs. 92, 129, 308, 411
  Brown (fetal), Fig. 76
  Marrow, Fig. 91
Fetal
  Adrenal, Fig. 324b
  Bone, Fig. 418
  Cochlea, Figs. 254, 255
  Dorsal root ganglion, Fig. 130
  Eye, Fig. 241
  Head, Fig. 241
  Kidney, Figs. 261, 262
  Liver, Fig. 135
  Lund, Figs. 176, 301-303
  Membranes, Figs. 173, 174
  Placenta, Fig. 418
  Striated muscle, Fig. 109
  Testis, Fig. 278
  Thorax, Fig. 144
  Thymus, Fig. 422
  Tongue, Fig. 160
  Tooth, Fig. 398
  Villi, Fig. 136
Fiber tracts, CNS, Fig. 82-84
Fibers
  Axion, Figs. 78, 104, 105
  Collagen, Figs. 123, 124, 127
  Conducting, Figs. 388-393
  Elastin, Figs. 125, 231, 232
  Muscle, Figs. 109-119
  Sharpey, Fig. 397
  Tomes, Fig. 396
Fibrocartilage, Figs. 87, 403
Fibrocytes, Figs. 123, 126, 127
Filiform papillae, Fig. 158
Finger, Figs. 148, 394
Follicles
  Atretic, Figs. 267, 269
  Graffian, Figs. 270-272
  Hair, Figs. 318, 319
  Lymph, Figs. 425-429
  Primordial, Fig. 268
  Spleen, Fig. 420
  Thyroid, Figs. 293-296
Forehead, Fig. 151
Foreskin, Fig. 147
Formats
  Fibrillary, 23
  Inlaid, 22
  Mosaic, 22
  Punctate, 23
  Tesselated, 21
  Tissue, Figs. 9-13
Fovea, eye, Fig. 250
Foveolae gastricae, Figs. 56, 189, 190

G
Gallbladder, Figs. 57, 187, 188
Ganglion cells
  Coeliac, Fig. 106
  Dorsal root, Figs. 107, 130, 377
  Myenteric plexus, Fig. 108
  Retina, Fig. 246

  Spiral, cochlea, Fig. 254
Gennari, stria, Figs. 353, 354
Germinal center, Figs. 138, 139, 428
Giannuzzi, crescents, Fig. 316
Gingiva, Fig. 155
Glands
  Anterior lingual, Fig. 317
  Apocrine, Fig. 306
  Areolar, Fig. 331
  Bartholin, Figs. 54, 55, 323
  Bowman's olfactory, Fig. 170
  Bronchial, Fig. 220
  Brunner's, Figs. 194, 321
  Bulbourethral, Fig. 322
  Ceruminous, Figs. 216, 217
  Cervix uteri, Figs. 214, 215
  Cowper, Fig. 322
  Eccrine, Fig. 307
  Endometrial, Figs. 206-213
  Esophageal, Fig. 166
  Gastric, Fig. 189-192
  Lacrimal, Fig. 314
  Littre, Fig. 238
  Mammary, Figs. 152, 239, 308-313, 331
  Mandibular, Fig. 316
  Meibom, Figs. 153, 330
  Mixed, Figs. 220, 316, 320
  Montgomery, Fig. 331
  Mucous, Fig. 317
  Parathyroid, Fig. 333, 334
  Pancreas, Figs. 318, 319
  Parotid, Fig. 315
  Pineal, Figs. 378-380
  Pituitary, Figs. 70, 338-342
  Prostate, Figs. 286-289
  Pyloric, Fig. 195
  Salivary
    Major, Figs. 314-317
    Minor, Figs. 161, 164, 166, 169, 172, 320
  Sebaceous, Figs. 151, 153, 329-331
  Serous, Figs. 314, 315
  Sublingual, Fig. 317
  Sweat, Figs. 306, 307
  Thyroid, Figs. 293-296
  Trachea, Fig. 320
  Uterine, Figs. 206-213
  Vestibular, Fig. 323
Globus pallidus, Figs. 83, 345, 346
Glomerulosa, adrenal, Figs. 287, 324
Glomerulus, renal, Figs. 261, 263, 265, 266
Glomus, Fig. 234
Glycocalyx, Fig. 199
Glycogen, Figs. 46, 63, 64, 209
Glycoprotein, Figs. 199, 340
Goblet cells, Figs. 47, 58, 201-205
Graffian follicles, Figs. 270-272
Granules
  Alpha cells, Fig. 340
  Argentaffin, Fig. 201
  Argyrophil, Fig. 202
  Basophil, Figs. 70, 340
  Beta, Figs. 70, 335, 336, 340
  Eosinophil, Figs. 70, 340
  Glycogen, Fig. 64

Juxta-glomerular, Fig. 266
Keratohyaline, Figs. 44, 328
Lipofuscin, Figs. 279, 283, 285, 289, 290, 325
Melanin, Figs. 45, 81, 242, 244-246, 380
Nissl, Fig. 79
Paneth cells, Fig. 200
Zymogen, Figs. 191, 319
Granulocytes, Fig. 134
Granulosa, Fig. 51

H
Hair, Figs. 19, 327, 328
    Cells, Figs. 159, 257-260
Hassall's corpuscles, Figs. 423, 424
Haversian system, Fig. 88
H bands, Fig. 114
Heart
    Conducting system, Figs. 388-393
    Fetal, Fig. 144
    Muscle, Figs. 117-119
    Valve, Fig. 184
    Walls, Figs. 179, 180
Henle layer, Fig. 328
Henle loop, Figs. 261, 262, 264
Hepatic cells, Figs. 63, 64
Hertwig's sheath, Fig. 398
Hippocampus, Figs. 132, 347-349
His, bundle, Figs. 391-393
Histiocytes, Figs. 137-139
Hofbauer cells, Fig. 408
Huxley's layer, Fig. 328
Hyaline cartilage, Figs. 85, 169, 417
Hyman, Fig. 156
Hypophysis, Figs. 338-342

I
I bands, Fig. 114
Identification
    Anuclear elements, 12
    Cells, 15
    Parts, 57
    Principles, 3
    Tissues, 18
Inclusions, nuclear, Fig. 223
Incus, Fig. 404
Inferior vena cava, Fig. 183
Intercellular bridges, Figs. 44-48, 385
Internal capsule, Figs. 100, 101, 343, 344
Interstitial cells
    Ovary, Fig. 73
    Testis, Figs. 72, 279
Intervertebral disc, Figs. 98, 99, 415
Intestine
    Large, Figs. 204, 205
    Small, Figs. 58, 196-203
Iris, Figs. 240, 242, 244, 245
Island of Reil, Figs. 347, 348
Islets of Langerhans, Figs. 68, 335-337
Isthmus, cerebral, Figs. 360, 361

J
Juxtaglomerular apparatus, Figs. 263, 265, 266

K
Keratin, Figs. 18, 44, 148, 149

Kidney, Figs. 261-266
Kupffer cells, Figs. 332

L
Labia minora, Fig. 146
Lacrimal gland, Fig. 314
Lamellar bone, Figs. 88-93
Lamina cribosa, Fig. 243
Langhans layer, Fig. 407
Langheran's islets, Figs. 68, 335-337
Larynx, Fig. 171
Lateral geniculate body, Fig. 347-349
Lens, Figs. 21, 240-242, 244
Leptomeninges, Figs. 175, 410
Leydig cells, Figs. 72, 279
Lieberkuhn, crypts, Figs. 200, 201
Ligament
    Flava (nuchae), Fig. 125
    Pectinate, Fig. 244
    Round, Fig. 400
Lineate sections, 60, Figs. 140, 145-215
Lingual glands, Fig. 317
Lip, Fig. 154
Lipid, Figs. 65-67, 274
Lipochrome, Figs. 279, 283, 285, 289, 290, 325
Littre's glands, Fig. 238
Liver
    Adult, Figs. 63, 64, 332
    Fetal, Fig. 135
Locus caeruleus, Figs. 360, 361
Lung, Figs. 176, 301-305
Lymph node, Figs. 137, 428
Lymphatic tissue, Figs. 137-139, 227, 228, 419-430
Lysochromes, 3, Fig. 66

M
Macula densa, Figs. 263, 265
Macula lutea, Fig. 250
Macula sacculi, Figs. 259, 260
Malpighii
    Corpuscles
        Renal, Figs. 261, 263, 265, 266
        Spleen, Fig. 420
    Stratum, Figs. 44, 45
Mammary gland, Figs. 239, 308, 309, 331
Mammillary bodies, Figs. 345, 346
Mandibular gland, Fig. 316
Marrow, bone, Figs. 91-93, 133, 134
Mastoid, Figs. 96, 251, 252
Matrix, 21
Medulla
    Adrenal, Figs. 324, 326
    Bone, Figs. 133, 134
    Brain, Figs. 366-369
    Hair root, Figs. 327, 328
    Kidney, Figs. 262-264
Meibomian gland, Figs. 153, 330
Meissner's corpuscles, Figs. 148, 384, 385
Meissner's plexus, Figs. 196, 204
Melanin, Figs. 45, 81, 242, 244-246, 380
Melanocytes, Fig. 45
Membrane
    Basement, Figs. 264, 265
    Bowman, Figs. 48, 242
    Bruch, Fig. 247

Descemet, Fig. 242
Diamnionic, Fig. 173
Dichorionic, Fig. 173
Fetal, Figs. 61, 173, 174
Granulosa, Fig. 51
Otolithic, Figs. 259, 260
Periodontal, Fig. 397
Reissner (tectorial), Figs. 255, 256
Synovial, Fig. 186
Tympanic, Figs. 251-253
Meninges, Figs. 175, 351, 355
Meniscus, Figs. 87, 403
Mesencephalon, Figs. 356, 357
Mesothelium, Figs. 179, 180, 185
Metaphysis, Fig. 418
Microglia, Fig. 79
Modiolus, Fig. 254
Montgomery, tubercles, Fig. 331
Multiperforate sections, 111, Figs. 142, 251-323
Muscle
    Cardiac, Figs. 117-119
    Conducting, Figs. 388-393
    Fetal, Fig. 109
    Nonstriated, Figs. 120-122
    Skeletal, Figs. 109-119
    Slow acting, Fig. 116
    Spindle, Figs. 111, 386, 387
Muscularis mucosae, Figs. 165, 166, 189, 190, 196-199, 204, 205
Myelin, Fig. 105
Myeloid tissues, Figs. 133, 134
Myenteric plexus, Figs. 196, 204
Myocardium, Figs. 117-119, 179, 180
Myoepithelium, Figs. 239, 306, 307, 309
Myxoid tissue, Figs. 52, 128

N
Nail, Figs. 20, 149, 394
Nasal musoca, Figs. 169, 170, 300
Nerve
    Cranial, Figs. 356, 357, 362-365
    Endings, Figs. 383-385
    Ganglia, Figs. 106, 107, 130, 254, 377
    Optic, Figs. 102, 382
    Peripheral, Figs. 103-105, 381
    Structure, Figs. 103-105, 381, 382
Neurones
    Small, Figs. 246, 247, 376
    Types, Figs. 77, 79-81, 131, 132, 246
Nipple, Fig. 152
Nissl bodies, Fig. 79
Nitabuch, layer, Fig. 409
Nodes
    Atrioventricular, Figs. 390-393
    Lymph, Figs. 137, 428
    Sinu-atrial, Figs. 388-390
Nomenclature, cells, 18-20
Nose, Figs. 169-170, 300
Nuclei
    Cells, 15, Figs. 38-42
    CNS, Figs. 349, 352, 356-369
Nucleus pulposus, Figs. 97, 98, 415

O
Odontoblast, Fig. 396

Olfactory bulb, Fig. 376
Olfactory mucosa, Fig. 170
Oligodendroglia, Figs. 79, 100
Olive, Fig. 366
Optic disc, Fig. 243
Optic nerve, Figs. 102, 240, 343, 344, 382
Ora serrata retainae, Fig. 249
Organization, 7
    Levels, Fig. 1-4
Organ of Corti, Figs. 254, 255, 257, 258
Ossicles, Figs. 95, 251, 252, 404
Osteoblasts, Fig. 418
Osteoclasts, Fig. 418
Osteon, Figs. 88-90
Otolith, Figs. 259-260
Ovary, Figs. 51, 67, 73, 99, 126, 267-275, 416
Oviduct, Figs. 224, 226
Ovum, Figs. 268, 270-272
Oxyphil cells, Figs. 69, 191

P
Pacinian corpuscle, Fig. 383
Palate, Fig. 164
Pampinniform plexus, Fig. 299
Pancreas, Figs. 68, 318, 319, 335-337
Paneth cells, Fig. 200
Papilla
    Circumvallate, Fig. 159
    Dermal, Figs. 148, 155
    Filiform, Fig. 158
    Hair, Fig. 327
    Renal, Fig. 262
Paracrine cells, Figs. 201-203, 295, 296
Paraganglia, Fig. 71
Parathyroid, Figs. 69, 333, 334
Parotid, Fig. 315
Pars intermedia, pituitary, Fig. 339
Pars nervosa, pituitary, Figs. 338, 342
Pars plana retinae, Fig. 248
Pars tuberalis pituitary, Fig. 341
Parts, construction, 7, 57, Figs. 5-8
Penis, Figs. 238, 298
Pericardium, Figs. 179, 180, 185
Peripheral nerve, Figs. 103-105, 381
Peritoneum, Fig. 178
Peyer's patch, Fig. 430
Pharynx, Fig. 161
Pineal gland, Figs. 16, 378-380
Pinna, Figs. 86, 145
Pituitary gland, Figs. 70, 338-342
Placenta, Figs. 136, 407-409
Pleura, Figs. 176, 301
Plexus
    Auerbach, Figs. 108, 196, 204
    Choroid, Fig. 405
    Meissner, Figs. 196, 204
    Pampinniform, Fig. 299
Polarization, Figs. 89, 113, 118
Pons, Figs. 84, 360-365
Position, 4
Precipitates, 3
    Formazan, Fig. 116
    Silver, Figs. 45, 78, 104, 201, 202, 296
Prepuce, Fig. 147
Prostate, Fig. 17, 286-289

Pulp
    Finger, Fig. 148
    Spleen, Figs. 419-421
    Tooth, Figs. 395, 396
Purkinje cells, Figs. 80, 355b
Putamen, Figs. 82, 345, 346
Pyloric glands, Figs, 193, 195
Pyloric sphincter, Fig. 193
Pyramids, Figs. 366-369
Pyriform fossa, Fig. 161

R
Reil, island, Figs. 347, 348
Reinke, crystals, Fig. 72
Reissner, membrane, Figs. 255, 256
Renal cortex, Figs. 261, 263, 265, 266
Renal medulla, Figs. 262, 264
Renal papilla, Fig. 262
Rete testis, Figs. 277, 291, 292
Reticulum, stellate, Figs. 398, 399
Retina, Fig. 246-250
Rods, Fig. 247
Round ligament, Fig. 400

S
Saccule, Figs. 251, 252
Salivary glands
    Major, Figs. 315-317
    Minor, Figs. 161, 164, 166, 169, 172, 320
Sand granules, Figs. 16, 380
Scala media, Figs. 254-256
Scala tympani, Figs. 254-256
Scala vestibuli, Figs. 254-256
Scalp, Fig. 150
Schlemm, canal, Fig. 245
Schmidt-Lanterman clefts, Fig. 105
Schwann, sheath, Fig. 103
Sclera, Figs. 124, 246, 248, 249
Sebaceous glands, Figs. 146, 151, 153, 329-331
Sections, microscopic forms, 57, Figs. 140-143
Semicircular canals, Figs. 251, 252
Semilunar cartilage, Fig. 87
Seminal vesicle, Fig. 209
Seminiferous tubules, Figs. 50, 276-281
Septum pellucidium, Figs. 343, 344
Sertoli cells, Figs. 280, 281
Shape, 4
Sharpey, fibers, Fig. 396
Sheath
    Hertwig, Fig. 398
    Schwann, Fig. 103
Silver reactions, 3, Figs. 45, 78, 104, 201, 202, 296, 381
Sinu atrial node, Figs. 388-390
Sinus, longitudinal, Fig. 410
Sinusoids
    Liver, Fig. 332
    Spleen, Fig. 420
Size, 4
Skin, Figs. 145-154
Small intestine, Figs. 58, 196-203
Solids
    Connective tissue, 148, Figs. 394-430
    Epithelia, 147, Figs. 324-342
    Muscle, 148, Figs. 386-393
    Neural, 147, Figs. 343-385
Space of Disse, Fig. 332
Spermatogonia, Fig. 280
Spermatozoa, Figs. 50, 280, 281, 283
Spindle, Figs. 111, 386, 387
Spinal cord, Figs. 370-375
Spleen, Figs. 419-421
    Accessory, Fig. 429
Stapes, Figs. 95, 251
Stellate reticulum, Figs. 398, 399
Sterocilia, Figs. 223, 259, 260, 283
Stomach, Figs. 56, 189-193
Stratified columnar epithelium, Figs. 54, 222, 223, 238
Stratified squamous epidermis, Figs. 144-154
Stratified squamous mucosa, Figs. 154-166
Stratified transitional epithelium, Figs. 48, 167, 168, 218, 219
Stratum corneum, Figs. 44, 45, 148
Stratum germinativum, Figs. 44, 45
Stratum granulosum, Figs. 44, 45
Stratum lucidum, Fig. 148
Stratum Malphigi, Figs. 44, 45, 148
Stria of Gennari, Figs. 353, 354
Stria vascularis, Figs. 255, 256
Striated muscle, Figs. 109-119
Subiculum, Fig. 349
Sublingual glands, Fig. 317
Submaxillary gland, Fig. 316
Substantia nigra, Figs. 81, 356-359
Substantia propria, cornea, Figs. 240, 242, 244
Substructure, 4
Summary, 202
Sweat glands
    Apocrine, Fig. 306
    Eccrine, Fig. 307
Synovial membrane, Fig. 186

T
Tarsal plate, Figs. 153, 330
Taste buds, Fig. 159
Taste hairs, Fig. 159
Tectorial membrane, Figs. 255-256
Temporal bone, Fig. 96
Tendon, Fig. 123, 401
Testis, Figs. 50, 72, 276-281
Testis, appendix, Fig. 406
Thalamus, Figs. 345, 346
Theca interna, Figs. 51, 271
Theca externa, Fig. 269
Thoracic duct, Fig. 237
Thorax, fetus, Fig. 144
Thymus, Figs. 422-424
Thyroid, Figs. 293-296
Tissues
    Connective, 21-23, Figs. 71-76, 85-99, 123-129
    Elastic, Figs. 86, 125, 163, 171, 181, 182, 216, 231
    Epithelial, 18, 21
    Epithelioid, Figs. 71-76
    Erectile, Figs. 238, 297, 298
    Fibrillary, Figs. 100-129
    Formats, Figs. 9-13
    Identification, 18
    Inlaid, Figs. 77-99
    Lymphatic, Figs. 137-139, 419-430
    Mosaic, Figs. 71-76

Muscle, 23, Figs. 109-122
Myeloid, Figs. 98, 99, 133-136
Neural, 22-23, Figs. 77-84, 100-108, 130, 132
Punctate, Figs. 130-139
Tessellated, Figs. 21, 44-70
Tomes' fibers, Fig. 396
Tongue, Figs. 115, 157-160
Tonsils, Figs. 425, 426
Tooth, Figs. 395-399
Tooth bud, Fig. 398
Trachea, Figs. 53, 172, 320
Tracts
    Cortico spinal, Figs. 360-373
    Spinal V, Figs. 366, 367
    Spinocerebellar, Figs. 370-375
    Spinothalamic, Figs. 370-375
Triads, liver, Fig. 332
Tricuspid valve, Fig. 184
Transitional epithelium, Figs. 49, 167, 168, 218, 219
Trophoblast, Figs. 52, 136, 173, 174, 407, 409
Tube, fallopian, Figs. 59, 224-226
Tubercle, Montgomery, Fig. 331
Tubules
    Convoluted, Fig. 263
    Dentine, Fig. 396
    Renal, Figs. 261-266
    Seminiferous, Fig. 278-281
Turbinates, Figs. 169, 300
Tympanic membrane, Figs. 251-253

U

Umbilical cord, Figs. 128, 402
Ureter, Fig. 49, 218, 219
Urethra, Fig. 238
Urinary bladder, Fig. 167, 168
Uterus, Figs. 74, 75, 122, 206-215, 400
Utricle, Figs. 251, 252
Utriculus masculinus, Fig. 286

V

Vagina, Fig. 162
Vallate papillae, Fig. 159
Valves, cardiac, Fig. 184
Vasa vasorum, Fig. 181
Vas deferens, Figs. 222, 223
Vein, Figs. 62, 235, 236

Vena cava, Fig. 183
Ventricle
    Brain, Figs. 343, 344, 349c
    Heart, Fig. 180
Vermis, Fig. 350
Veru montanum, Fig. 286
Vesicle
    Optic, Fig. 241
    Seminal, Fig. 290
Vessels
    Arteries
        Aorta, Figs. 181, 182
        Carotid, Figs. 231, 232
        Glomus, Fig. 234
        Muscular, Fig. 233
    Lymphatics, Fig. 237
    Veins
        Adrenal, Fig. 324
        Endothelium, Fig. 62
        Hepatic, Fig. 332
        Longitudinal sinus, Fig. 410
        Nasal mucosa, Fig. 300
        Pampinniform plexus, Fig. 299
        Portal, Fig. 332
        Structure, Figs. 235, 236
        Vena cava, Fig. 183
Villi
    Arachnoid, Figs. 382, 410
    Chorionic, Figs. 52, 136, 407-409
    Intestinal, Figs. 198, 199
Vitreous chamber, Figs. 240, 241
Vocal cord, Fig. 171

W

Wharton's jelly, Figs. 128, 402
Woven bone, Figs. 94-96, 404

Z

Z bands, Fig. 114
Zona fasciculata, adrenal, Figs. 324, 325
Zona glomerulosa, Figs. 324, 325
Zona pellucidum, ovum, Fig. 271
Zona reticularis, adrenal, Figs. 324, 325
Zymogen granules
    Pancreas, Fig. 319
    Stomach, Figs. 191, 192